Your *Clinics* subscription j

D0919057

You can now access the FULL TEXT of this publication online at no additional cost! Activate your online subscription today and receive...

- Full text of all issues from 2002 to the present
- Photographs, tables, illustrations, and references
- Comprehensive search capabilities
- Links to MEDLINE and Elsevier journals

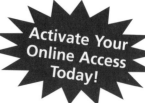

Activate Your Online Access Today!

Plus, you can also sign up for E-alerts of upcoming issues or articles that interest you, and take advantage of exclusive access to bonus features!

To activate your individual online subscription:

1. Visit our website at **www.TheClinics.com**.

2. Click on "Register" at the top of the page, and follow the instructions.

3. To activate your account, you will need your subscriber account number, which you can find on your mailing label (note: the number of digits in your subscriber account number varies from six to ten digits). See the sample below where the subscriber account number has been circled.

This is your subscriber account number

```
*******************************************3-DIGIT 001
FEB00   J0167   C7   (123456-89)  10/00   Q: 1

J.H. DOE, MD
531 MAIN ST
CENTER CITY, NY  10001-001
```

4. That's it! Your online access to the most trusted source for clinical reviews is now available.

theclinics.com

ELSEVIER

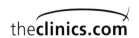

NEUROLOGIC CLINICS

Toxic and Environmental Neurology

GUEST EDITORS
Michael R. Dobbs, MD
Matthew P. Wicklund, MD

May 2005 • Volume 23 • Number 2

SAUNDERS

An Imprint of Elsevier, Inc.
PHILADELPHIA   LONDON   TORONTO   MONTREAL   SYDNEY   TOKYO

W.B. SAUNDERS COMPANY
A Division of Elsevier Inc.

The Curtis Center • Independence Square West • Philadelphia, Pennsylvania 19106

http://www.theclinics.com

NEUROLOGIC CLINICS
May 2005
Editor: Robert Gardler

Volume 23, Number 2
ISSN 0733-8619
ISBN 1-4160-2830-7

Reprints. For copies of 100 or more of articles in this publication, please contact the Commercial Reprints Department, Elsevier Inc., 360 Park Avenue South, New York, New York 10010-1710. Tel.: (212) 633-3813, Fax: (212) 462-1935, e-mail: reprints@elsevier.com

The ideas and opinions expressed in *Neurologic Clinics* do not necessarily reflect those of the Publisher. The Publisher does not assume any responsibility for any injury and/or damage to persons or property arising out of or related to any use of the material contained in this periodical. The reader is advised to check the appropriate medical literature and the product information currently provided by the manufacturer of each drug to be administered to verify the dosage, the method and duration of administration, or contraindications. It is the responsibility of the treating physician or other health care professional, relying on independent experience and knowledge of the patient, to determine drug dosages and the best treatment for the patient. Mention of any product in this issue should not be construed as endorsement by the contributors, editors, or the Publisher of the product or manufacturers' claims.

Neurologic Clinics (ISSN 0733-8619) is published quarterly by Elsevier. Corporate and editorial offices: 170 S Independence Mall W 300 E, Philadelphia, PA 19106-3399. Accounting and circulation offices: 6277 Sea Harbor Drive, Orlando, FL 32887-4800. Periodicals postage paid at Orlando, FL 32862, and additional mailing offices. Subscription prices are $175.00 per year for US individuals, $275.00 per year for US institutions, $88.00 per year for US students, $214.00 per year for Canadian individuals, $325.00 per year for Canadian institutions, and $113.00 per year for Canadian students. To receive student/resident rate, orders must be accompanied by name of affiliated institution, date of term, and the *signature* of program/residency coordinator on institution letterhead. Orders will be billed at individual rate until proof of status is received. Foreign air speed delivery is included in all *Clinics* subscription prices. All prices are subject to change without notice. POSTMASTER: Send address changes to *Neurologic Clinics*, W.B. Saunders Company, Periodicals Fulfillment, Orlando, FL 32887-4800. **Customer Service: 1-800-654-2452 (US). From outside of the US, call 1-407-345-4000.**

Neurologic Clinics is also published in Spanish by Nueva Editorial Interamericana S.A., Mexico City, Mexico.

Neurologic Clinics is covered in *Current Contents/Clinical Medicine*, *Index Medicus*, *EMBASE*/Excerpta Medica, and *PsycINFO*, and *ISI/BIOMED*.

Printed in the United States of America.

GUEST EDITORS

MICHAEL R. DOBBS, MD, Major, United States Air Force Medical Corps, Chief of Neurological Research, Wilford Hall Medical Center, Lackland Air Force Base, San Antonio, Texas

MATTHEW P. WICKLUND, MD, Col (sel), United States Air Force Medical Corps, Chairman, Department of Neurology, Wilford Hall Medical Center, Lackland Air Force Base, San Antonio, Texas

CONTRIBUTORS

ANTHONY A. AMATO, MD, Vice-Chairman, Department of Neurology; Chief, Neuromuscular Division; and Director, Clinical Neurophysiology Laboratory, Brigham and Women's Hospital; Associate Professor of Neurology, Harvard Medical School, Boston, Massachusetts

ELEANOR AVERY, MD, Lt Col, United States Air Force, Staff Neurologist and Chief of Geriatrics, Wilford Hall Medical Center, San Antonio, Texas

ALLISON CABAN-HOLT, PhD, Postdoctoral Fellow, Sanders-Brown Center on Aging, University of Kentucky Medical Center, Lexington, Kentucky

GREGORY COOPER, MD, PhD, Assistant Professor, Sanders-Brown Center on Aging: Alzheimer's Disease Research Center; Department of Neurology, University of Kentucky Medical Center; and Division Chief, Lexington Clinic Department of Neurology, Lexington, Kentucky

MICHAEL R. DOBBS, MD, Major, United States Air Force Medical Corps, Assistant Professor of Neurology, Uniformed Services University of the Health Sciences, Bethesda, Maryland; and Chief of Neurological Research, Wilford Hall Medical Center, Lackland Air Force Base, San Antonio, Texas

TRACY EICHER, MD, Captain, United States Air Force, Chief Resident, Neurology, Wilford Hall Medical Center, Lackland Air Force Base, San Antonio, Texas

R. BRENT FURBEE, MD, Medical Director, Indiana Poison Center, Department of Emergency Medicine, Division of Medical Toxicology, Indiana University School of Medicine, Indianapolis, Indiana

PATRICK M. GROGAN, MD, Associate Program Director, Department of Neurology, Wilford Hall Medical Center, Lackland Air Force Base, San Antonio, Texas

GARY S. GRONSETH, MD, Associate Professor and Vice Chair of Neurology, The University of Kansas, Kansas City, Kansas

MICHAEL HOFFMANN, MD, Professor, Department of Neurology, University of South Florida; and Director, Stroke Program, Tampa General Hospital, Tampa, Florida

MICHAEL S. JAFFEE, MD, Lt Col, United States Air Force, Neurology Program Director, Wilford Hall Medical Center, San Antonio, Texas; and Neurology Consultant to the United States Air Force Aeromedical Consult Service, Brooks Air Force Base, San Antonio, Texas

JONATHAN S. KATZ, MD, Associate Professor, Neurology, Stanford University Medical Center; and Department of Neurology, Palo Alto Veterans Affairs Health Care System, Palo Alto, California

ALI R. MALEK, MD, Assistant Professor, Department of Neurology, University of South Florida; and Director, Neurocritical Care Unit, Tampa General Hospital, Tampa, Florida

MICHELLE MATTINGLY, PhD, Assistant Professor, Department of Neurology, University of Kentucky Medical Center, Lexington, Kentucky

JONATHAN NEWMARK, MD, Col, MC, USAR, United States Army Medical Research Institute of Chemical Defense, Aberdeen Proving Ground, Maryland; Office of the Assistant Secretary for Public Health Emergency Preparedness, United States Department of Health and Human Services, Washington, DC; F. Edward Hebert School of Medicine, Uniformed Services University of the Health Sciences, Bethesda, Maryland

PETER J. OSTERBAUER, MD, Captain, United States Air Force, Department of Neurology, Wilford Hall Medical Center, Lackland Air Force Base, San Antonio, Texas

ERIC J. PAPPERT, MD, Assistant Professor of Neurology, Director, Parkinson's Disease and Movement Disorders Program, Department of Medicine, Division of Neurology, University of Texas, Health Science Center, San Antonio, Texas

ROBERT PASCUZZI, MD, Department of Neurology, Indiana University School of Medicine, Indianapolis, Indiana

L. CAMERON PIMPERL, Lt Col, United States Air Force, MC, Radiation Oncologist, Department of Radiation Oncology; Chairman, Neuro-Oncology Conference; Chairman, Cancer Clinical Activities Committee, Wilford Hall Medical Center, Lackland Air Force Base, San Antonio, Texas

JOSHUA S. ROTENBERG, MD, MMS, Chief, Pediatric Neurology, Departments of Pediatrics and Neurology, Wilford Hall Medical Center, Lackland Air Force Base, San Antonio, Texas

DANIEL E. RUSYNIAK, MD, Department of Emergency Medicine, Division of Medical Toxicology, Indiana University School of Medicine, Indianapolis, Indiana

CARRIE SCHMID, MD, Departments of Pediatrics and Neurology, Wilford Hall Medical Center, Lackland Air Force Base, San Antonio, Texas

FREDERICK A. SCHMITT, PhD, Professor, Department of Neurology, Sanders-Brown Center on Aging: Alzheimer's Disease Research Center; Departments of Psychiatry, Psychology, and Behavioral Science, University of Kentucky Medical Center, Lexington, Kentucky

DAVID R. WALLACE, PhD, Associate Professor of Pharmacology and Forensic Science, Oklahoma State University Center for Health Sciences, Tulsa, Oklahoma

RONAN J. WALSH, MD, Fellow, Neuromuscular Division, Department of Neurology, Brigham and Women's Hospital, Boston, Massachusetts

MATTHEW P. WICKLUND, MD, Col (sel), Chairman, Department of Neurology, Wilford Hall Medical Center, Lackland Air Force Base, San Antonio, Texas

CONTENTS

As the number of drugs and environmental and bacterial/viral agents with potential neurotoxic properties has grown, so has the need for additional testing. This article provides an overview of neurotoxicology on a molecular, cellular, and genetic level. These aspects of neurotoxicology are not mutually exclusive but intimately inter-related. The article discusses molecular and cellular changes that occur following exposure to exogenous agents that may provide protection and the molecular and cellular environments that may facilitate neurotoxicity. The genetic effects of toxic agents are discussed from the perspectives of genetic alterations following exposure and genetic alterations or defects present before exposure that may predispose an individual to a toxic insult following exposure.

This review offers basic principles for the clinician faced with a potential developmental neurotoxin. Normal central nervous system development is described, with particular emphasis on known vulnerable periods for toxic exposures. This article details three prevalent nervous system teratogens and the controversy regarding mercury exposure and the hypothesized link to autism.

Many unexplained neurologic disorders are believed to have a neurotoxic cause. Although uniquely protected by the blood-brain barrier, the central and peripheral nervous systems are vulnerable to a variety of toxins, as demonstrated by several historical outbreaks. This article reviews four of these unique outbreaks and their neurotoxic manifestations and relevance to modern neurologic problems, including ginger jake and peripheral neuropathy, Minamata disease and neurodevelopmental disorders, 1-methyl-4-phenyl-1,2,3,6-tetrahydropyridine poisoning and Parkinsonism, and, lastly, ergot poisoning and psychiatric disturbances.

Effective brain function is dependent on precise and complex interactions among neurotransmitters, hormones, enzymes, and electrolytes. Many of the chemically complex substances with which we come into contact can disrupt this intricately balanced system. Toxic substances, whether ingested, inhaled, or absorbed through the skin, may cause an encephalopathic state directly by affecting the brain itself or indirectly by compromising the brain's supportive systems. This article focuses on neurotoxins (heavy metals, solvents and vapors, pesticides, and natural neurotoxins) that directly induce an encephalopathic state.

Toxic exposure to a wide variety of substances may result in the development of clinical neuropathy syndromes. This review synthesizes the current information available on the relationship between various neuropathies and exposures to heavy metals, organic chemicals, prescription medications, substances of abuse, toxic marine and plant organisms, and venomous animals. The clinical phenotype, electrodiagnostic and histopathologic workup, prognosis, and available treatments of each neuropathy are discussed.

Muscle tissue is highly sensitive to drugs and toxins because of its high metabolic activity and potential sites for disruption of energy-producing pathways. Early recognition of toxic myopathies is important, as they potentially are reversible on removal of the offending toxin, with greater likelihood of complete resolution the sooner this is achieved. Clinical features range from mild muscle pain and cramps to severe weakness with rhabdomyolysis, renal failure, and even death. The pathogenic bases can be multifactorial. This article reviews drugs responsible for common types of toxic myopathy and their clinical and histopathologic features and illustrates possible underlying cellular mechanisms.

toxins to the development of GWS. This article reviews the evidence regarding the possible role of toxin exposure in causing GWS.

This article provides a brief overview of the environmental factors encountered in aviation, underwater, and space environments that are most implicated in neurologic dysfunction. Environmental factors unique to the aviation environment are hypoxia and acceleration. Common environmental factors that affect aviation and underwater environments are effects of pressure and decompression. A unique factor of the underwater environment is the effect of gases at depth. The distinguishing feature of the space environment is microgravity.

With increased access to once remote regions of the planet and renewed interest in exploring natural surroundings, previously geographically isolated and rare neurologic conditions can be encountered in any patient population. Rare envenomations and poisonings, once the purview of the tropical neurologist, now can be encountered by travelers to areas where creatures that have developed specialized defenses are endemic. Recognition, therefore, of the potentially neurotoxic fauna and flora in these areas holds value, even for the urban neurologist.

Neurotoxicity from radiation can range widely and produce effects that may include (1) small absolute increases in cancer risks, (2) subtle effects on higher level functioning in some individuals, (3) severe cognitive impairment in some individuals, (4) severe focal injury that may include necrosis or irreversible loss of function, and (5) overwhelming and rapidly fatal diffuse injury associated with high-dose, whole-body exposures. An understanding of the implications of nervous system exposure to radiation can guide efforts in radiation protection and aid in the optimization of the medical uses of radiation.

The threat of biological warfare and terrorism continues to be a growing concern. It is important for the neurologist to be acutely aware of biological and toxic agents that target the nervous system, because it is likely that a neurologist will be the first practitioner to see victims of a biological attack with certain agents. This article comprehensively reviews biological and biotoxic agents that may present with symptoms and signs referable to the central and peripheral nervous system.

Of the major classes of chemical warfare agents, nerve agents are of the most particular neurologic interest. These poisons act primarily as inhibitors of synaptic acetylcholinesterases, causing a rapidly progressive cholinergic crisis. The speed of onset can be so rapid, and so likely fatal in large doses, that emergent treatment becomes crucial. Although neurologists are unlikely to be the first responders providing emergent treatment, neurologists should be familiar with the pathophysiology and neurologic ramifications of the nerve-agent poisoning syndromes, not only to provide effective neurologic care but also to assist in the training of first responders.

FORTHCOMING ISSUES

RECENT ISSUES

NEUROLOGIC
CLINICS

ELSEVIER
SAUNDERS

Neurol Clin 23 (2005) xiii–xiv

Preface

Toxic and Environmental Neurology

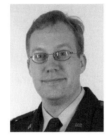
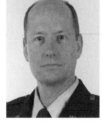

Maj Michael R. Dobbs, MD   Col (sel) Matthew P. Wicklund, MD
Guest Editors

Environmental conditions and toxins are important and under-recognized causes of neurologic disease. In addition to chemical toxins, extremes of cold, heat, and altitude all can have adverse effects on our bodies and nervous systems. As medical and scientific knowledge increases, more toxic and environmental causes of diseases are discovered.

Society continues to advance technologically. As it progresses, we often place ourselves into new situations and environments exposing ourselves to new substances. Some of these environments and substances may be harmful. It is reasonable to expect that we will continue to experience diseases caused by toxins and environments throughout our foreseeable future as a species.

This work is divided into sections. The first section is an overview of toxic neurology, including basic science, embryology, and neurotoxins in history. The second section is a systems-based approach to neurotoxic disorders. Next is a section on controversies in neurotoxicology, such as that regarding Gulf War syndrome. There also is a section covering the dangers of specific environments, such as wilderness and high altitudes. Finally, the issue ends with a section on neurologic weapons, detailed reviews of biological and chemical weapons that target the nervous system.

We have tried to piece together a broad compilation of reviews of toxins, situations, and environments likely to be harmful to the nervous system. We are proud that many of our contributors are military clinicians. It is our hope that this issue of *Neurologic Clinics* will aid the reader in patient care, research, and education.

0733-8619/05/$ - see front matter. Published by Elsevier Inc.
doi:10.1016/j.ncl.2004.12.001   *neurologic.theclinics.com*

We would like to thank all of the authors who contributed to this issue. We appreciate Sarah Barth and Bob Gardler at Elsevier for their patience in dealing with inexperienced Guest Editors. Most of all, however, we want to thank our wives, Betsy and Beth, for bearing with us as we completed this task.

Maj Michael R. Dobbs, MD
Wilford Hall Medical Center
2200 Bergquist Drive
Suite 1/MMCN
Lackland Air Force Base, TX 78236, USA

E-mail address: michael.dobbs@lackland.af.mil

Col (sel) Matthew P. Wicklund, MD
Wilford Hall Medical Center
2200 Bergquist Drive
Suite 1/MMCN
Lackland Air Force Base, TX 78236, USA

E-mail address: matthew.wicklund@lackland.af.mil

ELSEVIER
SAUNDERS

Neurol Clin 23 (2005) 307–320

NEUROLOGIC
CLINICS

Overview of Molecular, Cellular, and Genetic Neurotoxicology

David R. Wallace, PhD

*Department of Pharmacology and Physiology, Oklahoma State University Center for Health
Sciences, 1111 West 17th Street, Tulsa, OK 74107-1898, USA*

The field of neurotoxicology has grown immensely in the last 2 decades. One indication of this expansion is the ever-growing list of societies related to neurotoxicology or a neurotoxicologic field (eg, the International Neuro-toxicology Association and the Society of Toxicology, with the latter having subsections for those individuals with interest in neurotoxicology or a related field). Increased interest is due in part to the growth of pharmaceuticals with central nervous system (CNS) activity. The list of agents that have the po-tential to cause neurotoxic insult is continually growing. Not only are prescription/illicit pharmaceuticals of concern but the increasing number of agents that can be found in the environment (heavy metals, pesticides, ionizing radiation, and so forth) and in the workplace (industrial pollution, combustion by-products, and so forth) also suggests that the broad area of neurotoxicology will only continue to grow. Recently, there has been height-ened interest in the actions of toxins from bacterial or viral sources in the CNS. In late-stage AIDS, one clinical manifestation is AIDS-related dementia. At least in part, this clinical manifestation may be due to the toxic effects of two HIV-associated proteins. Thus, microbial toxins are another source of potential neurotoxic insult. In addition to the aforemen-tioned areas, the field of alternative medicine, which includes herbal and other "natural" products, has greatly contributed to the need for further neurotoxicologic studies. In most cases, alternative remedies are relatively benign, but through interactions with other exogenous agents or through their own bioaccumulation, CNS toxicity can be observed. The newest area of neurotoxicologic focus has been on the effects of biological weapons or weapons of mass destruction. As the specter of terrorism shadows everyday life, the need to understand the mechanism or mechanisms of action for

This work was supported by Grant DA13137 from the National Institutes of Health.
E-mail address: walladr@chs.okstate.edu

recognized bioweapons is significant. To understand the agents used for these devices would also provide insight into the actions of other neurotoxic agents.

Another complicating issue in the field of neurotoxicology is that some agents at "normal" concentrations are harmless and do not elicit any overt neurologic symptoms. In healthy adults, most exogenous agents are metabolized to inactive compounds, eliminated, or both. In some instances, however, agents may accumulate over time or dose to levels that are toxic, which could be due to chronic exposure or to inadequate metabolism or elimination. In addition, brief exposure may initiate changes that are not clearly observed early in exposure but may appear much later. This effect could interfere with the appropriate diagnosis of exposure versus a neurodegenerative disease that exhibits similar neurologic symptoms.

Thus, the current catalog of agents that may result in neurologic insult is significant and growing daily. As a population, we continue to lengthen our life span, which increases our exposure to toxins that may exert neurologic effects. In addition, as the population increases, our generation of pollutants also increases. Increased levels of pollutants that may be found in the home, workplace, and environment could produce unforeseen neurologic effects. In this situation, we enter a complex and possibly vicious cycle that could potentially become self-limiting. To break this cycle, we need to research further the mechanism of action, diagnosis, and potential treatment following exposure to these agents. Therefore, the need to examine and understand these agents is vital. As our understanding of these agents grows, our ability to develop and provide potential pharmacotherapies increases.

An issue that has plagued neurotoxicology research has been the use of appropriate and comparable animal or nonanimal model systems [1]. There are numerous factors and issues that need to be considered when selecting an animal model. The first is applicability to the human CNS. Neuronal systems studied must exhibit some commonality to human systems. Rodents are commonly used. In some instances, however, rodents are used to the exclusion of other systems, even when it is understood that their use is not the best model for the system in question [2]. Efforts from outside sources and agencies are forcing this dogma to change. Regulatory agencies such as the Food and Drug Administration and funding agencies such as the National Institutes of Health and the National Science Foundation are emphasizing a reduction in the number of animals used in research and are encouraging researchers to find alternative models for research [3,4]. Research into other species (*Drosophila* and *Caenorhabditis elegans*) has more fully elucidated their neural systems, and it has become evident to the neurotoxicology community that these species can provide powerful model systems to study specific interactions of toxic agents within the CNS. The human genome project has revealed that many human genes are similar, if not exact, to our ancient ancestors. Therefore, many species previously thought of as being too "primitive" are now known to express the genes of interest in neurotoxicity testing. Ballatori and Villalobos [1] provide an excellent review of alternative species used in neurotoxicity testing. Another concern with extrapolating in vitro work to in vivo work is the conditions in which the in vitro work is performed. Caution must be exercised when interpreting in vitro concentrations to in vivo effects, the use of immortalized cell lines to primary neuronal culture, and the employment of newly developed techniques without fully understanding the connection between in vitro and in vivo studies. In most cases, parallel in vitro and in vivo studies is most advantageous [5].

The intent of this review is to provide a current overview to neurotoxicology on a molecular, cellular, and genetic level. Examination of these topics clearly demonstrates that molecular, cellular, and genetic aspects of neurotoxicology are not mutually exclusive but are intimately inter-related. The molecular and cellular changes that occur following exposure to exogenous agents that may provide protection and the molecular and cellular environments that may facilitate neurotoxicity are discussed. The genetic effects of toxic agents are also discussed from the perspectives of genetic alterations following exposure and genetic alterations or defects present before exposure that may predispose an individual to a toxic insult following exposure.

Molecular neurotoxicology

Past work in the field of neurotoxicology has emphasized the outcomes following exposure to a toxic agent. This emphasis was due in part to the limitations of the technology available at the time. Most work was categorized into three groups: molecular-mechanistic, correlative, and "black box" [6]. The superficial nature of this work led to questions and concerns from the more established fields of neuroscience. This trend has slowly evolved and changed with the acceptance of the interdisciplinary nature of the neurotoxicology field. Areas of neurophysiology, neurochemistry, neuroscience, and molecular biology have demonstrated areas of overlap that have assisted in furthering our understanding of neurotoxicology. Further advances in neurotoxicology will come from additional molecular research and increased understanding of CNS injury from endogenous and exogenous agents [7].

Recently, there has been a substantial expansion and diversification in technology that has facilitated the study of neurotoxicology on molecular and cellular levels. Previous work in "molecular biology" has emphasized the studies of mRNA and gene expression. For this review, these topics are addressed in the genetics section, the rationale being that measurement of gene and mRNA expression is more a phenomenon of the gene and may not accurately represent the molecular function of the intracellular proteins.

One area of study that has gained significant attention in the past few years has been the field of proteomics. Lubec et al [8] provides a review of the potential and the limitations of proteomics. The *proteome* is the protein outcome from the genome. Genetic expression leads to the synthesis and degradation of proteins that are integrally involved in normal neuronal function. Agents that interfere with this protein processing could lead to neuronal damage, death, or predisposition to further insults. Oxidative or covalent modification of proteins could lead to alterations in tertiary structure and loss of protein function. The advantage to proteomics over "classical" protein chemistry is that proteomics examines multiple steps in the cycle of protein synthesis, function, and degradation, whereas protein chemistry focuses on the sequence of amino acids that form the protein. Therefore, proteomics focuses on a more comprehensive view of cellular proteins and provides considerable more information about the effects of toxins on the CNS [9]. Effects of possible toxic agents can be detected at the post-translational level following exposure [10,11]. The most applicable use for proteomics in assessing the effects of a possible toxin is mapping post-translational modifications of proteins [9]. Post-translational processing involves many processes including protein phosphorylation, glycosylation, tertiary structure, function, and turnover. Modifications of proteins in-fluence protein trafficking, which could have significant impact on the movement and insertion of proteins such as neurotransmitter receptors and transporters. In addition to alteration in post-translational processing, many potential toxic agents are electrophilic and covalently bind to groups on proteins, such as thiol groups, thus altering their structure, function, and subsequent degradation and elimination [12,13]. Oxidation of proteins is believed to be involved in many toxic insults and degenerative diseases of the CNS [14,15]. The measurement of oxidized proteins, or carbonyls, is an accepted method for the determination of oxidized proteins in brain tissue [16]. In addition to post-translational modifications, protein-expression profiling and protein-network mapping can also be employed. Protein-expression profiling can identify all proteins from a particular tissue or cell. This method is beneficial when comparing the "profile" of proteins within control tissues/cells to toxin-exposed tissues/cells and yields a greater amount of information on how multiple, potentially interacting proteins are affected following exposure. The method of protein-expression profiling has been used to assess protein changes in head trauma, hypoxia, and during the aging process [17–19]. A limitation for the use of protein-expression profiling is the amount of protein being measured. The protein of interest would have to be in substantial quantities and the difference would have to be great enough to be detected. An improvement on this method was described by Gygi et al [20] who used liquid chromatography-mass spectrometry detection of isotope-labeled proteins.

Protein-network mapping is an enormously powerful tool for identifying changes in multiprotein complexes induced by exposure to a possible toxin.

There are two approaches to measuring protein-network mapping. First, the "two-hybrid" system uses a reporter gene to detect the interaction of protein pairs within the yeast cell nucleus. The two-hybrid system can be used to screen potential toxic agents that disrupt specific protein–protein interactions. This method is not without limitations regarding data interpretation. Second, "pull-down" studies use immunoprecipitation of a protein that, in turn, precipitates associated or interactive proteins. Collectively, each method (post-translational modification, protein-expression profiling, and protein-network mapping) builds on each of the previous methods. Taken together, these methods provide a more complete and powerful image of protein modifications following potential toxin exposure.

Cellular neurotoxicology

The area of cellular neurotoxicology is relatively ubiquitous and may involve many cellular processes. These processes could include alterations in cellular energy homeostasis, ion homeostasis, intracellular signaling function, and neurotransmitter release, uptake, and storage. Finding an appropriate measurement following toxin exposure has been difficult. Ideally, the desired biomarker is one that could easily be measured in a living subject and would accurately represent the toxin exposure. It is widely recognized that a "single" marker probably does not exist, and that a combination of markers, examined together, would provide a more accurate assessment of toxin exposure. Further complicating the interpretation of toxicant-CNS effects are the various classifications of biomarkers. There are biomarkers of exposure, effect, and susceptibility [21]. Finding the appropriate biomarker for a particular toxin is a daunting task.

Developmental neurotoxicology is one of the more difficult disciplines to assess for toxin exposure. Initially, there is fetal development, when the CNS is most susceptible to toxins that cross the placental barrier. Postnatal development is also a vulnerable period, although much less so than fetal development. Lastly, prepubescent and adolescent development periods are also temporal time points that warrant monitoring and investigation. Barone et al [22] reviewed the biomarkers and methods used for assessing exposure to pesticides during these periods of development. A difficulty that requires attention is the use of an appropriate model system and interpretation of databases at the appropriate stages of development [22]. The use of oligodendrocytes, or oligodendroglia, has attracted attention due to the influence of some environmental toxins such as lead that affect the myelination of neurons [23]. Alterations in myelination change conduction speeds of myelinated neurons and thus affect neuronal function. Oligodendrocytes possess a variety of ligand- and voltage-gated ion channels and neurotransmitter receptors. The best characterized of the neurotransmitters that assist in shaping the developing oligodendrocytes population is glutamate [24,25]. The primary receptor classes expressed in oligodendrocytes are the ionotopic glutamate receptors (α-amino-3-hydroxy-5-methyl-4-isoxazolepropionic acid and kainate). In addition to glutamate receptors, γ-aminobutyric acid, serotonin, glycine, dopamine, nicotinic, β-adrenergic, substance P, somatostatin, and opioid receptors are also expressed. Calcium, sodium, and potassium channels have also been identified in oligodendrocytes (see reference [23] and references cited within). It has been established that crosstalk between neurons and glia exists [26]. Therefore, changes in glia, or oligodendrocyte, function may have a profound impact on neuronal function. In addition, the use of oligodendrocytes may provide a useful model system for the study of toxicant-CNS action.

Biomarkers of exposure include such combinations (biomarker/toxin) as mercapturates/styrene, hemoglobin/carbon disulfide, and porphyrins/metals [21,27]. The advantage to these biomarker/toxin combinations is they can be detected and measured shortly following exposure and before overt neuroanatomic damage or lesions. Intervention at this point, shortly following exposure, may prevent or attenuate further damage to the individual [28]. Biomarker combinations for effect include acetylcholinesterase/organophosphates, monoamine oxidase B/styrene and manganese, dopamine-β-hydroxylase/manganese and styrene, and calcium/mercury [27]. Susceptibility markers include δ-aminolevulinic acid dehydratase for lead and aldehyde dehydrogenase for alcohol [21,27]. Although these biomarkers can be used for examining toxin exposure in the CNS, they are difficult to measure directly. Therefore, there is a need for establishing biomarkers that can be easily measured in the periphery and that are similar to the targets of toxic substances in the CNS [29]. Parameters that can be measured in the periphery include receptors (muscarinic, β-adrenergic, benzodiazepine, σ- and α_2-adrenergic), enzymes (acetylcholinesterase, monoamine oxidase B), and signal transduction (calcium, adenylyl cyclase, phosphoinositide metabolism) and uptake systems (serotonin), which can be found in human blood cells [27,29]. Most commonly, the blood cell types that have been studied are lymphocytes, platelets, and erythrocytes. Of particular interest in the author's laboratory and in others is the dopaminergic system. The dopaminergic system is directly or indirectly involved in the neurotoxicity elicited by multiple compounds including the heavy metals manganese, lead, and mercury, and industrial solvents and toxins. Indices of dopaminergic function include measurement of dopamine-β-hydroxylase activity, monoamine oxidase activity, and the dopamine transporter function. For example, exposure to manganese results in dopamine autoxidation, free radical generation, followed by neuronal damage. This damage results in neurologic symptoms that resemble Parkinson's disease and have been referred to as "manganism." Although dopamine-β-hydroxylase and monoamine oxidase activity have been shown to be reliable markers of manganese exposure, Smargiassi and Mutti [30] reported that the measurement of prolactin levels is just as reliable and can be used to measure early exposure.

The use of peripheral biomarkers to assess toxin damage in the CNS has numerous advantages: time-course analysis may be performed, ethical concerns with the use of human subjects can be partially avoided, less invasive procedures to acquire samples can be used, and in general, peripheral studies are easier to perform. The use of the appropriate biomarker is extremely valuable and may signal the exposure to a toxin before clear clinical symptoms become present. Yet, several significant obstacles must be first overcome for a peripheral biomarker to reflect an accurate representation of CNS effects. First, CNS and peripheral markers must exhibit the same pharmacologic and biochemical characteristics under control situations and following toxin exposure. Second, time-course response profiles must be performed to determine whether the peripheral tissue responds in the same fashion as the CNS tissue [31,32]. Third, the complexity of the CNS allows for adaptation that may not be present in the periphery. Other neuronal systems or neurotransmitters may adapt or compensate for toxin-related CNS changes following exposure [33]. Finally, inherent in many human studies is inter- and intragroup variability that may in some instances be large. These factors must be considered when attempting to accurately determine whether a potential biomarker has been changed.

In most instances, hypothesis-driven research is the preferred modality. Research that is purely mechanistic has been frowned on by most funding agencies, yet mechanistic research still has a place in the field neurotoxicology and its importance cannot be underestimated. Work on the actions of organophosphate pesticides and their mechanisms of action are probably the best described [34–36]. The value of mechanistic studies in neurotoxicology is to facilitate the development of biomarkers for future use in detecting toxin exposure [36]. When one considers the thousands of toxins and the additional thousands of potential toxins that an individual may be exposed to in his or her lifetime, it is startling that only a handful of reliable biomarkers exist. The reason for this, at least in part, is the complexity of the CNS, which makes finding and characterizing an appropriate biomarker very difficult. Increased use of mechanistic studies, in a fashion similar to what has been accomplished with organophosphate exposure, would further advance our understanding of toxin effects and could lead to earlier detection of exposure [32,36]. In addition to mechanistic studies to identify and characterize biomarkers, use of existing data to formulate nonhuman studies characterizing the actions of a toxin could be extremely valuable. Slikker et al [37] used existing information on exposure of domoic acid, a glutamate agonist, in a population in which toxicity to this endogenous toxin was reported. Their findings suggest that a quantitative approach, which uses all data that are available, would yield an accurate dose-response model for domoic acid toxicity that is biologically based [37]. Using the method described by Slikker et al [37] would allow the use of nonhuman experimental units and provide information comparable to a comprehensive human study.

A cellular extension of the protein–protein interactions discussed in the previous section on molecular neurotoxicology involves the release of neurotransmitters. It is possible to measure neurotransmitter release in vitro using synaptosomal, brain slice, and culture methodologies. A drawback with this method is that it requires the removal of all or part of the brain from the subject. Westerink [38] reported the use of amperometry and a carbon microelectrode to measure the release of neurotransmitters from the synapse. The use of amperometry focuses on presynaptic effects of toxins and alterations of neurotransmitter release. Numerous protein–protein interactions (docking, exocytosis) must occur for proper release of neurotransmitters after stimulation (see reference [39] for review). Some of the proteins involved in the stimulation–exocytosis process are soluble N-ethylmaleimide sensitive fusion protein attachment protein receptors (SNARE), vesicle-associated SNARE proteins (synaptobrevins), and plasma membrane–associated SNARE proteins (syntaxin and synaptosomal-associated protein-25). Disruption of the activity of any of these proteins could result in robust changes in transmitter release. There is an increasing body of evidence that certain classes of drugs affect presynaptic release of neurotransmitters. Drugs of abuse, most notably amphetamine, have been shown to increase dopamine release and elicit toxicity in part through a presynaptic mechanism. Toluene has also been reported to increase the presynaptic release of dopamine in a calcium-dependent manner [38]. Polychlorinated biphenyls and heavy metals (lead, mercury, and manganese) have also been reported to increase presynaptic neurotransmitter release through calcium-dependent and calcium-independent mechanisms [38]. One difficulty in assessing the precise mechanism of action for some of these toxins is the diverse actions that each toxin displays. Therefore, with the use of amperometry, only catecholamine and indolamine release can be measured [38]; however, interactions of a toxin at a different neurotransmitter site may in turn alter the release of the catecholamine or indolamine being measured.

Collectively, evidence for biomarkers in cellular neurotoxicology is lacking compared with the number of potential toxins that a person may be exposed to during his or her lifetime. Recently, the tools to study protein–protein interactions have begun to catch up to the need for such tools. By examining the effect of a potential toxin on protein–protein interactions on an intracellular level, one can begin to describe the cellular changes that occur following toxin exposure that are devoid of obvious clinical symptoms. It is clear that additional work is needed, but research methodologies are now available to expand the current mechanistic literature and develop valuable and reliable biomarkers for particular toxins.

Genetic neurotoxicology

The purpose of this section is to present an overview of current literature available regarding the area of genetic neurotoxicology. For the sake of brevity, discussion on changes in mRNA and cDNA expression is minimized. Discussion on polymorphisms and genetic changes that may be present, however, is examined more thoroughly. The general area of genetic neurotoxicology can be subdivided into two subclasses: (1) toxin-induced alterations in genetic expression, and (2) genetic alterations that affect toxin metabolism, distribution, and clearance. These differences can be beneficial or toxic.

A sizable body of work is accessible regarding causal peripheral effects of toxins, genetic polymorphisms, and cancer [40–42]. This work has focused on peripheral cancers of the breast, lung, and bladder, among other organs. The cytochrome P450 enzymes (CYPs) are fairly ubiquitous, being found in the periphery and in the CNS. Numerous polymorphisms exist within the P450 family of enzymes. Polymorphisms have been identified in human CYP1A1, CYP1B1, CYP2C9, CYP2C18, CYP2D6, and CYP3A4. Together, CYP2D6 and CYP3A4 are responsible for >95% of the metabolizing activity of the CYP family. CYP3A4 is the principal human CYP responsible for the oxidation of parathion. Therefore, the potential for variations in the metabolism of the pesticide parathion and other organophosphates exists within the human population. In addition to polymorphisms in CYP3A4, a polymorphic change in glutathione S-transferase has been described. Thus, polymorphic changes in CYP3A4 or in glutathione S-transferase may increase or decrease an individual's susceptibility to organophosphate pesticides [43]. Organophosphates are not metabolized by only CYP3A4 and glutathione S-transferase. The organophosphate paraoxon is activated by the P450 enzymes first, followed by metabolism of its oxygenated active metabolite (oxon) by paraoxonase. Paraoxonase has been demonstrated to be polymorphic in human populations and may predispose an individual to not only altered organophosphate metabolism but also increased risk for heart disease [44]. Previously accepted dogma has stipulated that a toxin must be mutagenic/genotoxic for symptoms to occur. Trosko et al [45] present compelling arguments that a toxin can be epigenetic and still be damaging. An epigenetic event can be a stable or reversible alteration in the expression of the genomic information at the transcriptional, translational, or post-translational level [45]. In a manner similar to what was described for protein–protein interactions, a toxin interruption of extra-, inter-, or intracellular communication would disrupt the homeostatic regulation of the cells and may be an underlying cause for toxin-induced disease [45]. Another example of epigenetic toxicity is oxidative stress. Agents that cause oxidative stress do not always fit within the genotoxic paradigm, and the data from these studies are often open to interpretation [46]. Numerous compounds (2,3,7,8-tetrachlorodibenzo-p-dioxin, hydrogen peroxide, phenobarbital, polychlorinated biphenyls, DDT, and saccharin, among others) have been reported to elicit epigenetic events without being cytotoxic. These epigenetic agents can affect the expression of proteins that can stimulate (p53 and so forth) or inhibit (IκB) transcription [45,47,48]. Toxins that are not genotoxic but that cause an epigenetic event could be as important in the field of neurotoxicology as agents that are genotoxic or cytotoxic.

Genetic techniques have advanced to include the sequencing of the entire human genome and the mapping of the rodent genome. By identifying particular genes within the genome, it may be possible to determine susceptibility or resistance to a particular toxin. Currently, mapping tools that are available for the human genome include the genetic linkage map, the physical map, and the human transcript map [49]. The primary usage of this information is the identification of susceptibility genes. Using the mouse map, two strains with differing susceptibility to ozone were compared and a quantitative trait locus was identified [50,51]. As progress in this area proceeds, it is obvious that the use of the human genome map will be a powerful tool for the prediction of toxin effects and may provide new avenues to treat toxin exposure before clinical symptoms become relevant. Presently, the use of microarray technology has demonstrated immense usefulness in toxicity studies [52]. Vrana et al [52] describe the use of the microarray technology in an excellent review of the methodology. In addition to peripheral effects of toxins and alteration in DNA expression using microarray technology, recent work has examined the effects of toxic compounds on DNA expression in the CNS. A group of genes that may contribute to methamphetamine-induced toxicity in the ventral striatum of the mouse has been identified [53,54]. In addition, the use of microarray technology has demonstrated alterations in gene expression in animals exposed to the dopaminergic toxin, N-methyl-4-phenyl-1,2,3,6-tetrahydropyridine, and chronic alcoholism (see reference [52] and references cited within). It is clear that the microarray technology is an extremely powerful tool, but more work needs to be done to refine the method. Currently, a great deal of information is gathered from a microarray, but interpretation of the findings can be elusive. As the method becomes more refined and DNA analysis becomes more toxin specific, it could be possible to develop arrays for particular classifications of drugs or toxins.

Summary

It has become increasingly evident that the field of neurotoxicology is not only rapidly growing but also rapidly evolving, especially over the last 20 years. As the number of drugs and environmental and bacterial/viral agents with potential neurotoxic properties has grown, the need for additional testing has increased. Only recently has the technology advanced to a level that neurotoxicologic studies can be performed without operating in a "black box." Examination of the effects of agents that are suspected of being toxic can occur on the molecular (protein–protein), cellular (biomarkers, neuronal function), and genetic (polymorphisms) level. Together, these areas help to elucidate the potential toxic profiles of unknown (and in some cases, known) agents.

The area of proteomics is one of the fastest growing areas in science and particularly applicable to neurotoxicology. Lubec et al [8] provide a review of the potential and limitations of proteomics. Proteomics focuses on a more comprehensive view of cellular proteins and provides considerably more information about the effects of toxins on the CNS [9]. Proteomics can be classified into three different focuses: post-translational modification, protein-expression profiling, and protein-network mapping. Together, these methods present a more complete and powerful image of protein modifications following potential toxin exposure.

Cellular neurotoxicology involves many cellular processes including alterations in cellular energy homeostasis, ion homeostasis, intracellular signaling function, and neurotransmitter release, uptake, and storage. The greatest hurdle in cellular neurotoxicology has been the discovery of appropriate biomarkers that are reliable, reproducible, and easy to obtain. There are biomarkers of exposure, effect, and susceptibility [21]. Finding the appropriate biomarker for a particular toxin is a daunting task. The advantage to biomarker/toxin combinations is they can be detected and measured shortly following exposure and before overt neuroanatomic damage or lesions. Intervention at this point, shortly following exposure, may prevent or at least attenuate further damage to the individual [28]. The use of peripheral biomarkers to assess toxin damage in the CNS has numerous advantages: time-course analysis may be performed, ethical concerns with the use of human subjects can partially be avoided, procedures to acquire samples are less invasive, and in general, peripheral studies are easier to perform.

Genetic neurotoxicology comprises two focuses—toxin-induced alterations in genetic expression and genetic alterations that affect toxin metabolism, distribution, and clearance. These differences can be beneficial or toxic. Polymorphisms have been shown to result in altered metabolism of certain toxins (paraoxonase and paraoxon). Conversely, it is possible that some polymorphisms may be beneficial and help prevent the formation of a toxic by-product of an exogenous agent (resistance to ozone-induced lung inflammation). It has also become clear that interactions of potential toxins are not as straightforward as interactions with DNA, causing mutations. There are numerous agents that cause epigenetic responses (cellular alterations that are not mutagenic or cytotoxic). This finding suggests that many agents that may originally have been thought of as nontoxic should be re-examined for potential "indirect" toxicity. With the advancement of the human genome project and the development of a human genome map, the effects of potential toxins on single or multiple genes can be identified.

Although collectively, the field of neurotoxicology has recently come a long way, it still has a long way to go to reach its full potential. As technology and methodology advances continue and cooperation with other disciplines such as neuroscience, biochemistry, neurophysiology, and molecular biology is improved, the mechanisms of toxin action will be further elucidated. With this increased understanding will come improved clinical interventions to prevent neuronal damage following exposure to a toxin.

References

[1] Ballatori N, Villalobos AR. Defining the molecular and cellular basis of toxicity using comparative models. Toxicol Appl Pharmacol 2002;183:207–20.

[2] Olson H, Betton G, Robinson D, et al. Concordance of the toxicity of pharmaceutics in humans and animals. Regul Toxicol Pharmacol 2000;32:56–67.

[3] Goss LB, Sabourin TD. Utilization of alternative species for toxicity testing: an overview. J Appl Toxicol 1985;5:193–219.

[4] Bonaventura C. NIEHS Workshop: unique marine/freshwater models for environmental health research. Environ Health Perspect 1999;107:89–92.

[5] Tiffany-Castiglioni E, Ehrich M, Dees L, et al. Bridging the gap between in vitro and in vivo models for neurotoxicology. Toxicol Sci 1999;51:178–83.

[6] Lotti M. Neurotoxicology: the Cinderella of neuroscience. Neurotoxicol 1996;17(2): 313–21.

[7] Verity MA. Introduction: a coming of age for molecular neurotoxicology. Brain Pathol 2002;12:472–4.

[8] Lubec G, Krapfenbauer K, Fountoulakis M. Proteomics in brain research: potentials and limitations. Prog Neurobiol 2003;69:193–211.

[9] LoPachin RM, Jones RC, Patterson TA, et al. Application of proteomics to the study of molecular mechanisms in neurotoxicology. Neurotoxicol 2003;24:761–75.

[10] Ficarro SB, McCleveland ML, Stukenburg PT, et al. Phosphoproteome analysis by mass spectrometry and its application to Saccharomyces cerevisiae. Nat Biotechnol 2002;20: 301–5.

[11] Goshe MB, Conrads TP, Panisko EA, et al. Phosphoprotein isotope-coded affinity tag approach for isolating and quantitating phosphopeptides in proteome-wide analysis. Anal Chem 2001;73:2578–86.

[12] Harding JJ. Nonenzymatic covalent post-translational modification of proteins in vivo. In: Anfinsen CB, Edsall JT, Richards FM, editors. Advances in protein chemistry. New York: Academic Press; 1985. p. 247–334.

[13] Hinson JA, Roberts DW. Role of covalent and noncovalent interactions in cell toxicity: effects on proteins. Annu Rev Pharmacol Toxicol 1992;32:471–510.

[14] Butterfield DA, Stadtman ER. Protein oxidation processes in aging brain. Adv Cell Aging Gerontol 1997;2:161–91.

[15] Butterfield DA, Drake J, Pocernich C, et al. Evidence of oxidative damage in Alzheimer's disease brain: central role for amyloid beta-peptide. Trends Mol Med 2001;7:548–54.

[16] Castegna A, Aksenov M, Aksenov M, et al. Proteomic identification of oxidatively modified proteins in Alzheimer's disease brain. Part I. Creatine kinase BB, glutamine synthase and ubiquitin carboxy-terminal hydrolase L-1. Free Rad Biol Med 2002;33:81–91.

[17] Jenkins LW, Peters GW, Dixon CE, et al. Conventional and function proteomics using large format two dimensional gel electrophoresis 24 h after controlled cortical impact on postnatal day 17 rats. J Neurotrauma 2002;19:715–40.

[18] Gozal E, Gozal D, Pierce WM, et al. Proteomic analysis of the CA1 and CA3 regions of rat hippocampus and differential susceptibility to intermittent hypoxia. J Neurochem 2002; 83:331–45.

[19] Fountoulakis M, Hardmaier R, Schuller E. Differences in protein level between neonatal and adult brain. Electrophoresis 2000;21:673–8.

[20] Gygi SP, Rist B, Gerber SA, et al. Quantitative analysis of complex protein mixtures using isotope-coded affinity tags. J Neurochem 1999;17:994–9.

[21] Costa LG, Manzo L. Biochemical markers of neurotoxicity: research strategies and epidemiological applications. Toxicol Lett 1995;77(1–3):137–44.

[22] Barone S Jr, Das KP, Lassiter TL, et al. Vulnerable processes of nervous system development: a review of markers and methods. Neurotoxicol 2000;21(1–2):15–36.

[23] Deng W, Poretz RD. Oligodendroglia in development and neurotoxicity. Neurotoxicol 2003;24:161–78.

[24] Gallo V, Ghiani CA. Glutamate receptors in glia: new cells, new inputs and new functions. Trends Pharmacol Sci 2000;21:252–8.

[25] Matute C, Alberdi E, Domercq M, et al. The link between excitotoxic oligodendroglial death and demyelinating diseases. Trends Neurosci 2001;24:224–30.

[26] Aschner M. Neuron-astrocyte interactions: implication for cellular energetics and antioxidant levels. Neurotoxicol 2000;21(6):1101–7.

[27] Manzo L, Castoldi AF, Coccini T, et al. Assessing effects of neurotoxic pollutants by biochemical markers. Environ Res Sect A 2001;85:31–6.

[28] Manzo L, Castoldi AF, Coccini T, et al. Mechanisms of neurotoxicity: applications to human biomonitoring. Toxicol Lett 1995;77:63–72.

[29] Manzo L, Artigas F, Martinez M, et al. Biochemical markers of neurotoxicity: basic issues and a review of mechanistic studies. Hum Exp Toxicol 1996;15(Suppl 1):20–35.

[30] Smargiassi A, Mutti A. Peripheral biomarkers and exposure to manganese. Neurotoxicol 1999;20(2–3):401–6.

[31] Castoldi AF, Coccini T, Rossi AD, et al. Biomarkers in environmental medicine: alterations of cell signaling as early indicators of neurotoxicity. Funct Neurol 1994;9:101–9.

[32] Costa LG. Biomarker research in neurotoxicology: the role of mechanistic studies to bridge the gap between the laboratory and epidemiological investigations. Environ Health Perspect 1996;104(Suppl 1):55–67.

[33] Duman RS, Heninger GR, Nestler EJ. Molecular psychiatry: adaptations of receptor-coupled signal transduction pathways underlying stress- and drug-induced neural plasticity. J Nerv Ment Dis 1994;182:692–700.

[34] Lotti M. The pathogenesis of organophosphate polyneuropathy. Crit Rev Toxicol 1992;21: 465–88.

[35] Costa LG. Basic toxicology of pesticides. Occup Med State Art Rev 1997;12:251–68.

[36] Costa LG. Biochemical and molecular neurotoxicology: relevance to biomarker development, neurotoxicity testing and risk assessment. Toxicol Lett 1998;102–103:417–21.

[37] Slikker W Jr, Scallet AC, Gaylor DW. Biologically-based dose-response model for neurotoxicity risk assessment. Toxicol Lett 1998;102–103:429–33.

[38] Westerink RHS. Exocytose: using amperometry to study presynaptic mechanisms of neurotoxicity. Neurotoxicol 2004;25:461–70.

[39] Burgoyne RD, Morgan A. Secretory granule exocytosis. Physiol Rev 2003;83:581–632.

[40] Vineis P, Bartsch H, Caporaso N, et al. Genetic based N-acetyltransferase metabolic polymorphism and low-level environmental exposure to carcinogens. Nature 1994;369: 154–6.

[41] Millikan RC, Pittman GS, Newman B, et al. Cigarette smoking, N-acetyltransferases 1 and 2, and breast cancer risk. Cancer Epidemiol Biomarkers Prev 1998;7(5):371–8.

[42] Portier CJ, Bell DA. Genetic susceptibility: significance in risk assessment. Toxicol Lett 1998; 102–103:185–9.

[43] Eaton DL. Biotransformation enzyme polymorphism and pesticide susceptibility. Neurotoxicol 2000;21(1–2):101–11.

[44] Furlong CE, Li WF, Richter RJ, et al. Genetic and temporal determinants of pesticide sensitivity: role of paraoxonase (PON1). Neurotoxicol 2000;21(1–2):91–100.

[45] Trosko JE, Chang CC, Upham B, et al. Epigenetic toxicology as toxicant-induced changes in intracellular signaling leading to altered gap junctional intercellular communication. Toxicol Lett 1998;102–103:71–8.

[46] Trosko JE. Challenge to the simple paradigm that 'carcinogens' are 'mutagens' and to the in vitro and in vivo assays used to test the paradigm. Mutat Res 1997;373:245–9.

[47] Martinez JD, Pennington ME, Craven MT, et al. Free radicals generated by ionizing radiation signals nuclear translocation of p53. Cell Growth Diff 1997;8:941–9.

[48] Maniatis T. Catalysis by a multiprotein IκB kinase complex. Science 1997;278:818–9.

[49] Weissenbach J. Human genome mapping and sequencing: perspectives for toxicology. Toxicol Lett 1998;102–103:1–4.

[50] Kleeberger SR, Levitt RC, Zhang LY, et al. Linkage analysis of susceptibility to ozone-induced lung inflammation in inbred mice. Nat Genet 1997;265:2037–48.

[51] Prows DR, Shertzer HG, Daly MJ, et al. Genetic analysis of ozone-induced acute lung injury in sensitive and resistant strains of mice. Nat Genet 1997;17:471–4.

[52] Vrana KE, Freeman WM, Aschner M. Use of microarray technologies in toxicology research. Neurotoxicol 2003;24:321–32.

[53] Barrett T, Xie T, Piao Y, et al. A murine dopamine neuron-specific cDNA library and microarray: increased COX1 expression during methamphetamine neurotoxicity. Neurobiol Dis 2001;8:822–33.

[54] Xie T, Tong L, Barrett T, et al. Changes in gene expression linked to methamphetamine-induced dopaminergic neurotoxicity. J Neurosci 2002;22:274–83.

ELSEVIER
SAUNDERS

Neurol Clin 23 (2005) 321–336

Neurodevelopmental Toxicology

Carrie Schmid, MD, Joshua S. Rotenberg, MD, MMS*

*Departments of Pediatrics and Neurology, Wilford Hall USAF Medical Center,
San Antonio Military Pediatrics Consortium, 2200 Bergquist Drive, Suite 1,
Lackland Air Force Base, TX 78236, USA*

And the angel of the Lord said unto Manoah: Of all that I said unto the woman let her beware. She may not eat of any thing that cometh of the grapevine, neither let her drink wine or strong drink, nor eat any unclean thing...

Judges 13:13–14

Identical twin12-year-olds present to a pediatric neurology clinic with high-functioning autism manifesting as impaired social skills, impaired language, and stereotypic behaviors. The children have had developmental disability since infancy. Twin B has similar (although more severe) manifestations, with marked anxiety, violent outbursts, and Tourette's syndrome. The mother reports that the patients' father died at 37 years of age due to a glioblastoma multiforme. He had spent 19 years in the military working on nuclear weaponry. The father is described as "an odd duck" who had few friends. The mother recalls that he had a large head and hat size (it is common for military members to know their hat size). There is no history of accidental overexposure or a quantification of exposure.

The twins' head circumferences are at the 90% percentile. They make poor eye contact. They have frequent stereotypies with anxiety and have tics. Twin B clears his throat and both children have motor tics. The mother and maternal uncle (both are present) are noted to have poor eye contact, pressured speech, and somewhat bizarre affect.

The mother attributes the brain tumor and the subsequent autistic spectrum disorders on the occupational exposure. She asks for the physician's opinion.

Throughout history, medical practitioners have articulated scientific interest and medical concern about neurodevelopmental toxins. Because of

---

The opinions expressed are those of the authors and do not represent those of the United States Air Force or the Department of Defense.

* Corresponding author.

E-mail address: joshua.rotenberg@lackland.af.mil (J.S. Rotenberg).

0733-8619/05/$ - see front matter © 2005 Elsevier Inc. All rights reserved.
doi:10.1016/j.ncl.2004.12.010

the proliferation of environmental hazards and the concerns for their effects, the contemporary neurologist needs to have a familiarity with neurodevelopment and the agents that disturb its normal processes.

When a child is diagnosed with a neurologic disorder, it is common for parents to consider toxic exposures as a possible explanation. In addition, there is strong interest by educators, policy makers, community activists, lawyers, and scientists about possible associations between neurodevelopmental disorders and environmental exposures.

It is estimated that 3% of neonates have a central nervous system (CNS) or multiorgan malformation. Although it is estimated that only 3.5% of these insults can be attributed to environmental teratogens, new provocative agents are routinely discovered. In 60% of individuals, the cause of the malformation remains unknown. The Centers for Disease Control and Prevention reports that 17% of American children are diagnosed with developmental disabilities (eg, learning disabilities, behavioral/emotional impairments, mental retardation). Attention-deficit hyperactivity disorder affects up to 12% of school-aged children; learning disabilities affect up to 10% of children attending public school; autistic spectrum disorders increased in prevalence from 0.5 cases per thousand to 2 cases per thousand over the past 20 years [1–5].

The hazards of environmental toxins are significant and largely unstudied. The National Research Council estimated in 2000 that 3% of developmental disabilities are direct consequences of neurotoxic exposures and another 25% are due to environmental exposures plus genetic susceptibility [4]. Epidemiologic studies have identified in utero and childhood exposures to lead, mercury, polychlorinated biphenyls (PCBs), and pesticides that are associated with neurobehavioral disabilities.

According to the EPA's Office of Children's Health Protection, there have been over 80,000 commercial chemicals developed and used within the last century, and most have not been tested for hazardous properties [1]. There are 2800 chemicals produced in excess of 1 million pounds per year; fewer than half have been tested for toxicity to adults and children. In 1995, consumption of synthetic pesticides was estimated at 2.6 million metric tons with an expected increase of 1% per year thereafter. Exposure to lead today is 300 times that of the preindustrial era due to the proliferation of leaded products. Over 50 million plantation workers worldwide have direct contact with pesticides and over 500 million agricultural workers are exposed. Mining for precious metals in the Amazon River basin accounts for the release of 130 tons of methylmercury (MeHg) each year. In 1996, 3 to 4 million children living in the United States were within 1 mile of one of the 15,000 hazardous waste sites [1].

Causative links between putative toxins and neurobehavioral disorders are difficult to substantiate except in some well-studied instances. Most research has focused on the effects of teratogenic toxins in causing anatomic nervous system anomalies, whereas less research has focused on behavior.

Consequently, the clinician will have difficulty gleaning answers from the literature. Certain basic principles can guide the clinician, however, when evaluating patients and counseling families.

In this review, the authors offer basic principles for the clinician faced with a potential developmental neurotoxin. Normal CNS development is described, with particular attention to known vulnerable periods for toxic exposures. Three prevalent nervous system teratogens are discussed in detail. Finally, the controversy regarding mercury exposure and the hypothesized link to autism is addressed.

Neurodevelopmental toxicology—lessons from teratology

When a toxic exposure is a consideration for a pediatric neurologic disorder without a clear anatomic derangement, the problem is further complicated by the passage of time from exposure to presentation and the complexity of behavioral syndromes. Development, growth, medical illness, secondary psychiatric illness, and familial coping mechanisms are always the added dimensions in evaluating neurobehavioral syndromes in children. For instance, one might wonder if a flare of stereotypic behaviors in a teenage child with autism reflects the course of the primary condition, household psychosocial stressors, adolescence, or a manifestation of a coexistent medical problem (eg, sleep deprivation).

The detailed encounter, background scholarship, and clinical time for risk communication are often felt to be beyond the scope of the generalist. Such is not the case for most children with neurobehavioral disorders. Many principles of teratology can be applied to allay the fears of families. For instance, a single agent cannot cause many varied forms of developmental aberration in different individuals. One agent causes a recognized pattern of dysmorphism. As an illustration, nicotine alone has been linked to neurocognitive changes but not to spinal cord anomalies.

Clinicians should stress that agents with known teratogenic potential or adverse neurodevelopmental potential may be innocuous, depending on the scenario. There are several critical questions for assessing possible toxic exposures in the clinic.

1. What was the agent? Are there simultaneous coexposures? MeHg exposures from excessive fish consumption during gestation are more likely to be teratogenic than the ethylmercury in thimerasol-preserved vaccines. Fish with high levels of MeHg may also have high levels of PCBs.
2. At what age did the exposure take place? Some agents have a narrower window of possible effect than others. Although exposure to retinoic acid can cause spinal dysraphism, exposure in the ninth month of gestation could not cause such a malformation. Knowledge of the ontogeny of the nervous system allows a rational assessment of the likelihood of a putative teratogen effect.

3. What was the route of exposure? Oral exposures are more easily quantifiable than vapor exposures (usually a product of concentration and time).
4. What was the dose and duration of exposure? Any potential teratogens follow a dose-response curve, below which its effects are negligible. Several exceptions are discussed later.
5. Can a relevant biologic assay be performed? Although one can measure an instantaneous level of a toxin or its function, it may not be clinically relevant. For example, one can assay red blood cell acetylcholinesterase levels that can be suppressed following exposure to organophosphorus agents; however, there is a great variation in the activity of this enzyme in the population. A single measure in an adult individual is most valuable when it is compared with stable values before or weeks after an exposure. As a result, this assay is most useful for determining occupational exposures compared with a baseline. In addition, specific cholinesterase levels do not necessarily correlate with symptoms.

These considerations do not substitute for a detailed history of gestation, birth, development and a three-generation pedigree. Other significant variables include genetic variance in susceptibility, placental factors, and the pharmacokinetics of the individual agent. Of course, the physiology of pregnancy, the placenta, and the fetus will alter the dose and metabolism of the primary agent. It is difficult to extrapolate from adult or animal data to the prenatal human experience.

Especially with neurobehavioral syndromes, *stochastic* phenomena (in which damage to one cell causes a malformation that is an "all-or-nothing" event) are less common than *threshold* phenomena. Threshold phenomena are active at many biological sites over time; consequently, within a population, the severity and the prevalence increase with greater exposure. For instance, although all toxins have a threshold dose below which they are innocuous, the picture is not as clear for lead. The Centers for Disease and Control and Prevention set a maximal allowed blood level of 10 µg/dL, but subsequent studies have found adverse outcomes at levels below the set benchmark. In the case of lead, the threshold phenomenon for adverse neurodevelopmental outcome may be seen at minute amounts.

Finally, the clinician should keep the potential for neurodevelopmental toxins in context and avoid the hubris of certainty. Numerous factors affecting neurodevelopment are still poorly understood. Numerous confounders may be operative in clinical situations and uncontrolled studies. Viruses, physical factors, radiation, diet, and even stress can have untoward effects on prenatal and postnatal development. Underlying genetic susceptibilities may also be interacting with the environmental exposure. Consequently, parental claims and medical literature (especially unproven hypotheses, case reports, and uncontrolled studies) should be viewed with circumspection.

Central nervous system ontogeny

Classic teaching of CNS embryology describes visualized histologic changes divided into arbitrary phases that end at birth. In truth, the phases of CNS development overlap in sequence and continue postnatally. In addition, there is a molecular "new neuroembryology" [6]. Molecular biology and genetics have revolutionized this field, revealing the genes and their products that shape CNS development. Although the present article gives specific illustrative examples, the reader is referred elsewhere for details [6].

Even before the neural tube is seen on gestational day 21, critical events in the formation of the nervous system have taken place. Gastrulation establishes a midline, axes for dorsal–ventral and anterior–posterior orientation, and symmetry. The notochord and somites develop during this phase to induce the ectoderm to form the neural plate and to establish a segmental organization, respectively.

The development of the nervous system, per se, begins at 3 weeks' gestation as the ectoderm forms the neural plate. From the neural plate, the neural tube forms in axial fusion, with closure occurring in a simultaneous caudal and cranial progression. During this process of neurulation, the anterior and posterior neuropores close by gestational day 24 to 26 and gestational day 25 to 28, respectively.

After neurulation, subsequent processes are further divided into proliferation, migration, differentiation, synaptogenesis, apoptosis, and myelination. These processes start after gestational day 28 but continue postnatally. Glial and synapse formation continue to be robust until approximately 3 years of age.

Myelination begins prenatally and continues in the CNS throughout childhood and into adulthood. The vestibular system is primarily myelinated prenatally, whereas association cortices continue to be myelinated in the second decade. This progression is commonly seen on MRI scans of children's brains.

Newer research has focused on the ontogeny of neurotransmitter systems. These neurotransmitters have trophic functions in the developing brain and have function in synaptic neurochemical signaling. One line of inquiry has focused on the effects of stressors (eg, seizures, handling) on receptor development [7,8].

Given this complex progression, it is difficult to ascertain by way of animal and epidemiologic studies the precise cause of developmental aberration. Specific toxins have postulated mechanisms and they exploit certain periods in development. Table 1 illustrates some potential toxins and their corresponding vulnerable periods.

Neural proliferation is vulnerable to ethanol, organophosphates, and MeHg disruption. It follows that if proliferation is altered, migration may also be altered, leading to ectopic tissues [9]. Ethanol and MeHg are culprits in interfering with migration [4,10,11]. Neural cells receive multiple signals

Table 1
Potential neurotoxic agents and their teratogenic windows

Age	Process in development	Potential neurotoxic agents	Altered outcomes
0 to 4 weeks' gestation	Gastrulation—notochord and somite formation	Retinoic acid	Disordered polarity, malformations of the hindbrain and spinal cord
4 weeks' gestation	Neurogenesis in spinal cord and hindbrain	Hot tubs Folic acid antagonists	Anencephaly, hydrocephaly
28–35 weeks' gestation	Migration	Ionizing radiation MeHg	Ectopia Cerebral palsy Learning disorders
Middle-late pregnancy	Neuron proliferation Synaptogenesis	Lead PCBs MeHg	Neurobehavioral deficits
Third trimester	Neurogenesis in cerebellum, hippocampus Cell migration, myelination, synaptogenesis	Pesticides	Multiple: poor motor control, emotional lability, cognitive deficits and delays
Infant to 3 years of age	Development of executive functions in the prefrontal cortex	Lead, postnatal Alcohol, prenatal Cigarettes, prenatal	Behavioral impairments, possible increased criminality
4–17 years of age	Increase in fiber tracts of motor and speech functions	Organophosphates	Poor axonal outgrowth
	Ability to build on previous learning	Lead PCBs	Lowered IQ
	Improved sensory function, specifically auditory	MeHg Lead	Impaired concentration

directing the differentiation of the cells. The offenders of changing or interrupting the differentiation process include ethanol, nicotine, MeHg, and lead. Some of the same agents—ethanol, lead, MeHg, parathion, permethrin, di-isopropyl fluorophosphates, and PCB compounds—are involved in altering synaptogenesis [2,5,10,12–21].

The support network for neural elements is vulnerable to insults because its formation continues for several years. The genesis of the supporting cells (glia) begins at the time of neuron genesis (early gestation). The glia continue to differentiate and proliferate long after the migration of neural cells is complete. Myelination peaks during the third trimester in humans; however, it continues into the teenage and young adult years, accounting for its longer period of vulnerability. Myelination disturbances have been linked to malnutrition, iron deficiency, alcohol, and lead exposures [2,5,10,12–21].

Another important process for the developing nervous system is apoptosis (programmed cell death). Abnormal patterns of apoptosis are noted after toxic exposures. The hypothesis is that exposure leads to a shift in the balance of neurotrophic signals, resulting in an increase or decrease in the number of cells. Ethanol, lead, MeHg, and PCBs have been implicated in altered cell numbers [2,5,10,12–21].

Lead

Lead is a pervasive neurotoxin related to human industrial and chemical endeavors. Exposure was first recognized as a toxin among adults with occupations requiring use of lead-containing products (brass and bronze foundry workers, jewelry makers, painters, glassmakers, and potters). Today, humans are exposed despite increased regulation of its use in industrial products, leaded gasoline, and household interior paints. The major domestic sources of lead are dust and soil contaminated by lead-containing paint and industrial and vehicle emissions. Although there has been a dramatic decrease in lead levels, populations at risk have shifted from adult workers to pregnant mothers to toddlers and school-aged children.

In adults, the nervous system effects can be reversible, but in children, the outcome of lead encephalopathy is not good. Severe encephalopathy (seizures and coma) can be seen at high ($\geq$70 µg/dL) blood lead levels (BLLs). At low levels, lead is a significant neurodevelopmental toxin. In Europe, it is estimated that mild mental retardation resulting from lead exposure accounted for 4.4% of disability-adjusted life years [22]. Despite regulations and overall reduction in youth BLLs, significant concern exists regarding the loss of IQ points with chronic exposure, even at defined acceptable blood levels (<10 µg/dL) [5,11,23,43].

Children are vulnerable to exposures at various times of development due to their behaviors, socioeconomic factors, exposure to parental activities using lead (occupation or hobbies), use of folk remedies, malnutrition, neglect, or pre-existing developmental disorder. Fetuses may be exposed due to lead from maternal bone accumulation that is utilized during pregnancy. Toddlers are at risk due to hand-to-mouth activity. School-aged children may live and play in contaminated environments or use imported toys that contain lead. Children at high risk who should be tested for lead exposure are listed in Box 1.

When ingested, 40% of lead is absorbed, whereas 90% of inhaled lead is absorbed. This differential has implications for lead abatement programs that leave high levels of lead-containing dust.

Lead's mechanism of action is unknown. It affects multiple organ systems in the human body, including the bone marrow (specifically heme synthesis), the kidneys (specifically tubules), and the nervous system. It accumulates in

Box 1. Populations who should be tested for elevated blood lead level

After initial screening of children at risk (9–12 months old), assessment of BLLs should be repeated at 24 months when levels peak.

Universal screening
- In communities with inadequate data on the prevalence of elevated BLLs
- In communities with >27% of the housing built before 1950

Targeted screening
(Based on the assumption that universal screening is cost-effective in communities in which the prevalence of elevated BLL is at least 11%–14%)
- In communities in which <12% of children have BLLs of 10 µg/dL, or
- In communities with <27% of the housing built before 1950

Symptomatic screening/diagnostic testing
- Any child with an unexplained illness such as severe anemia, seizures, lethargy, or abdominal pain

Other groups to consider testing blood lead level
- Children 1 to 2 years of age living in housing built before 1950 situated in an area not designated for universal screening (especially if the housing is not well maintained)
- Children of ethnic or racial minority groups who may be exposed to lead-containing folk remedies
- Children who have emigrated (or been adopted) from countries where lead poisoning is prevalent
- Children with iron deficiency
- Children exposed to contaminated dust or soil
- Children with developmental delay whose oral behaviors place them at significant risk for lead exposure
- Victims of abuse or neglect
- Children whose parents are exposed to lead (vocationally, avocationally, or during home renovation)
- Children of low-income families who are defined as receiving government assistance (Supplemental Feeding Program for Women, Infants, and Children; Supplemental Security Income; welfare; Medicaid; or subsidized child care)

(*Data from* Screening for elevated blood lead levels. Pediatrics 1998; 101(6):1072. Available at: http://aappolicy.aappublications.org/cgi/content/full/pediatrics%3b101/6/1072.) Accessed October 1, 2004.

the bone and is released with high turnover (eg, during pregnancy). There are significant differences between the toxicity of lead in adults versus the fetus and child. Adults tend to have reversible toxicity, whereas the developing child is permanently affected [5,11,23]. One hypothesis for the mechanism of action in the developing nervous system is that lead substitutes calcium, leading to neuronal apoptosis, abnormal neurotransmitter release, and damage to endothelial and glial cells [5,11,23].

Animal studies provide the data for possible mechanisms. Animal nervous systems have shown changes in the N-methyl-D-aspartate glutamate receptors. These changes may account for the cognitive deficits observed in the exposed animals (eg, learning and memory). Further delineation of this mechanism of action and demonstration in vitro in human cell lines may provide another significant route of long-term damage [5,11,23].

BLL is the most frequent assay performed to assess lead exposure. A value greater than 10 µg/dL should be confirmed. In all cases of elevated BLL, a detailed environmental history should be performed. At mildly elevated levels, however, a source is often difficult to identify. Typically, treatment with chelation is not offered until levels are greater than 45 µg/dL. The American Academy of Pediatrics offers a detailed policy on screening and follow-up procedures [24].

When a lead exposure is identified, the emotional valence may be high for the family and the clinician. Before launching on a potential treatment (eg, chelation or environmental mitigation), risks and benefits should be considered.

Manmade substances: polychlorinated biphenyls and polybrominated diphenylethers and relatives

In the 1970s, the United States and European governments banned PCBs due to recognized dermal, fetal, and neurologic abnormalities. Nevertheless, they continue as toxic hazards due to environmental build-up. Widespread use of PCBs and their relatives—polychlorinated dibenzofurans and polychlorinated dibenzodioxins or dioxins—in insulators and industrial electronic equipment led to release into the environment. These chemicals were first noted to affect the environment in 1968 when birds tested positive for PCBs. Due to its ubiquitous presence in the environment and the resiliency of the chemical structures after disposal, PCB exposure is common, with the most common route occurring by ingestion of contaminated foods.

The disposed chemicals remain as oils that pollute the water supplies. Aquatic organisms consume them and the concentration is magnified up the food chain as they are subsequently consumed. Eating fish exposes most humans. Mass poisonings occurred in Japan in 1968 and in Taiwan in 1979 after contaminated cooking oil was used. The Japanese poisonings, approximately 2000 cases, were discovered when the population developed a skin disease named Yusho. The manifestations included severe acne in adults; however, the offspring of exposed women suffered diffuse damage. The most severe poisonings occurred in fetuses, and these children were born with subsequent ectodermal abnormalities including hyperpigmented skin, dilatation of eyelid sebaceous glands, neonatal teeth, discolored dentition, and growth retardation [25–27]. Infants continued to be exposed if breastfed; however, the significance of this exposure is unknown. In follow-up studies, children exposed in utero to maternal fat stores of PCBs demonstrated measurable behavioral and cognitive disabilities such as motor delays, lowered IQ, cognitive delays, lethargy, and apathy [16,25–27].

Similarly, polybrominated diphenylethers (PBDEs) have recently been more closely examined due to the structural relationship to PCBs and to the increasing concentrations in animal and human tissues. PBDEs are used as flame retardants and are still produced worldwide. Products containing PBDEs include electrical appliances, computer circuit boards, building materials, foam, carpet, upholstery, and vehicles. There is approximately 67,000 metric tons (148 million pounds) produced each year. They are slowly released as the plastics break down, and evidence suggests that exposure occurs by way of air dispersion and unintentional ingestion. Although no mass poisonings have identified teratogenic effects in humans, animal studies indicate that exposed newborn mice have permanent neurologic sequelae including abnormal motor behavior and reduced learning and memory capacity [25]. Due to the large environmental presence, the structural similarities to PCBs, and the animal data, there is concern for potential increases in human neurobehavioral disturbances due to exposure in utero and during childhood.

The proposed mechanism of action is endocrine disruption. Current focus includes evaluating thyroid hormone level and its function in relationship to these toxic exposures. Zoeller et al [28] report on the status of research and further delineate the proposed mechanism. Again, available data come from animal models. The interactions proposed to occur in utero include disruption of thyroid hormone–responsive genes, reduced circulating thyroid hormones, reduced thyroid responsiveness to thyroid-stimulating hormone, and increased clearance of T4 through enhanced liver metabolism [28,29]. The widespread exposures to PCB and PBDE contaminants, the negative impact of abnormal thyroid hormone action on the developing brain (ie, congenital hypothyroidism with severe mental retardation, motor abnormalities, and deafness), and the relationship between thyroid hormone and these contaminants lead to concern for neurodevelopmental hazards imposed on the vulnerable developing human.

Although many laboratories offer measurements of PCBs in breast milk or other samples, such assays have no clinical relevance. There are numerous differences in methods, quality assurance, and reference values. Outside of research studies, measurement of polychlorinated toxins is not recommended.

There is no effective treatment for PCB exposure. Hypothetically, lactating women may be counseled not to lose weight because the metabolism of fat stores liberates the toxin.

Pesticides: organophosphates and carbamates

As noted earlier, the potential exposure to pesticides is profound. Even humans not exposed by way of occupations are often exposed by way of household applications, residues on produce, and commercial applications, leading to dermal, gastrointestinal, or inhalational exposures. Whyatt and Barr reported in 2001 that 20 of 20 infants tested in New York City had positive organophosphate metabolites in their meconium. In addition, the Environmental Protection Agency surveyed American households and found that over 70% of respondents used at least one pesticide in or around the home [29a].

There is such concern for exposure, particularly with the developing child, that the United States Congress passed the Food Quality Protection Act of 1996. This law requires several actions on the part of governmental agencies to research and protect infants and children from toxic levels of exposure.

Much of the known consequences of human exposure to pesticides came about with acute poisonings in agricultural workers. Organophosphorus agents cause irreversible and reversible inhibition of acetylcholinesterase and other esterase enzymes. Excess acetylcholine causes a well-known cholinergic syndrome marked by nausea, vomiting, hypersecretion, bronchoconstriction, and CNS effects (ie, seizures, headache, vision changes, anxiety, ataxia). Miosis is often described as a hallmark sign of exposure but it can frequently be absent.

Acute exposures to organophosphorus agents can lead to chronic neurologic deficits including frequent headaches, difficulty with memory and concentration, mood alterations, and polyneuropathy. These effects can persist for months and even after acetylcholinesterase function has normalized.

In the CNS, pesticides affect more than the richly cholinergic areas of the brainstem and forebrain. The limbic system, hippocampus, basal ganglia, and cerebellum are also affected. In animal models, organophosphate exposure affects multiple neurotransmitters systems, second messengers, and neuronal proliferation. Additional evidence is accumulating in humans that chronic exposure during neurodevelopment may cause hyperactivity, poor attention span, and cognitive deficits [19–21,30–33,42]. Given the widespread use of these chemicals, however, there are relatively little data to further delineate the timing during development and amount of exposure needed for significant disabilities.

Treatment for acute organophosphate and carbamate poisoning should be instituted based on a clinical diagnosis of the cholinergic syndrome. In the United States, this treatment combines atropine and pralidoxime chloride. Seizures are treated with benzodiazepines because other anticonvulsants are ineffective. Organochlorine and pyrethroid exposures are treated with supportive measures.

Blood cholinesterase levels are useful for confirmation of acute exposure or for occupational monitoring, as discussed earlier.

Mercury

Human endeavors (eg, coal-fired power generation, waste incineration, mining, medical/dental uses) allow for exposures to inorganic mercury. Known for its occupational hazards, mercury has long been respected as a neurotoxin. There are three forms of mercury: (1) elemental—used in thermometers, dental amalgams, fluorescent light bulbs, and button batteries; (2) inorganic salts such as mercuric bichloride, also known as corrosive sublimate; and (3) organic compounds—MeHg, ethylmercury, and phenylmercury. Bacteria in the water produce organic mercury compounds.

Although the most commonly known form is elemental, the greater public health concern is for the organic form, as it is biomagnified by consumption along the food chain. Examples of fish with high levels of organic mercury are shark, tuna, and swordfish.

Toxic "epidemics" have occurred due to mercury contamination of waters supplying the fish for human consumption. In the 1950s and 1960s, the first large exposures were reported in Minamata and Niigata, Japan. The clinical syndrome, named Minamata disease, was recognized in adults with neurologic impairments including paresthesias, visual field constriction, ataxia, impaired hearing, and speech impairment. In offspring of the exposed Japanese women, who had minimal symptoms, there were 22 reports of congenital Minamata disease consisting of severe developmental disabilities (eg, cerebral palsy, mental retardation, and seizures). Another large exposure occurred in an Iraqi population who consumed grains treated with a fungicide containing MeHg. The exposures continued from 1959 to 1972, affecting over 6500 individuals including 83 pregnant women. Similar neurodevelopmental disabilities resulted [4,12,34–36].

Due to these disasters, scientists have studied multiple populations who depend on fish consumption for primary nutrition. In comparison to acute exposures, as in Japan and Iraq, these population studies usually involve significantly lower doses of chronic MeHg exposure, as measured in maternal peak hair mercury values. The population studies have been inconsistent; however, organic mercury easily crosses the blood-brain barrier and accumulates in the CNS. The threshold level established by the Environmental Protection Agency is 0.1 $\mu g/kg/d$, which is often exceeded in populations regularly consuming seafood (average hair mercury is often >10 $\mu g/g$ in fishing communities). The long-term sequelae of exposure to organic mercury in the developing nervous system include abnormal results on the Denver Developmental Screening Test, worse performance on the Wechsler Intelligence Scale for Children-Revised compared with controls, and neuropsychologic deficits (eg, language delays and attention and memory deficits) [34–36].

At the molecular level, MeHg has a high affinity for binding thiol groups such as found on proteins with cysteines. In vitro data from animal models demonstrate that high levels of MeHg (5–10 μmol) impair mitochondrial activity, leading to decreased energy sources and plasma membrane lysis and cell necrosis. Lower exposures (<1 μmol) cause apoptosis by way of activation of calpain and caspase-3 [34,35].

In addition to altering cell death mechanisms, MeHg affects the developing nervous system in other crucial mechanisms including the cytoskeleton, leading to errors in migration (eg, brain reduction, heterotopias in white matter, and abnormal neuronal arrangements); calcium homeostasis, leading to elevated intracellular calcium, which may lead to cell death; excitatory amino acid uptake inhibition, leading to extracellular accumulation of glutamate, which leads to neurodegeneration; and muscarinic cholinergic and dopaminergic systems with unknown long-term consequences. The reader is encouraged to read the in-depth review of the molecular consequences of MeHg exposure by Castoldi et al [34] and Davidson et al [35].

Mercury exposure can be diagnosed by a history and physical examination and confirmed with elevated blood mercury levels. A normal level does not rule out mercury exposure. For inorganic mercury, a 24-hour urine collection can be assayed. For inorganic mercury, whole blood mercury levels are recommended. For cumulative burden of mercury exposure, hair can be assayed, with a normal concentration being less than 1 part per million.

The most effective treatment is to curtail exposure. Although chelation regimens exist for inorganic mercury toxicity, no treatment exists for organic mercury exposure.

Area of controversy—autism

The apparent increase in autistic spectrum disorder, whether due to heightened awareness or an actual increase in prevalence, has attracted widespread public attention. The personal and social impact of this long-term disability has provoked much interest in determining its etiology and what, if anything, neurotoxins might contribute to this disorder. Autistic spectrum disorders commonly present at approximately 1 year of age, when verbal and social skills should be established.

In 1999, the Environmental Protection Agency published safe limits of mercury exposures. Although a level was specified, several other aspects of this policy should be noted. The primary exposures of concern were oral consumption of MeHG over time. Policy makers hypothesized that the ethylmercury in childhood vaccines might be as harmful as MeHG and contribute to autism. The measles-mumps-rubella vaccine contained thimerosal (approximately 50% ethylmercury) at the time. The doses of ethylmercury in the vaccines ranged from 12.5 to 25 µg/dose. In smaller infants, this could have exceeded the 0.1 µg/kg/d guideline. There were no data for a developmental impact of a single day's dose exceeding the guideline.

The hypothesis of the effects of ethylmercury had meager scientific evidence to validate it. Most pathologic studies of autism point to prenatal genetic factors causing changes in minicolumn organization or other anatomic findings. No postnatal exposures have been etiologically linked to autism.

Still, concern for a potential for developmental toxicity drove changes in immunization practices and vaccine production. The Food and Drug Administration requested that thimerosal, a preservative allowing for multidose vials, be removed from vaccines [37]. No vaccine in the United States currently contains thimerosal, but worldwide, many still do.

Since the initial hypothesis, research has concluded that the preponderance of the evidence negates this hypothesis. Further studies evaluating retrospective and prospective cohorts determined that there is no association between these vaccines and autism. In fact, two recent British epidemiologic studies with a combined number of over 120,000 participants not only found no adverse effects but also found protective effects on development with the thimerosal vaccines [38,39]. An excellent review of the epidemiologic studies has recently been published [40,41].

Summary

The fields of neurotoxicology and developmental toxicology are exploding in research and interest. Much of the data currently known are from epidemiologic human studies or studies of animal models. Each of these modes is difficult to translate to individual clinical encounters. It is often difficult to state with certainty which of the numerous chemical or physical agents in our environment are neurotoxic. Basic scientists will help with advances in molecular biology and toxicology. Improved clinical understanding of these issues may help patients to understand the medical issues; allay feelings of anxiety, guilt, or fear; and avoid unnecessary testing.

For exposures that manifest as threshold phenomena, such as lead, the risk to society is even greater than to an individual. Individual risk may be less of a concern than the population's risk because small elevations in the average BLL can cause profound shifts in the normative curve of intelligence, increasing the burden on our institutions and bankrupting the brain trust.

Good scholarship and interpersonal judgment are vital when counseling patients on the potential consequences of chemical exposures and are no less important when making policy. The challenge for the clinician reading the research is to remain aware of the limitations and biases of our science.

References

[1] Altshuler K, Berg M, Frazier LM, et al. Critical periods in development. OCHP Paper Series on Children's Health and the Environment 2003;3:1–31.

[2] Bearer CF. Developmental neurotoxicity: illustration of principles. Pediatric Clin N Am 2001;48(5):1199–213.

[3] Brent RL, Weitzman M. The current state of knowledge about the effects, risks, and science of children's environmental exposures. Pediatrics 2004;113(4):1158–66.

[4] Landrigan PJ, Kimmel CA, Correa A, et al. Children's health and the environment: public health issues and challenges for risk assessment. Environ Health Perspect 2003;112:257–65.

[5] Stein J, Schettler T, Wallinga D, et al. In harm's way: toxic threats to child development J Dev Behav Pediatr 2002;23(Suppl 1):S13–22.

[6] Sarnat HB, Menkes JH. Neuroembryology, genetic programming and malformations of the nervous system. In: Sarnat HB, Menkes JH, editors. Child Neurology. Philadelphia, PA: Lippincott Williams and Wilkins; 2000. p. 277–400.

[7] Zhang G, Raol YS, Hsu FC, et al. Long-term alterations in glutamate receptor and transporter expression following early-life seizures are associated with increased seizure susceptibility. J Neurochem 2004;88(1):91–101.

[8] Hsu FC, Zhang GJ, Raol YS, et al. Repeated neonatal handling with maternal separation permanently alters hippocampal GABAA receptors and behavioral stress responses. Proc Natl Acad Sci USA 2003;100(21):12213–8.

[9] Rice D, Barone S. Critical periods of vulnerability for the developing nervous system: evidence from humans and animal models. Environ Health Perspect 2000;108(S3):511–33.

[10] Gressens P, Mesples B, Sahir N, et al. Environmental factors and disturbances of brain development. Semin Neonatal 2001;6:185–94.

[11] Jacobson JL, Jacobson SW. Association of prenatal exposure to an environmental contaminant with intellectual function in childhood. Clin Toxicol 2002;40(4):467–75.

[12] Brent RL, Tanski S, Weitzman M. A pediatric perspective on the unique vulnerability and resilience of the embryo and the child to environmental toxicants: the importance of rigorous research concerning age and agent. Pediatrics 2004;113(4):935–44.

[13] Feldman RG, Ratner MH. The pathogenesis of neurodegenerative disease: neurotoxic mechanisms of action and genetics. Curr Opin Neuro 1999;12(6):725–31.

[14] Gitterman BA, Bearer CF. A developmental approach to pediatric environmental health. Pediatric Clin N Am 2001;48(5):1071–83.

[15] Kaplan A. Neurotoxicants threaten childhood development. Psychiatric Times 2001;28(3): 1–4.

[16] McDonald ES, Windebank AJ. Mechanisms of neurotoxic injury and cell death. Neuro Clin 2000;18(3):525–40.

[17] Rodier PM. Environmental causes of central nervous system maldevelopment. Pediatrics 2004;113(4):1076–83.

[18] Sun YE, Martinowich K, Ge W. Making and repairing the mammalian brain—signaling toward neurogenesis and gliogenesis. Semin Cell Dev Biol 2003;14:161–8.

[19] Tilson HA. Environmental health issues. Environ Health Perspect 1995;103(S6):147–51.

[20] Trask CL, Kosofsky BE. Developmental considerations of neurotoxic exposures. Neuro Clin 2000;18(3):541–62.

[21] Walker B. Neurotoxicity in human beings. J Lab Clin Med 2000;136:168–80.

[22] Valent F, Little D, Bertollini R, et al. Burden of disease attributable to selected environmental factors and injury among children and adolescents in Europe. Lancet 2004; 363(9426):2032–9.

[23] Bellinger DC. Lead. Pediatrics 2004;113(4):1016–22.

[24] Screening for elevated blood lead levels. Pediatrics 1998;101(6):1072.

[25] McDonald TA. A perspective on the potential health risks of PBDEs. Chemosphere 2002; 46:745–55.

[26] Miller RW. How environmental hazards in childhood have been discovered: carcinogens, teratogens, neurotoxicants, and others. Pediatrics 2004;113(4):945–51.

[27] Patandin S, Koopman-Esseboom C, DeRidder MA, et al. Effects of environmental exposure to polychlorinated biphenyls and dioxins on birth size and growth in Dutch children. Pediatr Res 1998;44(4):538–45.

[28] Zoeller RT, Dowling A, Herzig C, et al. Thyroid hormone, brain development, and the environment. Environ Health Perspect 2002;110(S3):355–61.

[29] Howdeshell KL. A model of the development of the brain as a construct of the thyroid system. Environ Health Perspect 2002;110(S3):337–48.

[29a] Whyatt RM, Barr DB. Measurement of organophosphate metabolites in postpartum meconium as a potential biomarker of prenatal exposure: a validation study. Enviro Health Perspect 2001;109(4):417–20.

[30] Sanborn MD, Cold D, Abelsohn A, et al. Identifying and managing adverse environmental health effects. 4. Pesticides. Can Med Assoc J 2002;166(11):1431–6.

[31] Schettler T. Toxic threats to neurologic development of children. Environ Health Perspect 2001;109(S6):813–6.

[32] Weiss B, Amler S, Amler RW. Pesticides. Pediatrics 2004;113(4):1030–6.

[33] Woodruff TJ, Axelrad DA, Kyle AD, et al. Trends in environmentally related childhood illnesses. Pediatrics 2004;113(4):1133–40.

[34] Castoldi AF, Coccini T, Ceccatelli S, et al. Neurotoxicity and molecular effects of methylmercury. Brain Res Bull 2001;55(2):197–203.

[35] Davidson PW, Myers GJ, Weiss B. Mercury exposure and child development outcomes. Pediatrics 2004;113(4):1023–9.

[36] Shanker G, Hampson RE, Aschner M. Methylmercury stimulates arachidonic acid release and cytosolic phospholipase A2 expression in primary neuronal cultures. Neurotoxicology 2004;25(3):399–406.

[37] Parker SK, Schwartz B, Todd J, et al. Thimerosal-containing vaccines and autistic spectrum disorder: a critical review of published original data. Pediatrics 2004;114(3):793–804.

[38] Heron J, Golding J, ALSPAC Study Team. Thimerosal exposure in infants and developmental disorders: a prospective cohort study in the United Kingdom does not support a causal association. Pediatrics 2004;114(3):577–83.

[39] Andrews N, Miller E, Grant A, et al. Thimerosal exposure in infants and developmental disorders: a retrospective cohort study in the United kingdom does not support a causal association. Pediatrics 2004;114(3):584–91.

[40] Parker SK, Schwartz B, Todd J, et al. Thimerosal-containing vaccines and autistic spectrum disorder: a critical review of published original data. Pediatrics 2004;114(3):793–804.

[41] Colosio C, Tiramani M, Maroni M. Neurobehavioral effects of pesticides: state of the art. Neurotoxicology 2003;24:577–91.

[42] Koler K, Brown T, Spurgeon A, et al. Recent developments in low-level lead exposure and intellectual impairment in children. Environ Health Perspect 2004;112:987–94.

[43] Schaumburg HH, Spencer PS. Classification of neurotoxic responses based on vulnerability of cellular sites. Neuro Clin 2000;18(3):517–24.

ELSEVIER
SAUNDERS

Neurol Clin 23 (2005) 337–352

NEUROLOGIC
CLINICS

Historical Neurotoxins: What We Have Learned from Toxins of the Past About Diseases of the Present

Daniel E. Rusyniak, MD[a],*, R. Brent Furbee, MD[b],
Robert Pascuzzi, MD[c]

[a]Division of Medical Toxicology, Department of Emergency Medicine,
Indiana University School of Medicine, Indianapolis, IN, USA
[b]Division of Medical Toxicology, Department of Emergency Medicine, Indiana Poison Center,
Indiana University School of Medicine, Indianapolis, IN, USA
[c]Department of Neurology, Indiana University School of Medicine,
Indianapolis, IN, USA

Responsible for our thoughts and actions, the nervous system, more than any other organ system in the body, defines us as individuals. Although well protected from the environment by the unique capillary system known as the blood-brain barrier, there are certain toxins that, nonetheless, specifically target the central and peripheral nervous systems. Several features make the nervous system uniquely susceptible to these toxins. Nerve cells and neurons with their long dendrites and axons have a large surface area for absorption and attack by chemicals. With a dry weight composed of 50% lipid, the brain and nervous tissue are particularly vulnerable to fat-soluble toxins. Once injured, neurons and nerve tissue have a limited capacity to regenerate, placing the emphasis for treatment on prevention. Along with affecting the adult nervous system, toxins also can have profound effects on the developing nervous system, resulting in neurodevelopmental disorders [1].

The increasing awareness of the neurotoxic potential of chemicals has resulted in congressional [2] and public emphasis placed on identifying those chemicals that have neurotoxic potential. In response to this increased awareness, several animal and cellular models have been developed to recognize neurotoxins better [3]. There are difficulties, however, in translating

---

* Corresponding author. Department of Emergency Medicine, Indiana University School of Medicine, 1050 Wishard Boulevard, Room 2200, Indianapolis, IN 46202-2859.
E-mail address: drusynia@iupui.edu (D.E. Rusyniak).

0733-8619/05/$ - see front matter © 2005 Elsevier Inc. All rights reserved.
doi:10.1016/j.ncl.2004.12.012

the findings of research to the public arena. A recent example of this is the concern about neurotoxic effects of household mold. Although studies show that certain fungal spores have potential for toxicity in high concentrations [4], there are no convincing scientific data to suggest that the quantities or exposure in everyday life cause neurologic effects [5]. Despite the lack of scientific support, several toxic tort cases regarding neurologic complications from environmental mold exposure have been tried in court. Although research on the neurotoxic effects of mold exposure is ongoing, it likely will be years before conclusive evidence is available. This delay between scientific discovery and the potential for public risk is one of the central problems in neurotoxicology. Epidemiologic studies from the 1960s to 1980s suggest that environmental toxins may be responsible for an increasing incidence in the United States of motor neuron disease and Parkinson's disease (PD) [6,7]. To date, however, no specific toxins have been identified. In fact, the majority of what has been learned about the neurotoxin potential of chemicals and compounds has come only after large neurotoxic outbreaks have occurred. The history of these epidemics can be instructive, however, in that they reveal potential hazards of certain classes of chemicals and shed insight into the mechanisms and treatments of common neurologic disorders.

This article reviews several unique historical neurotoxic outbreaks and discusses how knowledge from these has led to better understanding and prevention of neurologic disorders.

Ginger jake paralysis

In 1920, the 18th amendment prohibited the sale and importation of alcoholic beverages. A cottage industry subsequently arose to provide a legal means to purchase alcohol. Because an alcoholic extract of ginger had been considered a patent medicine and had been available since the 1800s, it provided a legally marketable source of ethanol. During Prohibition, a fluid extract of ginger, commonly called Jamaican ginger, or jake, could be sold legally. To curb its abuse, a standard formula for its manufacture was defined by the United States Pharmacopoeia requiring that the content of the extract contain 5 g of ginger per 1 mL of solvent (typically ethanol). This resulted in such a bitter concoction that it was deemed nonpotable [8]. The ginger extracts commonly were sold in pharmacies and roadside stands as remedies for a variety of ailments. With the alcohol content of jake as high as 80%, a 2-oz bottle could be mixed with a soft drink, making an intoxicating and palatable beverage. Agents of the United States Department of Agriculture occasionally monitored jake manufacturing by boiling samples down and measuring the weight of the remaining solids, which represented the powdered ginger root or oleoresin. In attempts to improve its palatability and reduce costs, many adulterants were used illegally as substitutes for the ginger solids, including molasses, glycerin, and, most commonly, castor oil [8].

In an attempt to find a cheaper alternative to castor oil, Hub Products (Boston, Massachusetts) began experimenting with a variety of commercially available solvents. Abandoning ethylene glycol and diethylene glycol as too volatile to survive the Department of Agriculture testing, Harry Gross, president of Hub Products, and his brother-in-law Max Reisman ultimately settled on using a previously believed nontoxic solvent called triorthocresyl phosphate (TOCP). Shortly after releasing their improved product in the spring of 1930, thousands of people, in Tennessee, Oklahoma, Kentucky, and Mississippi were stricken with a mysterious illness manifesting primarily as an ascending paralysis, with an estimated 50,000 persons in the United States becoming paraparetic or paraplegic [9].

Dr. Ephraim Goldfain was the first to recognize a case of ginger jake paralysis; in February of 1930 he described a man who had a rapidly progressive bilateral foot drop. The same day, another man presented with the same palsy and soon Dr. Goldfain had a list of 65 persons who had the mysterious affliction [9]. As these typically were poor workers known to imbibe jake, the notion soon came about that this illness was linked to the consumption of jake. Confirmation of the jake as the poison and the identity of the mysterious adulterant were solved ultimately in the laboratories of the National Institutes of Health (NIH) by Maurice Smith and Elias Elvove. Analyzing samples of jake collected from afflicted patients, Smith and Elvove determined that the toxic contaminant was a phenolic compound, later identified as TOCP, and were able to demonstrate that it caused a similar constellation of symptoms in a variety of experimental animals [10].

The prevalence of the ginger jake paralysis was such that it permeated popular music of the day, finding its way into 12 predominantly blues recordings between 1928 and 1934 [11]. Likewise, many organizations and societies were formed, including the United Victims of Jamaica Ginger Paralysis, which had 35,000 members [10]. The low socioeconomic status of the majority of jake victims resulted, however, in little public outcry or legislative action. It was not until 105 persons, including 34 children, died from poisoning by diethylene glycol, which had been used as a solvent for elixir of sulfonamide, that the Food, Drug, and Cosmetic Act of 1938 was passed. This Act prohibited the sale of medicine without proof of safety but came 8 years after the jake epidemic [12]. Because of the weak laws regarding patent medicines at the time, neither Gross nor Reisman initially served any jail time, despite paralyzing tens of thousands of persons. In the court case, it was learned that they had purchased enough TOCP to manufacture 640,000 2-oz bottles of jake. Ultimately, Gross was forced to serve some of a 2-year sentence after it was learned that he caused paralysis in 200 persons in California with the shipment of an additional two barrels of jake after the initial epidemic had been linked to his product [9].

Symptoms of ginger jake paralysis typically occurred within a week of consumption but in some cases could be delayed up to 30 days [13]. Symptoms consisted of cramping pains in the legs followed by a rapidly progressive ascending paralysis. Those patients who had mild severity developed symptoms only in their lower extremities, whereas severe cases involved the upper extremities also. Sensory symptoms were absent almost universally and only occasionally did bowel and bladder dysfunction occur. Physical examination was remarkable for a predominantly motor poly-neuropathy with weakness of the distal limb muscles (legs affected more often than arms), muscle atrophy, and a loss of reflexes [14]. Over time, flaccidity was replaced by hypertonicity, with a resultant spastic gait from permanent upper motor neuron damage [15]. Pathologic findings included peripheral nerve axonopathy with wallerian degeneration and spinal cord atrophy involving the anterior horn cells [13,16,17]. Those motor nerves with the longest and largest diameter were the most susceptible, with the sciatic being the most affected nerve. Electrophysiologic evaluation revealed evidence of sensorimotor polyneuropathy from a mixed process of axonal degeneration and secondary demyelination [18]. Many of the patients' symptoms were permanent, with only partial improvement in those areas that were least affected [15].

Although occurring almost 75 years ago, the epidemic of ginger jake paralysis still teaches important lessons in neurotoxicology. Before jake paralysis, many toxins were known to affect the peripheral nervous system but typically occurred in the setting of systemic toxicity. Notable examples include arsenic and lead, both of which caused peripheral neuropathies and other systemic effects. TOCP, alternatively, specifically targeted the periph-eral nervous system. Since the ginger jake poisonings, the ability of a variety of compounds have been shown to have isolated effects on the peripheral nervous system, including n-hexane and methyl-butyl-ketone [19]. Like TOCP, these compounds resulted in many cases of motor impairment after they were abused them as intoxicants.

Ginger jake paralysis is the result of phosphorylation and aging of a protein found in nervous tissue known as neuropathy target esterase (NTE) [20]. Like TOCP, other organophosphates are known to cause peripheral neuropathies by inhibiting NTE, a condition generally referred to as organophosphate-induced delayed peripheral neuropathy (OPIDP). Although present in all neurons except glia, the exact function of the NTE is not known. Studies in hens, however, show that more than 70% to 80% inhibition of NTE correlates strongly with the development of OPIDP [20]. Mice and rats, however, are relatively resistant to OPIDP, demonstrating the importance of screening neurotoxic compounds in a variety of animal species. The recognition of the role of NTE in OPIDP and the development of a reliable animal model in the hen has led to the better development of organophosphates with restricted toxicity likely preventing untold numbers of neuropathies [21]. Although the role of NTE in the development of

OPIDP is not known, TOCP offers insights into other peripheral nervous system neurotoxins. Like most chemical neuropathic agents, TOCP causes wallerian degeneration targeting axons predominantly, with myelin affected only secondarily. Like other toxic neuropathies, it affects the lower extremity long axons first in an ascending pattern, with motor function affected disproportionately. Patients who have rapidly ascending painful neuropathies are more likely, however, to have arsenic or thallium poisoning [22], whereas those who have cranial neuropathies have trichlorethyelene toxicity [23]. The rate of progression of TOCP also is indicative of a toxic neuropathy, as its symptoms rapidly progress in days to weeks, whereas metabolic disorders tend to occur over years.

Recognizing a toxic neuropathy is paramount when treating, because removing the patient from the source provides the only chance of improvement. Although the jake tragedy is one of the largest mass poisonings in history, several other outbreaks of neurotoxicity from alcohol and therapeutic drugs have occurred before and since its last case was reported. Among these have been peripheral neuropathies from arsenic-contaminated beer [24], encephalopathy and cerebral edema from triethyltin-contaminated antibiotics [25], and myoclonic encephalopathy mimicking Creutzfeldt-Jakob disease from gastrointestinal preparations containing bismuth [26]. In each of these cases, individual physicians associated the neurologic findings of patients with the use of products previously considered safe, resulting in dangerous products being pulled off the market and limiting the number persons severely affected. This highlights how important it is for a practicing neurologist to consider neurotoxins in the differential diagnoses for unexplained neurologic conditions.

Minamata Bay

In 1906, the company known today as Chisso Corporation established a factory in the small town of Minamata, a move that would forever change this picturesque fishing village. Located on the island of Kyushu in the Shiranui Sea, Minamata Bay was an ideal location for a large industrial plant. Chisso initially was set up as a carbide plant for the production of acetylene, and it added fertilizer production in the 1920s. In 1951, the plant began manufacturing acetaldehyde for the use in plastics, a process that used mercury oxide as a catalyst. Unbeknown to the company or scientists of the day, the inorganic mercury used in this process was methylated in an acetylene reaction tank, forming the toxic compound methyl mercury. As production increased, so did the waste runoff. As a result of the rising costs of recycling, the Chisso Corporation began dumping the mercury-laden waste directly into the bay [27]. When complaints were lodged, Chisso paid the local fisherman's union to keep quiet [28]. Their silence, along with the company's greed, ultimately led to more than 100 tons of mercury deposited into the bay, contaminating the waters and marine life within [29]. Unfortunately, many of the inhabitants of Minamata relied on fish caught from the bay as a primary dietary staple.

In 1956, a 5-year-old girl came down with a mysterious neurologic disorder. When 8 days later her 3-year-old sister was seen with similar symptoms, the town became concerned over the possibility of an epidemic of encephalitis [28]. At approximately the same time, Dr. H. Hosokawa, the hospital director and occupational health physician for Chisso, reported on four other cases of a degenerative neurologic condition to the Minamata Health Center [30]. Dr. Hosokawa and a local group of physicians from the Public Health Department and Chisso quickly determined that many other patients throughout the town were suffering similar neurologic problems; these became known simply as Minamata disease [28]. To investigate the cause of this mysterious illness, a team of physicians and researchers headed by Dr. Shoji Kitamura was called from Kumamoto University School of Medicine. At the time that they began their investigation, there were approximately 54 patients in whom symptoms had been noted [31]. Using epidemiologic tools, the investigators were able to deduce quickly many similarities in the cases. Nearly all the patients lived around the bay and were occupied in the fishing industry. It also was found that every patient had eaten either fish or shellfish from the bay. The illness struck adults and children and had a high mortality rate [32]. One of the most interesting early findings came from the townspeople who told the investigators about cats who walked around in circles, convulsed, stumbled around, salivated, and at times seemed to commit suicide by jumping into the bay [28,31]. This finding became one of the early breaks in the case, as cats in Minamata survived mostly on a diet of local fish. Although a cause was not yet identified, the cats seemed to show striking similarities to the human disease. Capitalizing on this, the Kumamoto investigators brought cats from a town 100 miles away from Minamata and fed them fish from the bay; all of them developed symptoms similar to the human cases [28]. Based on these initial findings, the investigators were able to confirm that the disease was neither infectious nor contagious, rather the result of eating fish from the bay. Furthermore, as the Chisso chemical factory was the only large industrial plant in the area, the investigators linked the illness to the factory wastewater dumped into the bay [30]. Unfortunately, the investigators' recommendation of banning fishing in the bay was not heeded [30]. This inaction sadly resulted in many other persons becoming ill. It was not until 1968, after another outbreak of neurologic illness from mercury dumping in the Japanese town of Niigata, that the Chisso Company halted its manufacturing of acetaldehyde under pressure from the public.

Although initially investigators were certain of the source of toxin, the actual toxin remained unidentified for several years. Initially, the investigators looked at a variety of potential agents, including manganese, zinc, copper, and selenium, but in none of these could they reproduce the illness in cats [30]. It was not until 3 years after the initial report linking the illness with the consumption of fish that the investigators discovered high levels of mercury in the fish and marine life from the bay [31]. The knowledge of elevated mercury and the similarity of the symptoms in the patients from Minamata to a report of methyl mercury poisoning from a seed company in Britain in 1940 [33] ultimately led to the discovery of methyl mercury as the causative agent in Minamata disease.

Over time it became clear that Minamata disease had two major victims, those who consumed large quantities of fish from the contaminated bay and, secondarily, their offspring. Acute Minamata disease, resulting from consumption of contaminated fish, presented most commonly with clinical findings consisting of marked concentric constriction of the bilateral visual fields, parasthesias of the extremities and mouth, ataxia, incoordination, tremor, dysarthria, and auditory impairments [28]. These symptoms in some patients were severe, progressive, and sometimes fatal. In those cases in which autopsies were performed, the pathologic findings most commonly consisted of neuronal damage in the cerebral and cerebellar cortex. The most affected areas were the calcarine region of the occipital lobe, the pre- and postcentral motor and sensory cortex, and the temporal cortex. In the cerebellum, there was loss of the granule cells with preservation of the neighboring Purkinje's cells [28,34]. The investigators also noted damage in the peripheral nerves largely in the sensory fibers [34,35].

Although initially believed to be protected by the maternal-fetal placental barrier, it was soon realized that the children born to mothers exposed to methyl mercury would come to bear brunt of methyl mercury's toxic effects. In 1958, Dr. Kitamura and his team began to notice an increasing number of cerebral palsy cases [36]. By 1964, autopsy and epidemiology studies clearly proved the association between intrauterine methyl mercury exposure and cerebral palsy–like symptoms (congenital Minamata disease). The most common symptoms seen in congenital Minamata disease included mental retardation (100%), primitive reflexes (100%), cerebellar ataxia (100%), limb deformities (100%), dysarthria (100%), chorea (95%), hypersalivation (95%), and microcephaly (60%) [27,28,36]. The incidence of congenital Minamata disease has been estimated to involve as many as 29% of children born between 1955 and 1958 in the Minamata area [36]. Pathologic changes in congenital Minamata disease are similar to the adult form, with general atrophy of the cortex, hypoplasia of the corpus callosum, demyelination of the pyramidal tracts, and hypoplasia of the granula cell layer of the cerebellum [36].

Although the findings from Minamata Bay are well known today, at the time they largely were ignored by persons outside of Minamata. Sadly, in the early 1960s, methyl mercury waste from a factory along the Agano River in Japan caused a second outbreak of Minamata disease in the town of Niigata [27]. In total, methyl mercury contamination in Japan resulted in a 2263 cases of adult and 63 cases of congenital Minamata disease recognized by the government [34]. Of those poisoned, 1368 patients who had acute and 13 patients who had congenital Minamata disease have died [34]. Recent research, however, showing impairment at lower levels of exposure than previously believed, may increase the estimate of affected persons to more than 20,000 [37]. Other cases of methyl mercury poisoning also have occurred since Minamata, including more than 6000 persons; 459 deaths occurred in Iraq after grain treated with a methyl mercury fungicide inadvertently was made into bread instead of planted [38].

Despite the magnitude of its tragedy, many lessons can be learned from the Minamata disaster. One of the most obvious is the consequences of unchecked and unregulated industrial pollution. In Minimata, the economic advantage of ocean dumping versus waste recycling pushed the Chisso Corporation into dumping massive amounts of industrial waste into the bay. The local fisherman and villagers who kept silent for a price ultimately paid a heavy toll, as the fishing industry in Minamata ceased to exist until the bay was reopened for fishing in 1997. The Chisso Corporation, whose cost-cutting waste management created the disaster, has paid out, to date, more than $2 billion in victim compensation and clean-up costs. The city also suffered greatly, losing more than 30% of its population and being associated forever with pollution and industrial greed. A memorial was completed in 1996 in Minamata as a remembrance of those who suffered and died from Minamata disease and as a warning to future generations.

Along with the environmental lessons learned from Minamata Bay, medicine also learned a valuable lesson in the susceptibility of the developing nervous system. Before Minamata, it was commonly believed that the fetus was protected from toxins by the placental barrier. As the mothers of these children who had congenital Minamata disease were comparatively unaffected and symptoms were unnoticed until 6 months of age and attributed initially to cerebral palsy, the magnitude and effect of methyl mercury on the developing fetus at first went unnoticed. To date, Minamata represents the best example of the sensitivity and risk of the developing central nervous system (CNS) to environmental and industrial toxins. The Minamata disaster has resulted in an increased search for other environmental causes of childhood developmental disorders. Most recently, ethyl mercury used as a preservative in vaccines has been a subject of intense debate as a possible cause of autism and other developmental disorders. To date, epidemiologic studies have not found any link between mercury and autism [39], although the subject still is argued.

The Minamata disaster underscores the importance of population-based surveillance of neurodevelopmental disorders. This, along with the appropriate epidemiologic studies, will help determine the role of other toxins in current and future neurodevelopmental disorders. Recognizing those toxins that have neurodevelopmental toxicity hopefully will result in successful screening and abatement programs, as has been demonstrated in childhood lead toxicity.

The frozen addicts

The historical data in this section is adapted from *The Case of the Frozen Addicts* by Langston and Palfreman [40] and the NOVA presentation by the same name, broadcast on February 18, 1986 [41].

Case report: Bethesda, Maryland, November 1976

Barry acquired his drug habit while living with his family in India. When they returned to Maryland, he decided to make his own drugs rather than buying them on the street. He searched for prospective compounds by reviewing chemistry literature. When synthetic opioids are developed, several related compounds often are made, but only one travels the complicated and expensive path through animal and human research to the marketplace. Many of those compounds are described in the scientific literature, and Barry took advantage of that. He set out to synthesize 1-methyl-4-phenyl-propionoxypiperidine (MPPP) a compound similar to meperidine. One day, in November of 1976, he overheated the mixture, which produced a slightly different compound, 1-methyl-4-phenyl-1,2,3, 6-tetrahydropyridine (MPTP), which contaminated the MPPP. Barry had unknowingly developed a compound that was, in effect, a bullet to the substantia nigra. When he injected the drug, he experienced severe burning at the injection site followed by euphoria. Within three days he was immobile and mute. He was taken to a hospital, where he was admitted with a diagnosis of catatonic schizophrenia and was administered phenothiazines. When that regimen failed, he underwent electroconvulsive therapy.

Barry eventually made his way to the NIH Clinical Center in Bethesda, Maryland. He was intelligent and cooperative. With his help, the NIH team began to focus on the drug he had injected just before the onset of his symptoms. It appeared that Barry had PD, but his age and the rapidity of onset suggested a toxic etiology. They began to wonder if their patient had stumbled onto a tremendous research tool, a means of rapidly producing Parkinsonism in animals.

A tiny amount of Barry's concoction remained. When tested, it yielded MPPP, 1-methyl-4-hydroxy-4-phenylpiperidine (a chemical intermediate), and MPTP. The team had come close to an answer, but the next step took their investigation off track. They injected the three compounds in rats. Although rats can demonstrate a temporary catatonic state when injected with opioids, they are not as susceptible to MPTP's effects as are primates. At that point, the only reported primate to have received MPTP was Barry.

The setback eroded some of the confidence that the drug and the symptoms were related. In 1979, the researchers published Barry's case report, suggesting a connection, but other cases were not forthcoming and the issue became dormant [42]. When undergoing L-dopa therapy, Barry improved significantly. His mobility and speech returned. His drug use continued, however, and in September of 1978 he died of a cocaine overdose.

Case report: San Jose, California, July 1, 1982

George's arm burned when he injected the heroin, but he experienced a remarkably good high, followed by hallucinations. Hours later, he began to stiffen slowly. It was imperative that he go to court that day or be sent back to jail on a parole violation for failure to appear. Unfortunately, as he entered the courthouse, his unsteady gate made him look drunk. He was arrested for public intoxication, a parole violation, and taken to jail. A physician was called to see him in jail because of his worsening stiffness. Four days after his arrest he was sent to the Santa Clara Valley Medical Center for evaluation. Initially, he was believed to have an extrapyramidal syndrome resulting from medication, because antipsychotics sometimes were administered to agitated patients, and the physicians could find no better explanation for what they were seeing. They tried diphenhydramine to no avail. He was given cogentin (Benztropine) and returned to his cell. The next morning George was back, stiff and mute. He was admitted to the psychiatric unit with an initial diagnosis of catatonic schizophrenia. Uncomfortable with that rare diagnosis, the psychiatrist requested a neurology consultation. Like the physicians before them, the neurologists had never seen a patient like George.

At approximately the same time that George's troubles began, David and Bill, two heroin dealers 30 miles to the south, were using what remained of their latest heroin acquisition. By July 5, they were paralyzed and may have died had their mother not found them lying in their living room. They later recalled a burning sensation when they injected the drug followed by a tremendous high. At the hospital, they were diagnosed as catatonic schizophrenics and admitted.

By the time Connie arrived at Stanford University Medical Center, she was motionless. For several days, her family had cared for her, suspecting that she was suffering from heroin withdrawal. She was not a long-term user, but her boyfriend Toby was a drug dealer and, eventually, she began to abuse heroin occasionally. Toby had been arrested and, while in jail, developed paralysis. He later was seen at Stanford. Connie initially was diagnosed as having hysterical paralysis, but Toby had been treated for some time with phenothiazines and they were blamed initially for his condition.

As these six patients in the San Jose area emerged, William Langston, a neurologist at Santa Clara Valley Medical Center, went to the media in an attempt to prevent further cases. With the help of police and laboratory researchers, the neurologists began to focus on MPTP as the source of the outbreak. At that point, the Bethesda case was buried in the medical literature. Along with Langston, Phil Ballard, a neurobehavioral fellow at Santa Clara, began to search for the connection. In a short time, they discovered the case report by Davis in 1979. During the next few years they, and many other scientists, began to piece together the mechanism by which MPTP causes such devastating neural damage [40,43].

Although not neurotoxic, MPTP is metabolized to a compound that is. It is oxidized to an intermediate, 1-methyl-4-phenyl-2,3-dihydropyridinium

(MPDP+) by monoamine oxidase type B (MAO-B) [44], then oxidized further to 1-methyl-4-phenylpyridinium (MPP+). Pretreatment with MAO-B antagonists has been shown to be protective by blocking the conversion of MPTP to MPP+ [45]. Although MPP+ cannot cross the blood-brain barrier, its parent compound, MPTP, crosses readily, thereby providing entry for the neurotoxic metabolite. It seems that once inside the CNS, MPTP is taken up by astrocytes, which contain the necessary MAO for conversion to MPP+. The toxic metabolite then is released into the extracellular space, where it is pulled specifically into dopaminergic neurons by the catecholamine reuptake system [46]. Studies demonstrate that dopamine reuptake blockers can prevent CNS damage in primates injected with MPTP.

Once inside dopaminergic neurons, MPP+ seems to be taken up into the mitochondria, where it interrupts electron transport in a fashion similar to rotenone [47,48]. Free radical formation and ATP depletion seem to account for cell death. A proposed final mechanism is that ATP depletion reduces the reuptake of excitatory amino acids, leading to depolarization of neuronal membranes and causing the firing of excitatory N-methyl-D-aspartate receptors and cellular demise [49]. The target cells are specific. Primate studies and autopsies on two affected patients (Barry and Bill) demonstrate extensive damage to the substantia nigra and little else.

All the patients improved when taking L-dopa. Movement and speech improved dramatically for most, but the improvement was short lived. Within a matter of months, they began to suffer dyskinesia and hallucinations that eventually were unbearable. For a time, drug holidays led to improvement, but, eventually, the window of time between reinstatement of the drug and onset of side effects closed to the point that some of the patients had to stop it entirely.

It seemed that the MPTP victims had no hope of recovery. Then, through the dogged efforts of Langston and his colleagues and some serendipitous events, the California neurologist came into contact with Anders Björklund and a Swedish research team that was studying Parkinsonism. The two patient groups had striking similarities. Eventually, through the collaboration of the United States and Swedish researchers, the first patient traveled to Lund, Sweden, for stereotactic implantation of fetal tissue. Specifically, George underwent injection of fetal substantia nigra cells into his putamen and caudate nucleus.

For several months, there seemed to be no progress. A year after surgery, slight improvement was noted, but after 2 years, George was improved markedly and Juanita, the next transplant patient, also was doing well. PET scans confirmed the production of dopamine by the transplanted fetal tissue. A third patient, Connie, also traveled to Lund for the surgery. She also demonstrated dramatic improvement in just 5 months.

Although seven MPTP patients have been well documented in the literature, Langston found others. They included scientists, pharmaceutical workers, and even the drug dealer who sold the California MPTP to six of the reported patients. It is believed that approximately 400 people were exposed to that batch. It is not known how many people suffered or will suffer damage as a result [40].

Because of its insidious onset and slow progression, PD had been nearly impossible to study in animals. The discovery of MPTP's effect on dopaminergic cells in the CNS made possible primate studies that have added immeasurably to the understanding of that disease. MAO-B antagonists were administered to patients who had PD and, although it did not reverse their symptoms, it did slow progression and delayed the need for higher doses of L-dopa [50].

For years, an etiology for PD has been elusive. Some twin studies suggest that there is not a genetic predilection for the disease [51], whereas others suggest there is [52]. The discovery of MPTP/MPP+ as a cause of Parkinson's-like disease is a strong support for at least some environmental role in the development of PD. Unlike other suggested environmental causes, such as manganese, MPTP can strike rapidly. Without question, the "frozen addicts," as they came to be known, suffered terribly as a result of their drug use. But, just as certainly, their misfortune has resulted in greater understanding of the disease process and management of Parkinsonism.

Ergotism

The witch trials in Salem, Massachusetts, in 1692, have been studied by many historians looking to explain a community event that led to the unfortunate deaths of 20 innocent Puritans [53]. In late 1691, eight young girls (mostly teenagers) presented with odd behavior, gesturing, posturing, altered speech, and convulsive seizures, then referred to as "unknown distempers." A doctor suggested the possibility that these girls had been bewitched, leading to allegations that witchcraft had been performed by residents of the village (including several Caribbean servants living in the households of the affected girls). Several of the affected girls testified that townspeople were conspiring with the devil and practicing witchcraft. In 1692, 20 residents of Salem were convicted of witchcraft and put to death (19 were hanged and one was crushed with rocks). An additional 150 innocent people were incarcerated and subsequently released in 1693 (at the direction of the incoming Governor). The notion that the affected young girls who had odd behavior and convulsions were the victims of ergotism, as opposed to witchcraft, has interested medical historians for decades. There is ample evidence to support this notion, including the physical symptoms of the girls, which parallel well known symptoms resulting from exposure to ergot-contaminated rye, induced by specific seasonal conditions [53]. Alternative explanations for the phenomenon at Salem include mass hysteria, fraud, politics, and social divisiveness.

Ergot alkaloids are derived from Claviceps purpurea, a grain fungus that has been implicated as a cause of epidemics of ergotism throughout the last millennium and is a proposed cause of the events of the Salem witch trials. Ergots thrive in the setting of cold winters followed by damp springtime. Ergotamine and dihydroergotamine are nonselective 5HT1 agonists that also have affinity for dopamine and norepinephrine receptors.

Acute ergot intoxication historically is referred to as convulsive ergotism, because of the acute and intense neurologic symptomatology. Patients may experience auditory and visual hallucinations, paranoia, mania, delirium, fever, diaphoresis, spasms, twitches, and jerks. The spasms suffered by ergot victims have at times been referred to as St. Vitus' dance (a term most neurologists associate with Sydenham's chorea). The clinical features of convulsive ergotism (muscle twitches and spasms, changes in mental status, hallucination, sweating, and fever lasting for several weeks) reflect serotonergic overstimualtion of the CNS (the serotonin syndrome) [54].

Often, chronic ergotism is referred to as the gangrenous form, also known as the holy fire or St. Anthony's fire (see later discussion), and is characterized by intense burning pain in the feet, hands, and limbs as a result of the vasoconstrictive properties of ergot. In severe cases, the affected tissues become dry, black, and mummified and limbs may drop off. Spontaneous miscarriage is common.

St. Anthony was an Egyptian ascetic in the third century who lived an austere life near the Red Sea [55,56]. His pious lifestyle was characterized by prolonged periods of fasting associated with hallucinations, visions, and various temptations that he believed to be the work of the devil. Although there is no evidence that St. Anthony had any direct association with ergot use or toxicity, his name was taken by an order of Hospitallers founded in France in approximately 1100. This order developed facilities around Europe for the purpose of caring for sufferers from ergotism. One therapeutic approach used by the Hospitallers involved drinking holy water that had been dripped over saints' bones. Although patients apparently improved in the setting of such treatment, it is logical to assume that that their improvement was related to consuming a diet free of contaminated grain. Amputated limbs often were left at shrines to St. Anthony as symbols of appreciation for cured patients.

Despite the known toxicity of this naturally occurring fungus, physicians have taken advantage of the vasocontrictive properties of these plants and drug users of its hallucinogenic effects. The use of ergot therapy during labor to accelerate parturition dates back to the 1600s, and it became accepted practice by the late 1900s. Early experience revealed the risk of stillbirth as a potential complication. In 1935, Dudley and Moir reported isolation of the active substance "to which ergot really owes its established reputation as the pulvis parturiens" [57]. They proposed the name, ergometrin. Thereafter, pure preparations of ergotamine, also known as ergonovine in the United States, were given intravenously or intramuscularly, pro-phylactically and for treatment of postpartum hemorrhage. In the 1920s, ergotamine was used for the treatment of migraine, an indication for which the drug still is prescribed in clinical practice.

Common adverse effects of ergotamine and dihydroergotamine include nausea, vomiting, abdominal pain, diarrhea, numbness and tingling, swelling in the limbs, nonspecific generalized fatigue and weakness, malaise, and peripheral and coronary arterial vasoconstriction. Therefore, ergots typically are contraindicated in patients who have known peripheral vascular disease, coronary artery disease, severe hypertension, stroke, or pregnancy. Ergotamine and dihydroergotamine are metabolized by the liver cytochrome P450 (P353A4) enzyme. Several medications are inhibitors of the cytochrome P450 systems and, therefore, predictably delay the metabolism of ergotamine, leading to potential toxic effects (discussed previously). Physicians should be particularly alert to the potential for adverse drug reactions from macrolyde antibiotics (erythromycin and clarithromycin), antifungal drugs (such as ketoconazole and fluconazole), protease inhibitors used commonly to treat HIV infection, and antidepressants (including fluoxetine) in patients who are taking ergot preparations [58].

Summary

Throughout history, humans have fallen victim to a variety of neurotoxins, with exposures coming in the form of tainted products, industrial pollution, drugs of abuse, and even the bread and water that sustain them. Despite this long and tumultuous history, neurotoxic outbreaks still occur with regular frequency. Although many difficulties currently exist in linking many of today's unexplained neurologic disorders to toxins, the past suggests a prominent role for neurotoxins in diseases (such as amyotrophic lateral sclerosis and PD), unexplained peripheral neuropathies, neurodevelopmental disorders, and many psychiatric disturbances.

References

[1] Nelson BK. Adult versus developmental neurotoxicology: an occupational perspective of similarities and differences. Neurotoxicol Teratol 1994;16:213–8.
[2] US Congress, Office of Technology Assessment, Neurotoxicity Identifying and controlling poisons of the nervous system, OTA-BA-436. Washington, DC: US Government Printing Office; April 1990.
[3] Eisenbrandt DL, Allen SL, Berry PH, et al. Evaluation of the neurotoxic potential of chemicals in animals. Food Chem Toxicol 1994;32:655–69.
[4] Fung F, Clark R, Williams S. Stachybotrys, a mycotoxin-producing fungus of increasing toxicologic importance. J Toxicol Clin Toxicol 1998;36:79–86.
[5] Lees-Haley PR. Toxic mold and mycotoxins in neurotoxicity cases: Stachybotrys, Fusarium, Trichoderma, Aspergillus, Penicillium, Cladosporium, Alternaria, Trichothecenes. Psychol Rep 2003;93:561–84.
[6] Lilienfeld DE, Chan E, Ehland J, et al. Two decades of increasing mortality from Parkinson's disease among the US elderly. Arch Neurol 1990;47:731–4.
[7] Lilienfeld DE, Chan E, Ehland J, et al. Rising mortality from motoneuron disease in the USA, 1962–84. Lancet 1989;1:710–3.
[8] Morgan JP. The Jamaica ginger paralysis. JAMA 1982;248:1864–7.

[9] Baum D. Jake leg. New Yorker 2003;15:50–7.

[10] Parascandola J. The Public Health Service and Jamaica ginger paralysis in the 1930s. Public Health Rep 1995;110:361–3.

[11] Morgan JP, Tulloss TC. The Jake Walk Blues. A toxicologic tragedy mirrored in American popular music. Ann Intern Med 1976;85:804–8.

[12] Wax PM. Elixirs, diluents, and the passage of the 1938 Federal Food, Drug and Cosmetic Act. Ann Intern Med 1995;122:456–61.

[13] Werden DH. Ascending paralysis resulting from the drinking of "Jamaica ginger"; a clinical study of fifty cases. Ann Intern Med 1932;5:1257–66.

[14] Lotti M, Becker CE, Aminoff MJ. Organophosphate polyneuropathy: pathogenesis and prevention. Neurology 1984;34:658–62.

[15] Morgan JP, Penovich P. Jamaica ginger paralysis. Forty-seven-year follow-up. Arch Neurol 1978;35:530–2.

[16] Sevim S, Aktekin M, Dogu O, et al. Late onset polyneuropathy due to organophosphate (DDVP) intoxication. Can J Neurol Sci 2003;30:75–8.

[17] Chuang CC, Lin TS, Tsai MC. Delayed neuropathy and myelopathy after organophosphate intoxication. N Engl J Med 2002;347:1119–21.

[18] Vasilescu C, Florescu A. Clinical and electrophysiological study of neuropathy after organophosphorus compounds poisoning. Arch Toxicol 1980;43:305–15.

[19] Spencer PS, Schaumburg HH, Sabri MI, et al. The enlarging view of hexacarbon neurotoxicity. Crit Rev Toxicol 1980;7:279–356.

[20] Glynn P. Neuropathy target esterase. Biochem J 1999;344:625–31.

[21] Lotti M, Johnson MK. Neurotoxicity of organophosphorus pesticides: predictions can be based on in vitro studies with hen and human enzymes. Arch Toxicol 1978;41:215–21.

[22] Rusyniak DE, Furbee RB, Kirk MA. Thallium and arsenic poisoning in a small midwestern town. Ann Emerg Med 2002;39:307–11.

[23] Lotti M, Becker CE, Aminoff MJ. Occupational peripheral neuropathies. West J Med 1982; 137:493–8.

[24] Reynolds ES. An account of the epidemic outbreak of arsenical pisoning occurring in beer drinkers in the North of England during the year 1900. Lancet 1901;i:166–70.

[25] Hryhorczuk DO, Aks SE, Turk JW. Unusual occupational toxins. Occup Med 1992;7: 567–86.

[26] Burns R, Thomas DW, Barron VJ. Reversible encephalopathy possibly associated with bismuth subgallate ingestion. Br Med J 1974;1:220–3.

[27] Kondo K. Congenital Minamata disease: warnings from Japan's experience. J Child Neurol 2000;15:458–64.

[28] Harada M. Minamata disease: methylmercury poisoning in Japan caused by environmental pollution. Crit Rev Toxicol 1995;25:1–24.

[29] Tedeschi LG. The Minamata disease. Am J Forensic Med Pathol 1982;3:335–8.

[30] Tsuchiya K. The discovery of the causal agent of Minamata disease. Am J Ind Med 1992; 21:275–80.

[31] Putman JJ. Quicksilver and slow death. National Geographic 1972;October:506–27.

[32] Harada Y, Noda K. How it came about the finding of methyl mercury poisoning in Minamata district. Congenital Anomalies 1988;28(Suppl October):S59–69.

[33] Hunter D, Bomford RR, Russell DS. Poisoning by methylmercury compounds. Q J Med 1940;9:193–213.

[34] Eto K. Minamata disease. Neuropathology 2000;20(Suppl):S14–9.

[35] Eto K, Tokunaga H, Nagashima K, et al. An autopsy case of minamata disease (methyl-mercury poisoning)–pathological viewpoints of peripheral nerves. Toxicol Pathol 2002;30: 714–22.

[36] Harada M. Congenital Minamata disease: intrauterine methylmercury poisoning. Teratology 1978;18:285–8.

[37] Watts J. Mercury poisoning victims could increase by 20,000. Lancet 2001;358:1349.

[38] Bakir F, Damluji SF, Amin-Zaki L, et al. Methylmercury poisoning in Iraq. Science 1973; 181:230–41.
[39] Hviid A, Stellfeld M, Wohlfahrt J, et al. Association between thimerosal-containing vaccine and autism. JAMA 2003;290:1763–6.
[40] Langston JW, Palfreman J. The case of the frozen addicts. New York: Pantheon Books; 1995.
[41] The case of the frozen addict [transcript]. "NOVA". PBS Television. February 18, 1986.
[42] Davis GC, Williams AC, Markey SP, et al. Chronic Parkinsonism secondary to intravenous injection of meperidine analogues. Psychiatry Res 1979;1:249–54.
[43] Langston JW, Ballard P, Tetrud JW, et al. Chronic Parkinsonism in humans due to a product of meperidine-analog synthesis. Science 1983;219:979–80.
[44] Chiba K, Trevor A, Castagnoli N Jr. Metabolism of the neurotoxic tertiary amine, MPTP, by brain monoamine oxidase. Biochem Biophys Res Commun 1984;120:574–8.
[45] Langston JW, Irwin I, Langston EB, et al. Pargyline prevents MPTP-induced parkinsonism in primates. Science 1984;225:1480–2.
[46] Chiba K, Trevor AJ, Castagnoli N Jr. Active uptake of MPP +, a metabolite of MPTP, by brain synaptosomes. Biochem Biophys Res Commun 1985;128:1216, 1228–32.
[47] Nicklas WJ, Vyas I, Heikkila RE. Inhibition of NADH-linked oxidation in brain mitochondria by 1-methyl-4-phenyl-pyridine, a metabolite of the neurotoxin, 1-methyl-4-phenyl-1, 2,5,6-tetrahydropyridine. Life Sci 1985;36:2503–8.
[48] Nicklas WJ, Youngster SK, Kindt MV, et al. MPTP, MPP + and mitochondrial function. Life Sci 1987;40:721–9.
[49] Loschmann PA, Lange KW, Wachtel H, et al. MPTP-induced degeneration: interference with glutamatergic toxicity. J Neural Transm Suppl 1994;43:133–43.
[50] Tetrud JW, Langston JW. The effect of deprenyl (selegiline) on the natural history of Parkinson's disease. Science 1989;245:519–22.
[51] Tanner CM, Ottman R, Goldman SM, et al. Parkinson disease in twins: an etiologic study. JAMA 1999;281:341–6.
[52] Piccini P, Burn DJ, Ceravolo R, et al. The role of inheritance in sporadic Parkinson's disease: evidence from a longitudinal study of dopaminergic function in twins. Ann Neurol 1999;45: 577–82.
[53] Woolf A. Witchcraft or mycotoxin? The Salem witch trials. J Trace Elem Electrolytes Health Dis 2000;38:457–60.
[54] Eadie MJ. Convulsive ergotism: epidemics of the serotonin syndrome? Lancet 2003;2: 429–34.
[55] Christopoulos S, Szilagyi A, Kahn SR. Saint-Anthony's fire. Lancet 2001;358:1694.
[56] De Costa C. St Anthony's fire and living ligatures: a short history of ergometrine. Lancet 2002;359:1768–70.
[57] Dudley HW, Moir C. The substance responsible for the traditional clinical effect of ergot. BMJ 1935;1:520–3.
[58] Baldwin ZK, Ceraldi CC. Ergotism associated with HIV antiviral protease inhibitor therapy. J Vector Ecol 2003;37:676–8.

ELSEVIER
SAUNDERS

NEUROLOGIC
CLINICS

Neurol Clin 23 (2005) 353–376

Toxic Encephalopathies

Tracy Eicher, MD, Eleanor Avery, MD*

*Wilford Hall Medical Center, 2200 Bergquist Drive, Suite 1/MMCN,
Lackland Air Force Base, TX 78236, USA*

Effective brain function is dependent on precise and complex interactions between neurotransmitters, hormones, enzymes, and electrolytes. Many of the chemically complex substances with which we come into contact can disrupt this intricately balanced system. Toxic substances, whether ingested, inhaled, or absorbed through the skin, may cause an encephalopathic state directly by affecting the brain itself or indirectly by compromising the brain's supportive systems. Because it would be impossible to address all of these substances, this article focuses on neurotoxins that directly induce an encephalopathic state.

Exposure to neurotoxins can produce a range of symptoms—all of which are nonspecific and may be confused with other conditions. Furthermore, the symptoms and acuity with which they present depends not only on the identity of the toxin itself but also on the extent and route of exposure. The baseline cerebral function and reserve of the exposed individual additionally impacts the clinical picture. A thorough history and awareness of key features of specific toxin-induced syndromes is therefore essential for timely diagnosis and treatment.

Acute toxic encephalopathies often present with symptoms of confusion, attentional deficits, seizures, and coma. Much of this constellation of symptoms is thought to be attributable to central nervous system (CNS) capillary damage, hypoxia, and cerebral edema in addition to indirect effects of the toxin on the body's supportive systems [1]. With the appropriate care, the neurologic symptoms may resolve completely; however, varying degrees of permanent deficits may remain, even in the setting of a one-time exposure.

With chronic, low-level exposure to a toxin, whether in the home or work environment, the symptoms may come on insidiously and may go unrecognized for some time. Symptoms tend to include mood disturbances,

* Corresponding author.
E-mail address: eleanor.avery@lackland.af.mil (E. Avery).

0733-8619/05/$ - see front matter © 2005 Elsevier Inc. All rights reserved.
doi:10.1016/j.ncl.2004.12.004
neurologic.theclinics.com

fatigue, and memory and cognitive complaints [1]. Although improvement may occur following removal of the toxin, permanent residual deficits more often remain if the encephalopathy was severe or the exposure prolonged. Time to peak recovery from a chronic toxin-induced encephalopathy may take months to years.

Heavy metals

The heavy metals represent a diverse group of elements with a range of toxic effects on neuronal function. The heavy metals are commonly encountered in a variety of environments, and their toxic effects have been shown to affect the CNS and the peripheral nervous system. Because of their variable presence in the environment, heavy metal toxicity may be limited to one individual or may result in exposures of epidemic proportion. Their mechanisms of neurotoxicity include interactions with cell nuclei, cytoplasmic structure, mitochondria, and the extracellular milieu [2].

Lead

Due to its extensive commercial use, lead has historically been one of the most common sources of heavy metal intoxication. Environmental and occupational regulations imposed in the last 2 to 3 decades, however, have substantially decreased the incidence of lead intoxication. Measures such as the removal of lead from gasoline, residential plumbing, and house paints and the reduction in the use of lead-soldered cans for food and beverages have resulted in a dramatic decrease in blood lead levels in the United States [3,4]. Continued sources of potential lead exposure include lead mining and smelters, manufacture and recycling of storage batteries, solder, lead-based paints, lead pipes, lead shot, ceramic glazes, crystal glass manufacturing, contaminated illicit whiskey, and lead compounds used in auto body repair and manufacturing [1]. In addition, lead contaminates in the air, soil, and water can reach dangerous levels in areas close to lead smelters and other industrial plants that use this metal in their manufacturing process [5–7].

Inorganic lead can be absorbed through the gastrointestinal (GI) or respiratory systems. In an industrial setting, inhalation of lead particles (*lead dust*) and absorption by way of the respiratory system is the most common route of intoxication, whereas nonindustrial toxicity tends to result from GI absorption. Ingestion of paint chips or contaminated soil makes children common victims. Moreover, children are at particular risk from oral ingestion because up to 50% of ingested lead is absorbed through the GI tract in children compared with only approximately 10% in adults [8]. Skin absorption of inorganic lead is very limited, whereas organic lead such as that found in leaded gasoline is readily absorbed by this route.

After it is absorbed, lead binds to erythrocytes and is distributed throughout the body. It is incorporated into the brain and other soft tissues where it may remain for weeks to months. Approximately 50%, however, makes its way to the bone matrix where it has a half-life on the order of years to decades. Lead is also able to cross the placenta, putting the developing fetal nervous system at risk [7]. There are several known mechanisms by which lead is toxic to the nervous system. It causes altered migration of neurons during development, interferes with neural cell adhesion molecules, and impairs the timed programming of cell–cell interactions. Lead interferes directly with certain neurotransmitter functions and disrupts calcium metabolism in a number of ways [8].

Acute lead encephalopathy is most commonly seen in children or in occupationally exposed adults. Children tend to present with lethargy, irritability, confusion, ataxia, and impaired motor functions. Adults display similar symptoms and often also complain of headache and fatigue. Systemic symptoms primarily consist of GI complaints such as anorexia, abdominal cramping, and constipation [1]. Chronic, low-level lead exposure also causes encephalopathy. The symptoms are similar to those of acute lead toxicity, but the insidious onset may cause them to be overlooked by family members and physicians. The long-term effects of chronic, low-level lead exposure have especially devastating effects on the still-developing nervous system of young children. Epidemiologic studies suggest that blood lead concentrations of less than 5 μg/dL may lead to lower IQ levels when the exposure occurs during the first few years of life [1,5]. The adult CNS is less sensitive to the effects of lead toxicity, and adults may tolerate higher levels of exposure before becoming notably encephalopathic. Accompanying symptoms of chronic lead encephalopathy in the adult include irritability, fatigue, headaches, arthralgias, myalgias, paresthesias, and sensory complaints. Many adults also complain of sleep disturbance, decreased libido, and anorexia. Blood lead levels between 30 μg/dL and 100 μg/dL result in symptoms ranging from mild confusion to stupor, coma, and death. In addition to elevated blood lead levels, laboratory indicators of lead-induced encephalopathy include anemia, decreased blood delta-aminolevulinic acid (ALA-D) and basophilic stippling on peripheral smear [1,7,8].

Treatment of lead toxicity should begin with removal of the individual from the source of exposure. The blood lead level at which chelation therapy is warranted has been debated; however, in the setting of lead encephalopathy following acute exposure, the use of chelating agents should be initiated immediately. Removal of the lead before it can be incorporated into the tissues is the goal. Due to the increased absorption and higher sensitivity of children to the effects of lead, exposures high enough to induce an encephalopathy also carry a high mortality rate. Even with chelation therapy, the mortality rate is as high as 25% to 38% if EDTA or 2,3-dimercaptopropanol (dimercaprol; British antilewisite) is used alone. The combination of EDTA and dimercaprol therapy, however, has been shown to reduce mortality. The oral chelating agent dimercaptosuccinic acid has been licensed by the Food and Drug Administration for reducing blood lead levels of 45 µg/dL or greater. It has been shown to be effective in temporarily reducing blood lead levels and has the advantage of being administered orally. Animal studies, however, indicate that it does not reduce the brain lead level beyond that which is expected from simply removing the source of exposure [9].

Mercury

Mercury exists in elemental, organic, and inorganic forms. Mercury in its various forms may be found in thermometers, barometers, batteries, electronic equipment, dental amalgams, disinfectants, bactericides, and fungicides. It is used in photography, as a preservative in latex paint and wood, and in the manufacture of felt. The extent to which mercury in most of these forms poses a health hazard is debated [7,9]. Mercury may be found in water supplies due to industrial pollution or as a result of leaching from rock or sediment where it occurs naturally. The 1950s exposure of over 2000 people in Minamata Bay, Japan, resulted from industrial dumping of mercury-containing waste into the water supply. After it is present in the water, mercury is methylated by microorganisms that in turn are ingested by aquatic species. Levels of methylmercury are thus bioamplified and can cause toxic exposures to those who eat affected seafood [10]. Neurologic manifestations of methylmercury toxicity range from paresthesias and tremor to ataxia, spasticity, visual and hearing loss, and encephalopathy. A range of cognitive and memory deficits can occur, and severe cases may result in coma and death [9].

Apart from methylmercury, acute mercury exposure is associated mainly with systemic effects on the lungs, kidneys, and GI systems (depending on the route of exposure), with any CNS effects occurring secondary to the systemic dysfunction. Chronic exposure to mercury, however, affects the CNS directly. Mercury toxicity secondary to chronic inhalation of mercury vapor, generally the result of occupational exposure, is the mechanism behind the *mad hatter* syndrome. This illness historically affected individuals who were chronically exposed during the manufacture of felt hats and consists of a fairly well defined set of neurologic and neuropsychiatric features including tremor, memory and cognitive dysfunction, social withdrawal, excitability, and emotional lability [11,12]. The combination of increased excitability, tremors, and gingivitis has been touted as the classic triad of long-term mercury exposure [13].

The ability of the different forms of mercury to cause encephalopathy and other neurologic symptoms depends on the rate at which they are metabolized peripherally and their ability to cross the blood–brain barrier. Mercury salts, for example, are not highly lipid soluble and therefore do not easily cross the blood–brain barrier; phenylmercury easily penetrates the blood–brain barrier but is metabolized quickly by the liver, greatly decreasing the number of toxic molecules entering the CNS [1,14].

Methylmercury, in contrast, is slowly metabolized and is actively trans-ported across the blood–brain barrier. Autopsy and imaging studies show that after it crosses the blood–brain barrier, mercury preferentially affects the cortex of the cerebrum and the cerebellum, with focal necrosis of neurons followed by phagocytosis and gliosis. Changes in the visual cortex and insula are especially prominent [15,16].

For the most part, treatment of acute mercury intoxication has focused on facilitating elimination of the mercury and providing supportive care. Dimercaprol causes redistribution of mercury from other body tissues to the CNS and should therefore be avoided. There are limited data suggesting that unithion and succimer may facilitate clearance of elemental mercury from the body and that these two agents and N-acetylcysteine (NAC) may increase clearance of methylmercury [7]. There is not enough information, however, to draw a conclusion regarding the effects of these agents on long-term neurologic outcomes.

Arsenic

Because it is odorless, tasteless, and highly toxic, arsenic has long been recognized for its potential as a homicidal agent. More frequently, it is used for more mundane purposes. Almost 75% of the arsenic and arsenic trioxide in the United States is used as an ingredient in wood preservatives. It is also used extensively in pesticides, herbicides, and in the production of glass, electronics, and computer microchips [1]. Arsenic is found in varying levels in soil, plants, and air. Groundwater contaminated by the leaching of arsenic from the ground is a major source of chronic toxic exposure in certain areas such as Bangladesh and West Bengal, India [1,17,18]. Most cases of acute arsenic poisoning are due to accidental ingestion of pesticides or insecticides or by inhalation in occupational settings. Encephalopathy is a common manifes-tation of acute exposure. Accompanying symptoms may include nausea, vomiting, bloody diarrhea, dizziness, diffuse muscle weakness, numbness, and paresthesias of the distal extremities. Respiratory symptoms can be seen in cases of inhalation exposure. Patients are often found to have hypotension, cardiac arrhythmias, myoglobinuria, and acute renal failure. In severe cases, seizures, coma, and death may follow. White transverse striations of the nails, also known as Mees' lines, appear 3 to 6 weeks following arsenic exposure, and may be an important diagnostic clue. It should be noted, however, that Mees' lines are nonspecific and can be seen following thallium poisoning, chemotherapy, and a variety of systemic disorders [9].

Chronic encephalopathy is more common after exposure to organic arsenic than inorganic arsenic. Careful questioning and neuropsychiatric testing, however, has shown cognitive and personality disturbances after exposure to inorganic arsenic [19–21]. The encephalopathy of chronic arsenic toxicity may manifest as confusion, irritability, paranoid delusions, or auditory or visual hallucinations [21,22]. Arsenic encephalopathy, whether acute or chronic, generally improves following removal of the exposure, although persistent deficits have been reported [22,23].

The extent of absorption of arsenic depends on the form in which it is encountered and the route of exposure. In general, soluble arsenic compounds are well absorbed by way of the lungs or GI tract. Arsenic is not well absorbed through the skin. It exerts its toxic effects on the nervous system by inhibiting mitochondrial function. It also binds to sulfhydryl groups of many proteins and interferes with several steps of oxidative metabolism in neurons and other cells [9].

Laboratory testing may show myoglobinuria, elevated liver enzymes, and increased cerebral spinal fluid protein (150–300 mg/dL). Arsenic binds to keratin, so levels can be detected in the hair and nails for weeks to months following an exposure. Because arsenic disappears rapidly from the blood, urine arsenic levels are the test of choice for confirmation of the diagnosis; however, urine levels may take days to weeks to return from the laboratory, and treatment should not be postponed if the suspicion is high. Treatment consists of decontamination of the gut if appropriate, aggressive supportive care, and chelation with dimercaprol, unithiol, or D-penicillamine [7,24].

Manganese

Manganese is an essential element and is present in all living organisms. It functions naturally in the human body as a cofactor for a number of enzymatic reactions. The principle source of this element to humans is in food; grains, fruits, nuts, and vegetables are rich in manganese [25].

Manganese is now widely used as a fuel additive in the form of methylcyclopentadienyl Mn tricarbonyl, replacing the previous lead-based additives. It is also used in fertilizers and in the manufacture of fireworks. Industrial uses include iron and steel manufacturing, metal-finishing operations, and as an alloy in welding [9,26]. Most commonly, manganese toxicity occurs in the occupational setting, with chronic exposure in mines, steel mills, and chemical industries.

In general, the classic presentation of manganese toxicity is parkinsonism; however, encephalopathy can occur with acute or chronic manganese toxicity. Acute to subacute exposure may result in acute psychosis, including auditory and visual hallucinations, compulsive behavior, euphoria, memory disturbance, and irritability. Headache is almost invariably present [27,28]. The classic motor features of tremor, increased tone, and gait abnormalities usually follow the onset of psychosis by 1 to 2 years. Masked facies and postural rigidity develop last [29]. Recovery from toxicity tends to be slow and minimal but depends somewhat on the duration and form of exposure. Chronic inhalation exposure appears to have a poor prognosis from the standpoint of the encephalopathy and motor symptoms; however, tremor tends to show some improvement. Case reports of shorter exposures and ingestion in drinking water indicate a somewhat better outcome except in young children, in whom even limited exposures can produce long-term developmental delays [27–31].

Absorption of manganese through respiratory systems may vary with the valence of the element and the size of the inhaled particles. GI absorption is less than 5% and occurs throughout the length of the small intestine. Manganese is transported in the blood and concentrates in mitochondria. It readily crosses the blood–brain barrier has a specific affinity for the subthalamic nucleus and globus pallidus. The putamen, caudate nucleus, cerebellum, pons, thalamus, and substantia nigra are also affected. The neurotoxicity of manganese is thought to relate in part to its ability to potentiate oxidation of substances such as catecholamines and fatty acids, resulting in an increased production of toxic free radicals that disrupt the integrity of neuronal membranes [1,9,32].

Due to rapid elimination of manganese from the blood, serum manganese levels are somewhat limited but often used for diagnosis. Urine levels provide a better means of assessing manganese levels in suspected toxic exposures; stool samples may also be used. Treatment is generally limited to removal of the toxic source. Chelation with calcium-EDTA has shown some benefit in cases of acute exposure. In cases of significant acute exposure, dialysis may also be used [1].

Aluminum

Aluminum is abundant in the natural environment and extensively used in packaging, construction, food containers, cooking utensils, and pharmaceuticals. Aluminum, however, is poorly absorbed following inhalation or ingestion. Despite this, aluminum toxicity occurs with certain high-level or prolonged exposures, and encephalopathy is a primary feature. The syndrome known as *potroom palsy* has been attributed to occupational exposure of workers in the manufacture of aluminum pots and in aluminum smelter workers [33–35]. Motor incoordination, poor memory, impaired cognition, and depression are hallmarks of this syndrome. *Dialysis dementia* is now attributed to toxic effects of aluminum in the dialysis fluid and in the phosphate binders used to regulate blood phosphate levels. The uremic state itself may increase aluminum retention, making these patients more sensitive to aluminum exposure. This syndrome arises in some patients after 3 to 7 years of dialysis. It often initially presents with isolated speech disorder. A progressive dementia ensues, followed by myoclonus, seizures, and death [9,36]. Deionization of the dialysate and avoidance of aluminum-containing phosphate binders have dramatically decreased the incidence of this disorder and may slow or stop progression of the syndrome when instituted in an already symptomatic patient.

Thallium

Although peripheral neuropathy is generally the predominant symptom of thallium toxicity, a debilitating encephalopathy may also occur. Thallium toxicity generally occurs after ingestion of thallium-containing chemicals, rat poison, or contaminated foods. Cases of exposure by depilatory agents and by pollutants of illicit drugs have also been reported [37–39]. Symptoms of thallium-induced encephalopathy include hallucinations, paranoia, and cognitive impairment. Alopecia, the classic diagnostic clue to thallium toxicity, generally does not occur for 2 to 3 weeks, and Mees' lines do not appear on the nails until 3 to 4 weeks following exposure. Blood and urine thallium levels may be used diagnostically.

Absorption and distribution of thallium may take up to 24 hours, and within this time frame, gastric lavage and laxatives may help reduce the toxic load. Absorption from the gut can also be inhibited by administration of potassium ferric hexacyanoferrocyanate III (Prussian Blue) or activated charcoal. Potassium chloride also enhances elimination of the toxin [24,39,40].

Tin

Tin is used extensively in canning, soldering, the electronics industry, and in the manufacture of certain plastics. Exposure in laboratory or occupational settings is most common. Exposure to inorganic tin as a particulate in dust or in gaseous form does not cause a neurologic syndrome. Organic tin, however, especially in the form of trimethyltin or triethyltin may cause severe encephalopathy with prominent cerebral edema. The symptoms consist of headache, apathy, memory loss, hallucinations, and confusion. Seizures, coma, and death often ensue [1,41–43]. Examination findings in organic tin encephalopathy may reveal abnormal eye movements. Papilledema is usually present and indicates the presence of cerebral edema. A case series by Besser et al [44] described a *limbic–cerebellar* syndrome that occurred in six workers following high-level exposure to trimethyltin vapors. These men presented with encephalopathy accompanied by variable combinations of hyperphagia, excessive thirst, and sexual aggressiveness, and with nystagmus, abnormal smooth pursuits, and ataxia [44].

Blood levels are not a good indicator of tin toxicity because trimethyltin and triethyltin have a low affinity for hemoglobin. Urine levels and urine absorption spectroscopy are more reliable. Urine levels generally peak at 4 to 10 days after exposure [41]. CSF studies tend to be normal.

There is limited information regarding successful treatment of organic tin toxicity with chelating agents. The case series by Besser et al [44], however, indicated that the combination of plasmapheresis and D-penicillamine may improve outcome.

Solvents and vapors

The question of whether long-term, low-level exposure to vapors from paints, solvents, or lacquers can cause a *chronic solvent encephalopathy* is a matter of some debate in the neurotoxicology literature [45–48]. There is no question, however, that acute, high-dose exposure, or moderate to high levels of prolonged exposure can cause CNS dysfunction. Hormes et al [49] reported on the long-term symptoms of 20 solvent-vapor abusers, finding that cognitive deficits including attention, memory, executive function, and visuospatial disturbances were present in 60%. Half of the patients displayed motor disorders and 45% had cerebellar dysfunction [49].

Toluene

Toluene is an aromatic alkylbenzene hydrocarbon compound used in paints, lacquers, glues, solvents, and many other products to which we are exposed daily. Gasoline contains up to 7% toluene by weight and represents the most significant source of toluene use in this country [1]. Accounts of acute and chronic encephalopathy due to intentional and accidental toluene inhalation have long been reported. In fact, the acute intoxicating effects of toluene-containing substances, together with their wide availability make this compound one of the most dangerous toxins in today's society. The recreational use of glues, gasoline, and paints is probably underestimated.

The acute effects of toluene toxicity include lightheadedness, confusion, euphoria, cognitive and memory difficulties, incoordination, and disequilibrium. Unconsciousness, coma, and death may occur with high levels of exposure. Findings of inappropriate behavior, fluctuating mood, nystagmus, and vacant staring are common acutely. The acute CNS effects of toluene are quickly reversed after cessation of exposure. After repeated exposures, however, intention tremor, motor incoordination, and cognitive deficits may become more marked and are less likely to fully resolve [50,51].

Toluene is highly lipid soluble. It crosses the blood–brain barrier easily and has an affinity for CNS white matter. The mechanism of toxicity to the CNS structures has not been firmly established; however, there is evidence that toluene causes breakdown of myelin and neuronal cell death directly or by way of production of free radicals during its metabolism. There is some evidence that toluene may also affect the neuronal response to certain neurotransmitters [48,49].

The American Conference of Governmental Industrial Hygienists (ACGIH) has set biologic exposure indices for workers at risk of toluene exposure. Urine hippuric acid levels at the end of shift are the recommended means of monitoring exposure. Blood toluene level may also be used [49]. Diagnosis in the setting of acute nonindustrial exposure is more likely to be based on history and findings at presentation. Treatment is limited to removal of the source of exposure and providing supportive care.

Trichlorethylene

Trichlorethylene (TCE) is an unsaturated chlorinated hydrocarbon widely used commercially as a degreasing solvent. It can also be found in cleaning solutions, flame retardant chemicals, and insecticides, and as a vehicle for paints, varnishes, and glues. Its release into the atmosphere by factories and into soil and water by improper waste disposal processes has been found to cause public exposures by way of air, water, and food products [52–54]. The Environmental Protection Agency has established recommended exposure limits for TCE; however, these levels are based on its carcinogenic properties. Minimal levels of exposure for its neurotoxic effects are less well established.

Occupational inhalation is the most commonly reported type of acute TCE exposure [1], whereas ingestion of TCE-contaminated drinking water has been a source of chronic exposure in several communities. Symptoms of acute toxicity generally include nausea, headache, dizziness, disorientation, stupor, and occasionally coma. Trigeminal neuropathy, with or without other cranial nerve dysfunction, is a prominent symptom of TCE toxicity, and peripheral neuropathy may occur. Recovery may be complete over hours to days if exposure time is limited. Long-term deficits resulting from more prolonged exposures include cranial nerve palsies and chronic encephalopathy. Short-term memory and attentional deficits, impaired visuospatial perfomance, and depressed mood or apathy commonly persist, although some improvement may be seen even years after the exposure [55–59]. With chronic, low-level exposure, changes in behavior or mood are often the first symptoms noted. Fatigue, dizziness, and headache often accompany the gradual onset of encephalopathy [60,61].

In addition to preventive measures, the ACGIH recommends using blood levels of the TCE metabolite trichloroethanol to monitor exposures in the occupational setting [62]. Treatment for acute inhalational exposure involves removing the victim from the area and providing fresh air or oxygen if available. Gastric lavage should be initiated for acute ingestion of TCE. Due to potential for cardiac arrhythmias and acute renal failure, cardiac monitoring is warranted and hemodialysis may be necessary. In addition, exposed individuals may become sensitized to TCE after an acute exposure and avoidance of even low-level exposures is recommended [1].

Perchlorethylene

Perchlorethylene (PCE), also known as tetrachlorethylene, is used as a degreasing agent in industrial settings. It has been used as an anesthetic and as an antihelmintic agent in the treatment of hookworm. Its ability to dissolve grease, wax, and oil without harming fabrics explains its extensive use in the dry cleaning industry [1]. Most reported toxic exposures to PCE occur by way of inhalation in occupational settings by industrial workers or dry cleaners. Users of coin-operated dry cleaning machines have also been victims of acute PCE intoxication. PCE contamination of soil, groundwater, and foods may lead to oral exposure, but the neurotoxicity of such low-level ingestions is not known.

Acute effects of high-level exposure to PCE produce an encephalopathy that typically resolves fully after exposure is stopped. Symptoms include headache, dizziness, a feeling of intoxication, and confusion. After prolonged acute exposure, personality changes, irritability, and outbursts of rage have been reported [1,63]. Chronic inhalation exposure may result in an encephalopathy that includes prominent memory impairment, chronic dizziness, drowsiness, and frequent fainting spells [64,65]. Intolerance to alcohol and increased sensitivity to multiple other chemicals have also been reported [1].

Recommended exposure limits for PCE in air and water have been established by various agencies including the Occupational Safely and Health Administration and the ACGIH. Safety levels for PCE, however, are based more on its carcinogenic properties than on neurotoxicity. Laboratory evaluation in exposed individuals can include levels of PCE in exhaled air or blood. Alternatively, urine levels of the PCE metabolite trichloroacetic acid may be used. Trichloroacetic acid is also a metabolite of TCE and other solvents, and potential exposure to these substances should be taken into account [1,62].

Treatment for acute PCE intoxication is similar to that described in the previous section for TCE, including eliminating the exposure, providing fresh air or oxygen if available, gastric lavage for oral ingestion, and aggressive supportive care. As in TCE exposures, the patient should be closely monitored for possible cardiac arrhythmias, acute renal failure, and pulmonary edema.

Carbon disulfide

Carbon disulfide is found in solvents, soil fumigants, insecticides, and varnishes. It is used in the production of perfumes, cellophane, viscose rayon, and certain types of rubber [66]. Toxic exposures occur most commonly in the occupational setting by way of inhalation, although it can also occur transdermally.

Although the mechanism of toxicity is uncertain, acute inhalation of concentrations exceeding 300 to 400 ppm causes an encephalopathy with symptoms ranging from mild behavioral changes and drowsiness to confusion, mania, marked mood swings and behavioral outbursts, and psychiatric disturbances. Long-term exposures to lower levels of carbon disulfide have been reported to cause minor mood and cognitive changes [67,68]. The chronic encephalopathy may be subtle and revealed only by neuropsychiatric testing or it may be more marked, with symptoms resembling those of acute toxicity. Other symptoms that may point to long-term carbon disulfide exposure include a peripheral neuropathy, parkinsonism, and retinopathy [66,67].

No specific treatment has been proved effective for minimizing effects of carbon disulfide toxicity. Avoidance of high levels or prolonged exposures is therefore essential. Due to variability in absorption of carbon disulfide, however, simply measuring air levels is not an adequate means of monitoring for potential occupational exposures. Individual blood or urine carbon disulfide levels should be checked. Carbon disulfide exists in the blood in bound and unbound forms. Elimination from the blood is therefore biphasic, with a half-life of 2 hours for unbound carbon disulfide and 43 hours for bound carbon disulfide. Alternatively, urine levels of carbon disulfide or its metabolite 2-thio-thiazolidine-4-carboxylic acid may be monitored [1].

Hexacarbon solvents

Of the hexacarbon solvents, n-hexane and methyl n-butyl ketone (MnBK) are the most neurotoxic. This toxicity is due in large part to their common metabolite (2,5-hexanedione) and to their lipophilic properties and the ease with which they cross the blood–brain barrier [1]. n-Hexane and MnBK occur naturally in the environment as products of the earth's natural gases. They are liberated in higher amounts during petroleum production and refining and are present in certain glues, paints, and solvents.

An acute encephalopathy with euphoria, dizziness, ataxia, decreased mentation, and hallucinations may result from acute, high-level exposures to these substances. Thus, products containing n-hexane and MnBK have high potential for recreational abuse. The acute encephalopathy appears to be fully reversible after cessation of the exposure; however, adequate studies have not been done regarding long-term neuropsychiatric sequelae. Chronic or repeated exposure to these hexacarbon compounds commonly results in a sensorimotor polyneuropathy. CNS involvement is evidenced by abnormalities of somatosensory evoked potentials; however, encephalopathy is not an established feature of chronic n-hexane or MnBK exposure [1,66,69].

Xylene and styrene

Xylene and styrene are structurally similar to toluene. Xylene is found in many solvents, paints, varnishes, and rust preventatives, and is present in a variety of industrial settings. Styrene is found in floor waxes, paints, varnishes, auto body putty, and polishes. It is frequently used in the manufacture of fiberglass-reinforced plastics (such as in boats). Both chemicals can produce an encephalopathy in the acute setting, with symptoms similar to those seen in toluene and other solvents. Chronic CNS dysfunction is less severe and full recovery of function more likely with exposure to these chemicals compared with toluene. Subjective complaints of memory and cognitive deficits, headache, fatigue, and irritability, however, may continue for weeks to months after cessation of exposure. Concommitant exposure to more than one neurotoxic agent is common with solvents, which complicates analysis of their individual effects [70–76].

Ethanol

The ability of ethanol (EtOH) to cause an acute encephalopathy is well known. Obviously, the most common circumstances of EtOH toxicity relate to ingestion in a recreational setting; however, EtOH may be found in many household products, pharmaceuticals, and industrial solvents. As the EtOH level increases, a variety of symptoms occur, ranging from euphoria to stupor and coma. Dysequilibrium, cognitive impairment, diplopia, and psychomotor slowing are common. The acute effects of EtOH exposure are secondary to its ability to bind nonspecifically to a number of neurotransmitter and neuromodulator receptors. Among other effects, it facilitates γ-aminobutyric acid type A receptor function and inhibits glutamate N-methyl-D-aspartate receptor function [77,78]. Of note, the presence of EtOH amplifies the toxicity of many other solvents due to its high affinity for alcohol dehydrogenase and CYP2E1, the same liver enzymes that are needed for the metabolism of other solvents [48]. This interaction is especially important in the setting of recreational inhalation of solvent vapors. In such settings, concomitant EtOH use is common and dramatically increases the chance of lethal outcome.

That chronic EtOH abuse can cause long-term cognitive and memory deficits is well established. Separating the direct neurotoxic effects of EtOH from the effects of nutritional deficits, electrolyte disturbances, polysubstance abuse, and general poor health habits, however, can be somewhat difficult. It is believed that EtOH exerts direct toxic effects on neural tissues. Animal studies that control for nutrition and other factors indicate that EtOH directly damages neurons and has the ability to cause pathologic cortical changes. Specifically, loss of neurons in the basal forebrain and hippocampus has been demonstrated. Imaging studies in humans indicate that the frontal lobes are especially vulnerable to EtOH toxicity [79].

The symptoms of chronic alcohol use are varied and no reliable predictors apart from certain vitamin deficiencies have been identified to indicate which set of symptoms is more likely to occur in any given individual. Moreover, the amount and duration of EtOH intake before symptom onset is markedly different from person to person. *Alcoholic dementia*, a common result of chronic EtOH use, consists of widespread cognitive dysfunction and is probably due to the direct neurotoxic effects of this substance. Alcoholic dementia is distinct from the Wernicke-Korsakoff syndrome, and its pathophysiology is not well understood. Although increased ventricle size and shrinkage of cerebral white matter are common findings on imaging, there is often poor correlation between the amount of atrophy and the degree of dementia [79]. Perceptual disturbances are also common in chronic alcohol users ($\sim$25%) and include visual illusions and visual, auditory, olfactory, and tactile hallucinations. These distortions of perception seem to be a separate issue from the cognitive dysfunction. They are usually brief and intermittent but may progress (albeit rarely) into frank and unremitting psychosis [80]. Cerebellar degeneration occurs with unknown prevalence in the alcoholic population. Selective atrophy of the anterior and superior parts of the cerebellar vermis with less involvement of the cerebellar hemispheres leads to truncal ataxia with milder limb ataxia.

Wernicke-Korsakoff syndrome

Although Wernicke's and Korsakoff's syndromes are clinically separate, both are linked causally to thiamine deficiency in alcoholics. Wernicke's encephalopathy is an acute encephalopathy that arises in chronic alcohol use and thiamine deficiency. The symptoms progress over days to weeks and consist of lethargy, ophthalmoplegia, impaired memory, decreased attentiveness, and perceptual disturbances. If untreated, it may progress to stupor and coma. If treated, the above symptoms may remit, or they may evolve into Korsakoff's syndrome. In Korsakoff's syndrome, the major impairment involves memory, but more subtle cognitive deficits may be identified on neuropsychiatric testing. A marked anterograde amnesia with inability to retain new information is present and accompanied by a more patchy and variable retrograde amnesia. Importantly, alertness and attentiveness are intact, and the individual appears behaviorally normal [80]. Pathologic changes in Wernicke-Korsakoff syndrome are most notable in the hypothalamus, medial thalamus, mammillary bodies, periaqueductal gray matter of the mesencephalon, and medial pons and medulla [79].

Marchiafava-Bignami disease

In 1903, Marchiafava and Bignami described a disease affecting middle-aged and elderly Italian men who were chronic consumers of red wine. The clinical features consisted of insidious onset of altered mental status, memory loss, ataxia, behavioral changes, and sometimes delusions. In addition, seizures and focal neurologic signs such as aphasia and apraxia were noted. Findings at autopsy invariably included the absence of inflammation, necrosis of the corpus callosum, and symmetric lesions throughout other regions of the brain. This disease has long been attributed to alcoholism and malnutrition; however, the mechanism and what part alcohol plays in the disease are unknown. Although chronic alcohol use continues to be an overwhelmingly common characteristic, Marchiafava-Bignami disease has been reported in rare cases in which there was not a significant history of alcohol use [80]. Thus, the question of whether EtOH plays a primary role in this disease process remains unanswered.

Carbon monoxide

Carbon monoxide (CO) is encountered frequently as a by-product of the burning of many different substances. It is present in automobile exhaust and cigarette smoke and is a metabolite of methylene chloride, which is commonly found in solvents. CO has long been known to cause both short- and long-term CNS effects. This toxic gas causes neural damage by way of tissue hypoxia and free radical production. It binds to hemoglobin in the blood, decreasing the ability of blood to deliver oxygen to body tissues. It also disrupts oxidative phosphorylation in mitochondria, leading to indirect damage to the brain and other tissues with high metabolic demands. CO exerts direct neurotoxic effects at the cellular level and has been shown to cause lipid peroxidation, leading to white matter destruction [81–83].

Headache, dizziness, confusion, and visual changes are common symptoms of CO exposure, but signs of cerebral dysfunction may be absent acutely. Nausea, abdominal pain, shortness of breath, and generalized weakness are commonly reported [81]. Delayed onset of encephalopathic features after apparent full recovery has been estimated to occur in up to 30% of CO victims. Symptoms of cognitive decline, personality changes, psychosis, and parkinsonism may begin anywhere from a few days to several months following the exposure. The mechanisms for this syndrome are not well defined, but recovery occurs in 50% to 75% of victims within a year [84,85].

CO levels in exhaled air can be measured by emergency personnel at the scene of exposure. Blood level of carboxyhemoglobin is the most sensitive marker for confirming the diagnosis and determining level of toxic exposure. It should be noted that smokers have elevated levels of carboxyhemoglobin at baseline. Furthermore, blood carboxyhemoglobin levels begin to decline quickly after removal of the exposure. Levels should therefore be drawn as soon as possible when an accurate estimation of level of exposure is needed [81]. Following stabilization of the victim, neuropsychologic testing is recommended and provides a means of following the clinical course thereafter. The Carbon Monoxide Neuropsychological Screening Battery is an easy-to-use test developed specifically for evaluation of CO victims [86].

After the source of exposure has been removed, providing fresh air is the first priority in treatment. Hyperbaric oxygen therapy greatly enhances recovery from acute symptoms; however, it is unclear whether it decreases the incidence of the delayed neuropsychiatric syndrome or improves long-term outcome. It is nonetheless recommended when the victim is unconscious for any period of time, has an abnormal score on the Carbon Monoxide Neuropsychological Screening Battery, has a carboxyhemoglobin level > 40%, or in the presence of certain other complicating medical factors [81].

Pesticides

Organophosphates

Organophosphate compounds are present in nearly 40% of the pesticides used in the United States. Most organophosphates are well absorbed through the skin, lungs, and GI tract [1]. Toxic exposures by way of inhalation or skin absorption occur each year in farmers, gardeners, crop dusters, and pesticide handlers. A fair number of toxic exposures also occur by ingestion—in suicide attempts or by children. Organophosphates inhibit acetylcholinesterase, thus creating an excess of acetylcholine by blocking its breakdown. The result is increased salivation, lacrimation, sweating, and diffuse muscle weakness. The acute CNS effects include confusion, dizziness, ataxia, blurred vision, hallucinations, and decreased memory and concentration. Seizures, coma, and death may ensue in severe cases. Certain CNS symptoms may predominate in exposures to different organophosphates, reflecting the distribution of different types of acetylcholinesterase throughout the brain [87]. Organophosphates are thought to have chronic CNS sequelae; specifically, studies have found that victims of high levels of exposure to organophosphates later score worse on mood inventories and on tests of sustained visual attention than their nonexposed counterparts [88,89]. Case reports suggest that executive function, memory, and certain domains of learning may be impaired for prolonged periods in some individuals, but slow recovery of most functions seems to be the trend [1,90–93]. Further studies are needed before conclusions can be drawn with regard to long-term brain dysfunction in chronic, low-level exposure to organophosphates.

Due to the ease of absorption of organophosphates through the skin and respiratory tract, use of protective masks, gloves, and proper clothing is paramount in preventing acute toxicity. Agents containing organophosphates should be kept well out of the reach of children and should remain in well-marked containers. In the event of exposure of the skin to organophosphate agents, the skin should immediately and thoroughly be washed. In cases of ingestion, gastric lavage should be performed unless the individual has vomited. In all forms of organophosphate exposure, maintaining the airway and minimizing aspiration may require suctioning or intubation. Atropine may be used to combat the muscarinic effects of organophosphates, but it will not reverse the nicotinic effects, and muscle weakness will not improve. The cause of organophosphate-induced seizures is cholinergic, and seizures should be treated with atropine because they will not respond to dilantin or other antiepileptics [1,94].

Carbamates

Carbamates are also used extensively as pesticides. Their mechanism of action, like organophosphates, is inhibition of acetylcholinesterase; however, they differ from organophosphates in that they have a shorter duration of action on acetylcholinesterase, making them less toxic. The toxicities of individual carbamates vary based on differences in their chemical structures. Certain carbamates such as disulfiram (Antabuse) and pyridostigmine are used medically [95].

The acute syndrome of carbamate toxicity can be identical to that seen with organophosphates, including acute encephalopathy. Despite their generally lower toxicity compared with organophosphates, seizures, coma, and death can occur. The CNS effects, however, tend to occur mainly in children [96]. Subjective symptoms of headaches, photophobia, memory problems, dizziness, and irritability have been reported to last for years following acute, high-dose exposures to carbamates, but whether these symptoms eventually remit is not clearly established [97,98]. Although case reports suggest that a chronic encephalopathy may result from long-term low-dose carbamate exposure, objective evidence is currently lacking [99].

Measures of erythrocyte acetylcholinesterase activity are suggested for documentation and monitoring of acute carbamate toxicity. Blood or urine levels of the specific compound and its metabolites may also be helpful, especially after blood cholinesterase activity has returned to normal. Treatment of acute carbamate exposure is similar to that discussed with organophosphate poisoning. Due to the shorter action of carbamates on acetylcholinesterase, caution should be used in the administration of atropine. Use of excess atropine after the effect of the carbamate has worn off can result in unwanted anticholinergic side effects including fever and delerium [1,95].

Natural neurotoxins

Many plant, insect, reptile, and animal species produce toxic agents as part of their natural defense against predators or as weapons for immobilizing and digesting prey. These toxins range in potency from those that cause only minor skin irritation to those that are potentially fatal to humans. Of the more potent substances, many are capable of causing an encephalopathic state indirectly by way of their effects on the body's supportive systems. This section is limited to natural neurotoxins that directly affect the CNS and in which encephalopathy is a predominant feature of the clinical syndrome.

Plant toxins

Many plants have neurotoxic potential. Many such plants and their extracts have long been used recreationally for their hallucinogenic properties. *Cannabis sativa* (marijuana), and *Lophophora williamsii* from which mescaline is derived are among the many hallucinogenic plants with potent acute CNS effects. *Juniperus macropoda* (juniper), *Nepeta cataria* (catnip), *Piper methysticum* (kava), *Mandragora officinarum* (mandrake), and *Catharanthus roseus* (Madagascar periwinkle) are just a few of the commonly encountered plants with hallucinogenic properties found in herbal preparations. Although benign in small doses, these substances produce an acute encephalopathy at higher doses. The commonly used spice *Myristica fragrans* (nutmeg) is also hallucinogenic in high doses. *Lobelia inflata* (lobelia) and *Argemone mexicana* (prickly poppy) are euphoriants, and *Nicotiana* (tobacco) species, *Passiflora incarnata* (passion flower), and *Catha edulis* (khat) are all strong CNS stimulants that can, at certain doses, produce an acute encephalopathic state, with confusion, agitation, and decreased concentration and cognition. Similarly, the sedating effects of *Artemisia absinthium* (wormwood), *Valeriana officinalis* (valerian), and *Rauwolfia serpentina* (snakeroot) can produce encephalopathy at moderate to high doses [100,101]. In general, the neurotoxic effects of these plants and their extracts are temporary and full recovery is expected.

Mushroom toxicity

There are around 5000 species of mushroom found in the United States. Most of these fungi are harmless; however, about 100 species are toxic if ingested. In general, poisonous mushrooms can be placed into two classes based on the time to onset of symptoms following ingestion. Mushrooms that predominantly affect the nervous system generally produce an immediate response, such as hallucinations, and include *Amanita muscaria*, *A panthirina*, and mushrooms in the *Psilocybe* genus. Exposure to these fungi is usually in the setting of intended recreational use [102]. The CNS toxicity of *A muscaria* and *A panthirina* is due to ibotinic acid and its derivative muscimol. Ibotinic acid is an excitatory amino acid that mimics the action of glutamate on the CNS. CNS symptoms vary somewhat but most often include alterations in mental status, visual changes, hallucinations, agitation, and ataxia. In severe cases, seizures and psychosis may occur. Muscle fasciculations and anticholinergic symptoms such as flushing, mydriasis, and urinary retention are commonly seen [102,103]. The *Psilocybe* mushrooms contain psilocybin and its more potent metabolite psilocin. These indolealkylamines are structurally similar to serotonin and interact with CNS receptors to produce a lysergic acid diethylamide–like syndrome, including visual illusions, vivid hallucinations, euphoria, and reckless behavior. Anxiety, drowsiness, and dysphoria commonly occur, as do flushing, hyperthermia, tachycardia, and hypertension. The acute neurotoxic effects of mushrooms typically resolve completely and without chronic sequelae [100,103].

Marine toxins

Several marine toxins are known to exert potent neurotoxic effects. Most are limited to peripheral nerve dysfunction (less frequently to brainstem dysfunction) and do not typically cause notable encephalopathy. Domoic acid, however, is an exception. Domoic acid is produced by *Nitzschia pungens* and certain *Pseudonitzschia* species of algae. It is bioamplified in mussels that ingest the algae and exert its neurotoxic effects on humans who consume these infected shellfish. This toxin was responsible for the 1987 outbreak of *amnestic shellfish poisoning* off the coast of Prince Edward Island and has since been identified in waters off the western coasts of California, Oregon, and Canada [104].

Domoic acid acts as an excitatory neurotransmitter and is over 30 times as potent as glutamic acid and 3 times more potent than kainic acid [104]. The neurologic effects of domoic acid are thought to be secondary to these powerful excitotoxic actions. Symptoms vary somewhat from individual to individual but may include headache, memory loss, confusion, and altered states of consciousness. Limbic seizures, myoclonus, and coma also occur. Diarrhea, vomiting, and GI cramping are variable in severity. Recovery from the CNS effects of domoic acid is gradual and most often complete over 2 to 3 months. Some patients, however, continue to have severe memory problems despite preservation of other areas of cognition and executive functions [104,105]. Development of temporal lobe epilepsy also is a reported sequela of domoic acid toxicity. Cendes et al [106] reported autopsy findings in one such patient that revealed extensive neuronal loss in the hippocampi and patchy neuronal loss in the medial and basal amygdala. It is believed that domoic acid binds to kainic acid receptors in these areas, causing excessive stimulation that results in cell death. This theory is supported by findings in laboratory animals [106].

The patient history should raise the suspicion of domoic acid poisoning but confirmation can be established using a mouse bioassay test. Treatment of domoic acid toxicity is symptomatic. The seizures tend to respond to antiepileptic drug therapy, but it has been suggested that diazepam and phenobarbital are superior to phenytoin in this patient population. This information is based on a limited number of cases [104].

Insect and animal toxins

Snake venoms

Snake venoms vary greatly with respect to their primary sites of action. In general, they contain numerous compounds, many of which are still under investigation. Neurotoxins can be found as components in the venom of several species of snake; however, most of these are neuromuscular blocking agents and do not directly cause encephalopathy. Coral snake venom is an exception and causes euphoria, drowsiness, tremors, and cranial nerve deficits such as slurred speech, dysphagia, and diplopia [107].

Spider venoms

Similarly, spider venoms are complex and may contain multiple systemic toxins in addition to neurotoxic agents. Despite the fact that various spider venoms have the ability to affect the CNS by altering neurotransmitter release or blocking certain channels, encephalopathy rarely occurs in adults. In severe cases, encephalopathy may occur acutely in children; however, it is difficult to determine to what extent that encephalopathy is caused by direct neurotoxicity and how much is secondary to systemic effects [108].

Scorpions

The venoms of most scorpions such as the common American scorpion *Vejovis spinigerus* do not exert significant neurotoxic effects on humans. The sting of some members of the *Centruroides* genus are an exception. The *Centruroides sculpturatus* and *C exilicauda*, found in the western United States, have been reported to produce neurologic symptoms in children. The neurologic symptoms are limited to peripheral and cranial nerves with motor restlessness, random movements of the head and neck, roving eye movements, tongue fasciculations, and dysphagia. Stings of the *C sculpturatus* have also been reported to cause nystagmus and oculogyrus [107,108]. These children may appear to be encephalopathic due to the apparent agitation and abnormal movements combined with immature psychologic and communication skills; however, no true changes in cognition, memory, or higher brain functions have been reliably documented in these patients.

References

[1] Feldman RG. Approach to diagnosis. Occupational and environmental neurotoxicology. Philadelphia: Lippincott-Raven; 1999.
[2] Anthony DC, Montine TJ, Valentine WM, et al. Toxic responses of the nervous system. In: Klaassen CD, editor. Casarett and Doull's toxicology: the basic science of poisons. 6th edition. New York: McGraw-Hill; 2001. p. 535–63.
[3] Second national report on exposure to environmental chemicals. Lead. Centers for Disease Control and Prevention; 2003 Available at: [http://www.cdc.govexposurereport/metals/pdf/lead.pdf]. Accessed October 9, 2004.
[4] Pinkle JL, Brody DJ, Ganter EW, et al. The decline in blood lead levels in the United States. JAMA 1994;272:284–91.
[5] Landrigan PJ, Baker EL, Feldman RG, et al. Increased lead absorption with anemia and slowed nerve conduction in children near a lead smelter. J Pediatr 1976;89:904–10.
[6] Kentner M, Fischer T, Richter G. Changes in external and internal lead load in different working areas of a starter battery production plant in the period 1982–1991. Int Arch Occup Environ Health 1994;66:23–31.
[7] Kosnett MJ. Heavy metal intoxication and chelators. In: Katzung BG, editor. Basic and clinical pharmacology. 9th edition. New York: McGraw-Hill; 1998. p. 970–81.
[8] Goyer RA. Results of lead research: prenatal exposure and neurological consequences. Environ Health Perspect 1996;104:1050–4.
[9] Goyer RA, Clarkson TW. Toxic effects of metals. In: Klaassen CD, editor. Casarett and Doull's toxicology: the basic science of poisons. 6th edition. New York: McGraw-Hill; 2001. p. 811–67.
[10] Eyl TB. Organic-mercury food poisoning. N Engl J Med 1971;284:706–9.
[11] Rowland LP. Occupational and environmental neurotoxicology. In: Rowland LP, editor. Merritt's neurology. 10th edition. Philadelphia: Lippincott, Williams and Wilkins; 2000. p. 940–8.

[12] Albers JW, Kallenbach LR, Fine LJ, et al. Neurologic abnormalities and remote occupational elemental mercury exposure. Ann Neurol 1988;24:651–9.

[13] Hunter D, Bomford RR, Russell DS. Poisoning by methyl mercury compounds. Q J Med 1940;9:193–7.

[14] Gutknecht J. Inorganic mercury (Hg2+) transport through lipid bilayer membranes. J Membr Biol 1981;61:61–6.

[15] Takeuchi T. Neuropathology of Minamata disease in Kumamoto: especially at the chronic stage. In: Roisin L, Shiaki H, Greeric N, editors. Neurotoxicology. New York: Raven Press; 1977. p. 235–46.

[16] Eto K. Pathology of Minamata disease. Toxicol Pathol 1997;25:614–23.

[17] Ratnaike RN. Acute and chronic arsenic toxicity. Postgrad Med J 2003;79:391–6.

[18] Chowdhury UK, Biswas BK, Chowdhury TR, et al. Groundwater arsenic contamination in Bangladesh and West Bengal, India. Envirom Health Perspect 2000;108:393–7.

[19] Abernathy CO, Lin YP, Longfellow D, et al. Arsenic: health effects, mechanisms of actions, and research issues. Environ Health Perspect 1999;107:593–7.

[20] White RF, Proctor SP. Clinico-neuropsychological assessment methods in behavioral toxicology. In: Chang LW, Slikker W, editors. Neurotoxicology: approaches and methods. New York: Academic Press; 1995. p. 711–26.

[21] Bolla-Wilson K, Bleeker ML. Neuropsychological impairment following inorganic arsenic exposure. J Occup Med 1987;29:500–3.

[22] Morton WE, Caron GA. Encephalopathy: an uncommon manifestation of workplace arsenic poisoning? Am J Ind Med 1989;15:1–5.

[23] Hotta N. Clinical aspects of chronic arsenic poisonings due to environmental and occupational pollution in and around a small refining spot. Jpn J Const Med 1989;53: 49–69.

[24] Sasser SM. Rodenticides. In: Viccellio P, editor. Emergency toxicology. 2nd edition. Philadelphia: Lippincott-Raven; 1998. p. 425–36.

[25] Prohaska JR. Functions of trace elements in brain metabolism. Physiol Rev 1987;67: 858–910.

[26] Mergler D. Manganese: the controversial metal. At what levels can deleterious effects occur? Can J Neurol Sci 1996;23:93–4.

[27] Mena I, Marin O, Fuenzalida S, et al. Chronic manganese poisoning: clinical picture and manganese turnover. Neurology 1967;17:128–36.

[28] Bencko V, Cikrt M. Manganese: a review of occupational and environmental toxicology. J Hyg Epidemiol Microbiol Immunol 1984;28:139–48.

[29] Huang C, Chu N, Lu C, et al. Chronic manganese intoxication. Arch Neurol 1989;46: 1104–6.

[30] Zhang G, Liu D, He P. Effects of manganese on learning abilities in school children. Chin J Prevent Med 1995;29:156–8.

[31] Bronstein AC, Kadushin FS, Riddle MW, et al. Oral manganese ingestion and atypical organic brain syndrome and autistic behavior. Vet Hum Toxicol 1988;30:346.

[32] Fuller GN, Goodman JC. Central nervous system toxic and metabolic disorders. Practical review of neuropathology. Philadelphia: Lippincott, Williams and Wilkins; 2001.

[33] Murray JC, Tanner CM, Sprague SM. Aluminum neurotoxicity: a reevaluation. Clin Neuropharmacol 1991;14:179–85.

[34] Longstreth WT, Rosenstock L, Heyer NJ. Potroom palsy? Neurologic disorder in three aluminum smelter workers. Arch Intern Med 1985;145:1972–5.

[35] White DM, Longstreth WT, Rosenstock L, et al. Neurologic syndrome in 25 workers from an aluminum smelting plant. Arch Intern Med 1992;152:1443–8.

[36] Alfrey AC, LeGendre GR, Kaehny WD. The dialysis encephalopathy syndrome: possible aluminum intoxication. N Engl J Med 1976;294:184–8.

[37] Thompson C, Dent J, Saxby P. Effects of thallium poisoning on intellectual function. Br J Psychol 1988;153:396–9.

[38] McMillan TM, Jacobson RR, Gross M. Neuropsychology of thallium poisoning. J Neurol Neurosurg Psychiatr 1997;63:247–50.

[39] Insley BM, Grufferman S, Ayliffe A. Thallium poisoning in cocaine abusers. Am J Emerg Med 1986;4:545–8.

[40] Thompson DF. Management of thallium poisoning. Clin Toxicol 1981;18:979–90.

[41] Aldridge WN, Brown AW, Brierley JB, et al. Brain damage due to trimethyltin compounds. Lancet 1981;2:692–3.

[42] Fait A, Ferioli A, Barbieri F. Organotin compounds. Toxicology 1994;91:77–82.

[43] Feldman RG, White RF, Eriator II. Trimethyltin encephalopathy. Arch Neurol 1993;50: 1320–4.

[44] Besser R, Kramer G, Thumler R, et al. Acute trimethyltin limbic-cerebellar syndrome. Neurology 1987;37:945–50.

[45] Cherry N, Hutchins H, Pace T, et al. Neurobehavioral effects of repeated occupational exposure to toluene and paint solvents. Br J Ind Med 1985;42:291–300.

[46] Arlien-Soborg P, Bruhn P, Gyldensted P, et al. Chronic painters' syndrome: chronic toxic encephalopathy in house painters. Acta Neurol Scand 1979;60:149–56.

[47] Schaumberg HH, Spencer PS. Organic solvent mixtures. In: Spencer PS, Schaumberg HH, editors. Experimental and clinical neurotoxicology. 2nd edition. New York: Oxford University Press; 2000. p. 894–7.

[48] Brackner JV, Warren DA. Toxic effects of solvents and vapors. In: Klaassen CD, editor. Casarett and Doull's toxicology: the basic science of poisons. New York: McGraw-Hill; 2001. p. 869–916.

[49] Hormes J, Filey C, Rosenberg N. Neurologic sequelae of chronic solvent vapor abuse. Neurology 1986;36:689–702.

[50] Lee BK, Lee SH, Lee KM, et al. Dose dependent increase in subjective symptom prevalence among toluene-exposed workers. Ind Health 1988;26:11–23.

[51] Lazer RB, Ho SU, Melen O, et al. Multifocal central nervous system damage caused by toluene abuse. Neurology 1983;33:1337–40.

[52] Fan AM. Trichlorethylene: water contamination and health risk assessment. Rev Environ Contam Toxicol 1988;101:55–92.

[53] Entz RC, Diachenko GW. Residies of volatile halocarbons in margarines. Food Addit Contam 1988;5:267–76.

[54] Burmaster DE. The new pollution—groundwater contamination. Environment 1982;24: 7–36.

[55] Perbellini L, Olivato D, Zedde A, et al. Acute trichlorethylene poisoning by ingestion: clinical and pharmacokinetic aspects. Int Care Med 1991;17:234–5.

[56] Feldman RG, White RF, Currie JN, et al. Long term follow up after single toxic exposure to trichlorethylene. Am J Ind Med 1985;8:119–26.

[57] Lawrence WH, Partyka EK. Chronic dysphagia and trigeminal anesthesia after trichlorethylene exposure. Ann Intern Med 1981;95:710.

[58] Leandri M, Schizzi R, Scielzo C, et al. Electrophysiological evidence of trigeminal root damage after trichlorethylene exposure. Muscle Nerve 1995;18:467–8.

[59] Szlatenyi CS, Wang RY. Encephalopathy and cranial nerve palsies caused by intentional trichlorethylene inhalation. Am J Emerg Med 1996;14:464–7.

[60] Bernad PG, Newell S, Spyker DA. Neurotoxicity and behavior abnormalities in a cohort chronically exposed to trichlorethylene. Vet Hum Toxicol 1987;29:475.

[61] Burg JR, Gist GL, Alldred SL, et al. The national exposure registry—morbidity analysis of noncancer outcomes from trichlorethylene subregistry baseline data. Int J Occup Med Toxicol 1995;4:237–57.

[62] American Conference of Governmental Industrial Hygienists (ACGIH). Threshold limit values (TLVs) for chemical substances and physical agents and biological exposure indices (BEIs). Cincinnati (OH): ACGIH; 1995.

[63] Garnier R, Bedouin J, Pepin G, et al. Coin-operated dry cleaning machines may be responsible for acute tetrachlorethylene poisoning: reports of 26 cases including one death. Clin Toxicol 1996;34:191–7.

[64] Freed DM, Kandel E. Long-term occupational exposure and the diagnosis of dementia. Neurotoxicology 1988;9:391–400.

[65] White RF. Differential diagnosis of probable Alzheimer's disease and solvent encephalopathy in older workers. Clin Neuropsychol 1987;1:153–60.

[66] Aminoff MS. Effects of occupational toxins on the nervous system. In: Bradley WG, Daroff RB, Fenichel GM, et al, editors. Neurology in clinical practice. 3rd edition. Boston: Butterworth-Heinemann; 2000. p. 1511–9.

[67] Huang CC, Chu CC, Chen RS, et al. Chronic carbon disulfide encephalopathy. Env Neurol 1996;36:364–8.

[68] Cassitto MG, Camerino D, Imbriani M, et al. Carbon disulfide and the central nervous system: a 15-year neurobehavioral surveillance of an exposed population. Environ Res 1993;63:252–63.

[69] Chang YC. Neurotoxic effects of n-hexane on the human central nervous system: evoked potential abnormalities in n-hexane polyneuropathy. J Neurol Neurosurg Psychiatry 1987; 50:269–74.

[70] Bakinson MA, Jones RD. Gassings due to methylene chloride, xylene, toluene, and styrene reported to Her Majesty's Factory Inspectorate 1961–1980. Br J Ind Med 1985;42: 181–90.

[71] Klaucke DN, Johansen M, Vogt RL. An outbreak of xylene intoxication in a hospital. Am J Ind Med 1982;3:173–8.

[72] Ruijten MWMM, Hooisma J, Brons JT, et al. Neurobehavioral effects of long-term exposure to xylene and mixed organic solvents in shipyard painters. Neurotoxicology 1994; 15:613–20.

[73] Uchida Y, Nakatsuka H, Ukai H, et al. Symptoms and signs in workers exposed predominantly to xylenes. Int Arch Occup Environ Health 1993;64:597–605.

[74] Bond J. Review of the toxicology of styrene. Crit Rev Toxicol 1989;19:227–49.

[75] Edling C, Anundi H, Johansson G, Nilsson K. Increase in neuropsychiatric symptoms after occupational exposure to low levels of styrene. Br J Ind Med 1993;50:843–50.

[76] Crandall MS, Hartle RW. An analysis of exposure to styrene in the reinforced plastic boat-making industry. Am J Ind Med 1985;8:183–92.

[77] Nestler EJ, Self DW. Neuropsychiatric aspects of ethanol and other chemical dependencies. In: Yudofsky SC, Hales RE, editors. The American Psychiatric Publishing textbook of neuropsychiatry and clinical neurosciences. 4th edition. Washington, DC: American Psychiatric Publishing; 2002. p. 899–921.

[78] Kumari M, Ticku MK. Regulation of NMDA receptors by ethanol. Prog Drug Res 2000; 54:152–89.

[79] Brust JCM. Persistent cognitive impairment in substance abuse. Continuum: neurologic complications of substance abuse. 2004;5(10):144–50.

[80] Brust JCM. Alcoholism. In: Rowland LP, editor. Merritt's neurology. 10th edition. Philadelphia: Lippincott, Williams and Wilkins; 2000. p. 921–9.

[81] Ernst A, Zibrak JD. Carbon monoxide poisoning. N Engl J Med 1998;339:1603–8.

[82] Thom SR. Carbon monoxide-mediated brain lipid peroxidation in the rat. J Appl Phys 1990;68:997–1003.

[83] Thom SR. Leukocytes in carbon monoxide-mediated brain oxidative injury. Toxicol Appl Pharmacol 1993;123:234–47.

[84] Choi IS. Delayed neurologic sequelae in carbon monoxide intoxication. Arch Neurol 1983; 40:433–5.

[85] Min SK. A brain syndrome associated with delayed neuropsychiatric sequelae following acute carbon monoxide intoxication. Acta Psychiatr Scand 1986;73:80–6.

[86] Messiers LD, Myers RAM. A neuropsychological screening battery for emergent assessment of carbon-monoxide poisoned patients. J Clin Psychol 1991;47:675–84.

[87] Finkelstein Y, Wolff M, Biegon A. Brain acetylcholinesterase after acute parathion poisoning: a comparative quantitative histochemical analysis post mortem. Ann Neurol 1988;24:252–7.

[88] Steenland K, Jenkins B, Ames RG, et al. Chronic neurologic sequelae to organophosphate pesticide poisoning. Am J Pub Health 1994;84(5):731–6.

[89] Rosenstock L, Keifer M, Daniell W, et al. Chronic central nervous system effects of acute organophosphate pesticide intoxication. Lancet 1991;338:223–7.

[90] Ames RG, Steenland K, Jenkins B, et al. Chronic neurologic sequelae to cholinesterase inhibition among agricultural pesticide applicators. Arch Environ Health 1995;50:440–4.

[91] Fiedler N, Kipen H, Kelly-McNeil K, et al. Long-term use of organophosphates and neuropsychological performance. Am J Ind Med 1997;32:487–96.

[92] Gershon S, Shaw FH. Psychiatric sequelae of chronic exposure to organophosphorus insecticides. Lancet 1961;1:1371–4.

[93] Namba T, Nolte CT, Jackrel J, et al. Poisoning due to organophosphate insecticides: acute and chronic manifestations. Am J Med 1971;50:475–92.

[94] Thiermann H, Mast U, Kimmeck R, et al. Cholinesterase status, pharmacokinetics and laboratory findings during obidoxime therapy in organophosphate poisoned patients. Hum Exp Toxicol 1997;16:473–80.

[95] Taylor P. Anticholinesterase agents. In: Goodman Gilman A, Rall TW, Nies AS, et al, editors. Goodman and Gilman's the pharmacological basis of therapeutics. 8th edition. Elmsford (NY): Pergamon Press; 1990. p. 131–49.

[96] Lifshitz M, Shahak E, Bolotin A, et al. Carbamate poisoning in early childhood and in adults. Clin Toxicol 1997;53(1):25–7.

[97] O'Malley M. Clinical evaluation of pesticide exposure and poisonings. Lancet 1997;349: 1161–6.

[98] Grendon J, Frost F, Baum L. Chronic health effects among sheep and humans surviving an aldicarb poisoning incident. Vet Hum Toxicol 1994;36:218–23.

[99] Branch RA, Jacqz E. Subacute neurotoxicity following long-term exposure to carbaryl. Am J Med 1986;80:741–5.

[100] Doctor SV. Neuropsychiatric aspects of poisons and toxins. In: Ydofsk SC, Hales RE, editors. The American Psychiatric Publishing textbook of neuropsychiatry and clinical neurosciences. 4th edition. Washington, DC: American Psychiatric Publishing; 2002. p. 891–8.

[101] Farnsworth NR. Hallucinogenic plants. Science 1986;162:1086–92.

[102] Shih RD. Mushroom poisoning. In: Viccellio P, editor. Emergency toxicology. 2nd edition. Philadelphia: Lippincott-Raven; 1998. p. 1081–6.

[103] Norton S. Toxic effects of plants. In: Klaassen CD, editor. Casarett and Doull's toxicology: the basic science of poisons. 6th edition. New York: McGraw-Hill; 2001. p. 965–76.

[104] So YT. Effects of toxins and physical agents on the nervous system: marine toxins. In: Bradley WG, Daroff RB, Finichel GM, et al, editors. Neurology in clinical practice. 3rd edition. Boston: Butterworth-Heinemann; 2000. p. 1535–9.

[105] Teitelbaum JS, Zatorre RJ, Carpenter S, et al. Neurological sequela of domoic acid intoxication due to the ingestion of contaminated mussels. N Engl J Med 1990;322:1781–7.

[106] Cendes F, Andermann F, Carpenter S, et al. Temporal lobe epilepsy caused by domoic acid intoxication: evidence for glutamate receptor-mediated excitotoxicity in humans. Ann Neurol 1995;37:123–6.

[107] Garcia-Prats VM. Reptilian envenomation. In: Viccellio P, editor. Emergency toxicology. 2nd edition. Philadelphia: Lippincott-Raven; 1998. p. 1035–48.

[108] Findlay ER. Toxic effects of terrestrial animal venoms and poisons. In: Klaassen CD, editor. Casarett and Doull's toxicology: the basic science of poisons. 6th edition. New York: McGraw-Hill; 2001. p. 945–64.

Toxic Neuropathies

Patrick M. Grogan, MD[a],*, Jonathan S. Katz, MD[b,c]

[a]Department of Neurology, Wilford Hall Medical Center, San Antonio, TX, USA
[b]Stanford University Medical Center, Palo Alto, CA, USA
[c]Department of Neurology, Palo Alto Veterans Affairs Health Care System,
Palo Alto, CA, USA

Peripheral nerve dysfunction can result from exposure to a wide variety of organic and nonorganic compounds. The incidence of toxic occupational exposures has been declining steadily, owing to a better understanding of various chemicals and their adverse effects on the body, a general appreciation of risk in society, and improvement of occupational health safety laws. Other toxic exposures associated with the development of a polyneuropathy include ingestion of certain toxic plants and animals, uncommon encounters between man and nature, recreational substance abuse, and medications prescribed by health care professionals. This article synthesizes the available published information on various toxins and their effects on the peripheral nerve in an effort to keep physicians aware of their existence, clinical presentations, diagnosis, and treatments.

Neuropathy secondary to alcohol and drugs of abuse

Alcohol

Chronic alcohol abuse is associated with a distal, symmetric, primarily sensory polyneuropathy. These cases typically present with painful dysesthesias and sensory loss affecting the distal lower extremities and, in more severe cases, the hands [1]. Neurologic examination reveals the distal sensory loss with hyporeflexia. There may be weakness in more advanced cases. Autonomic involvement usually accompanies the sensory features, resulting in distal skin atrophy, discoloration, and hair loss. Gait ataxia, or other features of cerebellar involvement, is present if there is concomitant

* Corresponding author. Department of Neurology/MMCN, Wilford Hall Medical Center, Lackland AFB, TX 78236.
   E-mail address: patrick.grogan@lackland.af.mil (P.M. Grogan).

0733-8619/05/$ - see front matter © 2005 Elsevier Inc. All rights reserved.
doi:10.1016/j.ncl.2004.12.003
neurologic.theclinics.com

alcoholic cerebellar degeneration. Other complications, including liver disease, poor nutrition, memory impairment, and social disorganization, are common, because peripheral polyneuropathy frequently is only one component of more generalized manifestations of alcohol toxicity.

Laboratory studies in the patient who has alcoholic neuropathy may detect a transaminitis with elevated gamma glutamyl transferase levels and elevated mean corpuscular volume. Serologic levels of thiamine and other B vitamins [2] are not reliable indicators of their intake in patients' diets [1]. Electrodiagnostic studies typically reveal an axonal polyneuropathy marked by reduced amplitudes of sensory nerve action potentials (SNAP) to a greater degree than compound motor action potentials. These features may be noted even in the absence of strong clinical evidence for a peripheral neuropathy [1–5]. Some reports identify significant conduction velocity slowing and F-wave prolongation, either with [2,5,6] or without [7] amplitude reduction, suggesting a wide spectrum of electrodiagnostic characteristics. Pathologic studies, however, consistently report axonal degeneration as the primary abnormality in alcoholic neuropathy [1,2,4,5].

Some controversy exists as to whether or not the neuropathy observed in alcoholic patients is a direct toxic effect of alcohol or a secondary phenomenon related to nutritional deficiencies. Several observations point to nutritional deficiency, specifically in thiamine and the B vitamins. First, alcoholic neuropathy clinically is similar to the neuropathy observed in patients who have thiamine deficiency [8], and progression of the neuropathy stabilizes and may even improve with thiamine and other vitamin replacement [9]. Thiamine deficiency in the absence of alcohol use also has been shown experimentally to induce axonal damage in animals [5,10], whereas alcohol use in nutritionally well-fed animals does not [1]. Finally, reduced blood levels of thiamine and other measurable B vitamins are reported in patients who have alcoholic neuropathy [11].

In contrast, the major argument for a direct toxic effect of alcohol on peripheral nerve comes from a study by Behse and Buchthal, in which patients who had alcohol-related neuropathy were compared with patients who had postgastrectomy and who developed neuropathy but had no history of alcoholism [2]. The neuropathies in these groups clinically were similar, but more than 60% of the alcoholic patients had no identifiable nutritional deficiency, and the postgastrectomy patients displayed prominent conduction velocity slowing, suggesting a different type of neuropathy than in the alcoholic group [2]. This study has been challenged, however, because nutritional deficiency was based on subjective weight loss and normal serologic levels of thiamine, which are unreliable indicators of proper nutrition levels [1]. Moreover, the electrodiagnostic studies on postgastrectomy patients were based on only 6 patients, whereas varying degrees of conduction slowing can be present in alcoholic patients [2,6,7].

The treatment of alcoholic neuropathy involves discontinuing alcohol consumption and resuming proper nutritional intake. Thiamine and

B-vitamin supplementation may have some beneficial effect [9]. Patients may hope for stabilization of the symptoms, because clearly, substantial improvement in these patients is uncommon and may relate to the typically chronic duration of the neuropathy and the irreversibility of ongoing axonal damage at the time of diagnosis. Studies looking at recovery patterns are limited.

Inhalants/nitrous oxide

Several neurologic disorders are caused by vitamin B_{12} or cobalamin deficiency, including subacute combined degeneration of the spinal cord, encephalopathy, and a predominantly large fiber, sensory polyneuropathy. Identical disorders are reported in patients exposed to nitrous oxide through general anesthesia or in inhalational abusers of nitrous oxide because of its disruptive effects on vitamin B_{12}–dependent biochemical pathways. Nitrous oxide oxidizes cobalamin, thereby disrupting the cobalamin-dependent methionine synthase reaction necessary to create methionine, which is a substrate for myelin production.

Neuropathic symptoms include progressive distal sensory loss with paresthesias and pain, often beginning in the hands. There is predominant vibratory and proprioceptive sensory loss on examination secondary to the involvement of large-fiber sensory nerves and the dorsal columns of the spinal cord. A reverse Lhermitte's sign, or a sharp electric sensation ascending from the toes with neck flexion, also may be seen [12]. Extremity weakness with spasticity and hyperreflexia indicates the additional presence of a myelopathy. Electrophysiologic studies demonstrate varying results, with generalized conduction slowing of motor and sensory fibers and preserved amplitudes seen in some cases [13] and a predominantly axonal polyneuropathy in others [14,15]. Replacement of vitamin B_{12} intramuscularly may be associated with improvement in the peripheral neuropathy [14,16], although this is not a universal feature [17].

Drugs of abuse: opiates, sedatives, and amphetamines

Various peripheral nerve disorders are reported in association with abuse and overdose of opiates, sedatives, and amphetamines, including mononeuropathies, brachial plexopathies, and Guillain-Barré syndrome (GBS) [18–22]. In one study of 198 heroin users, 49% were reported to have developed a peripheral neuropathy [21]. The diagnosis was based on a patient questionnaire, and the symptoms reported were consistent with transient mononeuropathies, which most likely developed secondary to prolonged limb compression that occurred during deep periods of unconsciousness. Such neuropathies likely are the most common peripheral nerve disorders encountered in patients abusing these drugs. Excluding compressive neuropathies, data in this area comes primarily from case studies or series and definitive evidence of causation between drug use and any specific peripheral nerve disorder generally is lacking.

Neuropathy secondary to drugs/iatrogenic neuropathy

Several medications may cause a peripheral neuropathy, the majority of which are consistent with a length-dependent, predominantly sensory axonopathy. A detailed review of each of these medications is not provided in this article, because several publications on this subject are available [15,23]. Table 1 provides a quick reference to those medications, with strong evidence substantiating an association with neuropathy development and a brief description of their clinical, electrophysiologic, and histopathologic characteristics.

Neuropathy secondary to heavy metals/organic chemicals

Arsenic

Exposure to potentially toxic levels of arsenic can occur from drinking contaminated groundwater, working in mining and ore-smelting plants, accidental ingestion of pesticides, and, most infamously, intentional suicidal or homicidal ingestions. The neuropathy is a painful, length-dependent, sensory (more than motor), peripheral axonopathy affecting all extremities [24]. Initial symptoms begin 2 to 3 weeks after initial exposure and start with pain in the distal lower extremities, which progresses to sensory loss and weakness and, eventually, involvement of the distal upper extremities [25,26]. Examination reveals distal sensory loss, hypo- or areflexia, and normal to mildly weak distal musculature. Systemic abnormalities that may serve as important clues to the diagnosis include weight loss, severe alopecia, and white horizontal striations on the nails (Mees' lines). Reports of the electrodiagnostic abnormalities vary and range from mild motor conduction slowing [27] to an axonal neuropathy marked by low amplitude sensory and motor action potentials with relatively preserved conduction velocities [26]. Higher levels of arsenic exposure are associated with a more severe, rapidly progressing polyneuropathy with electrodiagnostic demyelination, which can appear clinically and electrodiagnostically similar to GBS [28]. In its most extreme form, arsenic toxicity can progress to quadriparesis and ventilator dependence [29].

Diagnosis can be confirmed by detecting elevated arsenic levels in blood, urine, hair, or nail clippings. Elimination of continued arsenic exposure and use of sulfur chelators, including dimercaptosuccinic acid or penicillamine, are standard treatments [26]. Resolution of neuropathic complaints is dependent on the length and severity of arsenic exposure before initiation of therapy.

Lead

Lead toxicity may occur from occupational (metal soldering, ore smelting, battery manufacturing, or industrial painting) or nonoccupational (accidental ingestion of leaded paint by children or exposure to leaded water and food containers) exposures. Fortunately, the occurrence of lead toxicity has been reduced greatly as a result of improved public health. Peripheral neuropathy is one of the most common of the many different effects that lead toxicity may have on the nervous system. Reports describe a pure motor neuropathy affecting the upper more than the lower extremities, presenting as a symmetric or asymmetric wrist drop [30]. The weakness also may involve other muscle groups of the distal upper extremities. Lower extremity involvement, including isolated foot drop, also may occur. A length-dependent, painful, predominantly sensory polyneuropathy also is reported from lead exposure [31,32], although the clinical and electrophysiologic findings [31] from these reports leave open some questions as to the existence of this presentation. When sensory loss is noted by the patient or detected on clinical examination, it usually is minor in comparison to the motor abnormalities [30]. Abdominal pain, constipation, and a microcytic, hypochromic anemia are characteristically present in lead poisoning and serve as critical clues to the diagnosis. In fact, the absence of these systemic features should raise doubts regarding the diagnosis [30].

Electrodiagnostic studies in lead-induced neuropathy show abnormalities of nerve conduction begin to occur with lead levels in blood above 70 μg/100 ml [30]. These studies reveal a wide range of electrophysiologic abnormalities, from mild motor conduction slowing to axonal features with frank electromyographic (EMG) denervation. Peripheral nerve pathology studies in lead intoxication show increased paranodal demyelination and internodal remyelination with low-level lead exposure, whereas advanced neuropathies demonstrate axonal degeneration [30]. Detecting elevated blood lead levels above 70 μg/100 ml, an established level below which peripheral neuropathy is unlikely to occur [33], may further assist in the diagnosis.

Treatment of lead-induced neuropathy requires eliminating continued exposure and initiating therapy to enhance excretion with various chelating agents, such as EDTA, penicillamine, and British anti-lewisite. These agents are able to lower blood levels, but there is no conclusive evidence that this approach assists in the resolution of neuropathic symptoms [26,30].

Thallium

Thallium toxicity has become rare since thallium was banned from use in pesticides in the 1970s. Currently, this neuropathy is seen only in unintentional ingestions, usually linked to attempted homicides. Neuropathic and systemic symptoms are similar to arsenic exposure, with a painful,

Table 1
Medications causing peripheral neuropathy

Drug name	Neuropathy phenotype			Electrophysiology	Pathology	Additional characteristics
	Motor	Sensory	Pain			
Almitrine	–	+	+	Distal axonopathy	Axonal degeneration	Marked weight loss occasionally
Amiodarone[a]	+	+	+/–	Distal axonopathy + slowed conduction velocity	Axonal degeneration/ segmental demyelination	Optic neuropathy
Cisplatin	–	+	+/–	Distal axonopathy	Axonal degeneration	Ototoxicity
Dapsone	+	+	+/–	Distal axonopathy	Axonal degeneration	Pure motor variant reported
Dideoxynucleosides[a]	–	+	+	Distal axonopathy + slowed conduction velocity	Axonal degeneration/ myelin splitting	—
Disulfiram	–	+	+/–	Distal axonopathy	Axonal degeneration	Optic neuropathy
Etoposide	–	+	+/–	Distal axonopathy	—	—
Isoniazid	+	+	+/–	—	Axonal degeneration	Responds to pyridoxine replacement
Metronidazole	–	+	+/–	Distal axonopathy	Axonal degeneration	—

Misomidazole	−	+	+	Distal axonopathy	Axonal degeneration	—
Perhexiline	+	+	+	Slowed conduction velocity	Axonal degeneration/segmental demyelination	—
Phenytoin	−	+	+/−	—	Axonal degeneration	—
Pyridoxine	−	+	+	Distal axonopathy	Axonal degeneration	—
Suramin	+	+	+/−	Distal axonopathy + slowed conduction velocity	Axonal degeneration	Electrophysiologic conduction block
Taxol	+	+	+	Distal axonopathy	Axonal degeneration	—
Thalidomide[a]	−	+	+	Distal axonopathy	Axonal degeneration	Dorsal root ganglion degeneration
Vinca alkaloids[a]	+	+	+/−	Distal axonopathy	Axonal degeneration	Early autonomic features common

[a] Indicates neuropathy is commonly associated with the medication.

progressive, length-dependent, sensory (more than motor) axonopathy that develops within 1 to 2 weeks after exposure [26]. The pain and dysesthetic sensations in the limbs are severe and excruciating [25], typically beyond that seen in common sensory neuropathies from other causes. Examination findings include distal sensory loss, distal weakness, and hyporeflexia. Alopecia occurs similarly to arsenic toxicity. There also is a dark discoloration of the hair root under light microscopy, owing to gaseous inclusions induced by thallium, which cause light to diffract [34]. Electrodiagostic and nerve biopsy findings are consistent with axonal degeneration [26]. Diagnosis is made by thallium analysis in blood, urine, or hair samples. There is no specific therapy for the neuropathy, but gastric lavage, activated charcoal, hemodialysis, and Prussian blue all assist in blocking further absorption and accelerating removal of the toxin [26].

Acrylamide

Chronic inhalation or skin exposure to acrylamide monomers, used in the creation of grouting agents, adhesives, and flocculators, may induce a length-dependent, sensorimotor, peripheral axonopathy [26,35]. Exposure generally has been limited to specific occupations, although recently, interest in acrylamide exposure has resurfaced with the discovery that it can be formed unintentionally by cooking certain foods at high temperatures (particularly French fries) [36]. It is doubtful that consumption of such foods exposes an individual to neurotoxic doses.

Distal sensory loss with ataxia, weakness, and hyporeflexia, initially starting in the lower extremities and gradually spreading to the arms, is characteristic of this neuropathy [35]. Autonomic dysfunction with distal hyperhydrosis and cold skin temperature frequently also are noted. Central nervous system effects, in particular cerebellar dysfunction, may accompany the neuropathy, accentuating the sensory ataxia. Electrophysiologic studies reveal diffuse amplitude reduction of SNAP and minimal slowing of sensory and motor conduction velocities [35]. Peripheral nerve histopathology demonstrates distal axonal degeneration with large myelinated axons affected most severely [26]. Direct measurements of serum acrylamide levels are not available commonly.

Interest in acrylamide neuropathy also has surged because acrylamide neurotoxicity can be induced experimentally in rats. Experimental acrylamide neuropathy serves as a model of diffuse axonal polyneuropathy [37], and its histochemical similarities to streptozotocin-induced diabetic neuropathy in rats suggest new theories regarding a possible common mechanism [38]. Several treatments, including the immunosuppressant FK-506 and the neurotrophic factor NT-3, demonstrate promising results in prevention of neuropathy progression in these experimental models [36,37].

Carbon disulfide

Chronic, low-level, inhalational exposure to carbon disulfide, currently used in rayon and cellophane production, is linked to the development of a distal sensorimotor axonopathy [35]. Fortunately, improvements in occupational health safety have reduced carbon disulfide levels in certain workplaces from 100 to 200 ppm to 10 to 20 ppm [39]. Even with these reductions, concern remains that sensorimotor complaints can result directly from this toxin [35]. Typical features of a distal neuropathy, including sensory loss, weakness, and hyporeflexia, are noted on examination. Electrophysiologic studies demonstrate conduction velocity slowing in motor and sensory nerves [39] and fibrillations on EMG of lower extremity muscles [35]. Nerve histopathology demonstrates predominantly large-fiber axonal and myelin degeneration [40]. Despite removal from exposure, sensory and motor complaints and electrophysiologic changes may persist for years [39] and there are no reported treatments.

Dioxin/Agent Orange

Agent Orange is the code name given to a particular herbicide used extensively during the Vietnam War from 1962 to 1971 [41]. The herbicide contained an equal mixture of two phenoxy acids, one of which had an obligatory byproduct during its production, 2,3,7,8–tetrachlorodibenzo-p-dioxin, otherwise known as TCDD or dioxin. A variety of health issues in Vietnam War veterans became attributed, albeit with some controversy, to dioxin, including various cancers, birth defects in children fathered by veterans, cognitive and neuropsychiatric problems, and peripheral neuropathy.

Whether or not Agent Orange causes a neuropathy remains controversial. Neuropathic symptoms theoretically attributed to dioxin exposure typically are a distal sensory polyneuropathy affecting the lower extremities, with abnormal sensory findings and hyporeflexia on examination [42]. Most studies note that only individuals who have higher exposures, characterized as those who have dermatologic changes (chloracne) from direct contact with dioxin, have any significant increase in risk for developing a polyneuropathy [42,43]. Experimentally, electrodiagnostic and histologic evidence of a toxic polyneuropathy is observed in rats after an intraperitoneal injection of dioxin [44,45], but it is unclear how this correlates with dioxin exposures reported in the Vietnam War or in particular occupations.

The National Academy of Sciences Institute of Medicine report on Agent Orange exposure concludes there is inadequate evidence to determine that exposure causes a peripheral neuropathy, based on available Vietnam veteran studies [41]. These include studies of veterans involved in Operation Ranch Hand who were responsible in varying capacities for aerial spraying of Agent Orange and likely had the highest levels of exposure. Subsequent to the Institute of Medicine report, two other reports on the association between dioxin and neuropathy in Vietnam veterans were published. The first concluded an increased odds ratio (2.5–5.8) of a 'diagnosed' peripheral neuropathy in Operation Ranch Hand veterans who had high serum dioxin levels [46]. This study is severely limited, because no electrodiagnostic testing was used, minimal objective evidence for a peripheral neuropathy was used, and a 'diagnosed' neuropathy (their most conclusive definition for the presence of neuropathy) could be based purely on subjective sensory complaints. The second study assessed Korean military members who served in the Vietnam War and concluded that, in general, veterans were 2.39 times more likely to develop a peripheral neuropathy compared with non–Vietnam veterans [47]. It is unclear, however, what type of exposure any of their subjects had to Agent Orange, and there is no documentation of which variables were used to make the diagnosis of a polyneuropathy, although it seems that nerve conduction studies were used. Even taking these studies into account, there continues to be insufficient evidence to associate a peripheral polyneuropathy with prior exposure to Agent Orange.

Ethylene oxide

Ethylene oxide is a gas used for sterilization of medical equipment and is implicated as a cause of an axonal polyneuropathy in medical personnel and hospital sterilization workers [35]. It also is implicated as a potential cause for the neuropathy observed in patients who are on chronic dialysis [48]. The neuropathy reported predominantly is sensory, with or without objective sensory loss and hyporeflexia on examination. Mild motor and sensory conduction slowing is observed on electrophysiologic testing in some studies, although others find few abnormalities suggesting a peripheral neuropathy [49]. Nerve biopsy findings range from relatively normal [49] to evidence of axonal degeneration [35].

Hexane/hexacarbons

Awareness of hexacarbon neuropathy related to n-hexane exposure developed in the 1960s, when it was first reported [50]. N-hexane is a component of petroleum products, solvents, and glues and is associated with occupation-related neuropathies in automobile mechanics [50], shoe-makers [35,51], purse makers [52], and furniture finishers [35]. Recreational inhalant abuse also is associated with hexacarbon neuropathy [53].

The typical phenotype is a distal, ascending, sensorimotor polyneurop-athy with sensory loss, distal weakness and atrophy, and hyporeflexia on examination [35,54]. Weight loss and anorexia can be associated with the polyneuropathy in more severe cases. A subacute, predominantly motor phenotype also is reported [53]. Electrophysiologic testing may show decreased sensory amplitudes as the primary abnormality [55], but several recent reports document multifocal motor conduction block with prominent conduction slowing in exposed patients [51–53,56]. The latter electrodiagnostic features appear more commonly in those patients reported as having a predominantly motor phenotype. Nerve biopsy features include axonal loss with subperineurial edema, focal enlargement of axons, and paranodal myelin retraction [53,56].

Treatment includes removal from exposure to n-hexane–containing compounds, although the neuropathy may progress for several months [35,53] followed by gradual spontaneous improvement over months to several years [35,50]. Claims of improvement with B-complex vitamin administration and Chinese traditional medicines are reported [54], but there are no formal studies to support this.

Methyl bromide

Peripheral neuropathy is an uncommon side effect of chronic exposure to methyl bromide. Exposure to methyl bromide may occur with use of soil fumigants [57], but it also is used as a refrigerant and a component in fire extinguishers. The development of neuropathic symptoms usually is associated with chronic, low-level exposure, typically resulting from inhalation over several months [58], but a more acute presentation, within 1 week of exposure through abraded skin also is reported [57]. A distal, sensorimotor axonal polyneuropathy occurs that is similar to other toxic neuropathies, clinically and electrophysiologically [35,57]. With more acute exposures, the neuropathy can be accompanied by central nervous system deficits, including pyramidal signs, cerebellovestibular abnormalities, and encephalopathy [26,58]. The sensory loss and weakness gradually resolve after removal of the exposure [35], although minor sensory complaints may persist for several years [58].

Neuropathy secondary to marine toxins

Ciguatera neuropathy

Ciguatera initially was reported in patients who ate snails, but is now recognized that it may be associated with consumption of a variety of tropical fish, including red snapper, grouper, and barracuda [59,60]. The causative agent, ciguatoxin, is produced by the dinoflagellate, *Gambierdiscus toxicus*, found in algae, which is eaten by smaller fish and transmitted up the food chain [61]. Symptoms of nausea and vomiting develop within 3 to 12 hours of ingestion. The peripheral neuropathy usually is the most distressing neurologic symptom [59], although a broad spectrum of complaints, including myalgias, weakness, sensory abnormalities, headaches, tremor, and ataxia, commonly occur.

The neuropathy from ciguatera toxin is marked by the onset of acral and perioral paresthesias, dysesthesias, and pruritis that develop 12 to 48 hours after ingestion of contaminated fish [60–62]. Paradoxical temperature reversal is a common complaint relatively specific to this neuropathy

[61,63]. This reversal is marked by the experience of a warm, burning, and dysesthetic sensation when patients are exposed to cold temperatures on their skin. Less commonly, warm temperatures are perceived as normal or cold. Gross temperature perception using baths of varying water temperature is normal, but temperatures lower than 25°C reliably produce severe burning and parasthesias that do not develop with exposure to warmer temperatures [63]. It is suggested this phenomenon results from the toxin's preferential activity on small, unmyelinated, C-polymodal nociceptor fibers [61,63,64].

Examination findings suggestive of a peripheral neuropathy typically are limited to reduced light touch, pain, and vibration sensation and hyporeflexia [61–63]. Although subjective weakness and myalgias commonly are reported, objective weakness rarely is found. Diagnosis is based on the clinical presentation, and recognizing the temporal relation to fish ingestion. Electrophysiologic studies demonstrate a spectrum of characteristics, ranging from normal findings [61] to motor and sensory conduction slowing with preserved amplitudes [62]. Nerve biopsies show abnormalities of the myelin sheath, with prominent edema of the adaxonal Schwann cell cytoplasm in severe cases [65]. Bioassays are being developed to detect ciguatoxin levels in suspected fish tissues [66].

Treatment of ciguatera typically is supportive, and symptoms usually resolve within days to weeks, although they can last for several months after exposure [60,63]. Recurrent sensory abnormalities may be noted with alcohol ingestion or exercise [60]. Infusions of hyperosmotic mannitol (10 ml/kg of 20% mannitol solution) are reported to reduce the painful dysesthesias if administered within 48 hours of symptom onset, but this is based solely on empiric data from case studies [59]. A study evaluating the effect of mannitol on nerves exposed to ciguatoxin in rats demonstrates no improvement in the electrophysiologic abnormalities induced by the toxin [67].

Tetrodotoxin-related neuropathy

Tetrodotoxin is an exceptionally potent sodium channel blocker found in high concentrations in the skin and viscera of tetraodontiform fish, including puffer (*Fugu poecilonotus*) and porcupine fish (*Diodon hystrix*), and in blue-ringed octopus and certain amphibians [68,69]. The toxin is recognized best in tales of fatal poisonings after ingestion of improperly prepared fugu, an expensive Japanese delicacy of raw puffer fish that should be eaten only when prepared by a specially licensed chef.

Tetrodotoxin poisoning causes a rapidly progressive sensorimotor polyneuropathy that may affect bulbar and respiratory muscles. Acral and perioral paresthesias and sensory loss develop within minutes to hours of ingestion [68,69]. Limb weakness develops soon after and may result in flaccid quadriparesis [69]. Autonomic neuropathy symptoms, including hyperhydrosis, excessive salivation, hypotension, bradycardia, and temperature dysregulation are frequent. Clinical severity depends on the amount of the toxin ingested, and it is recommended that the skin, liver, gonads, and intestines be avoided, as these tissues contain the greatest concentrations of toxin [70].

The underlying pathophysiology of tetrodotoxin poisoning relates to sodium-channel blockade that impairs propagation of the nerve action potential. This conduction abnormality can be detected by electrophysiologic studies that disclose evidence of profound sensorimotor conduction velocity slowing (<30 m/s for upper and <23 m/s for lower extremities) without conduction block or temporal dispersion [69]. Prolonged terminal motor and F-wave latencies typically are the most notable electrodiagnostic features [69]. SNAP amplitudes may be reduced mildly, but motor studies retain normal amplitudes and morphology. These abnormalities resolve gradually as the toxin clears.

Treatment is supportive, and recoveries may be dramatic. The literature contains examples of rapid improvements from a dense quadriparesis with respirator dependency back to normal, provided adequate supportive care is initiated early [68,69].

Paralytic shellfish poisoning

Saxitoxin is a heat-stable, water-soluble compound found in various dinoflagellates that is concentrated in clams, mussels, and other shellfish that ingest the microorganisms. High concentrations of the dinoflagellates in water may discolor it black, pink, or red (ie, red tide), during which times shellfish harvesting must be avoided [70]. Saxitoxin blocks sodium transport by binding to voltage-sensitive sodium channels of susceptible cell membranes [71].

Ingestion of saxitoxin-contaminated shellfish may induce neuropathic complaints, typically including numbness and paresthesias of the distal extremities and the perioral region [72–74]. Symptoms develop within 1 to 2 hours of ingestion and resolve spontaneously without residual abnormalities in 1 to 2 days. Subjective weakness is reported in 30% to 70% of patients [73,74], but reports of objective limb weakness are unusual. The term, paralytic, reflects the respiratory depression that can occur in severe poisonings. This is attributed to blockade of diaphragmatic neurotransmission and is demonstrated experimentally using diaphragmatic EMG in rodents [75]. Electrophysiologic testing shows moderately prolonged F-wave latencies [76], with prolonged motor and sensory latencies and slow conduction velocities in more severe intoxication [77]. The latter are similar to the electrodiagnostic changes seen with tetrodotoxin poisoning, which likely reflect the common effect on sodium channels.

Treatment of paralytic shellfish poisoning is supportive with patients surviving even severe respiratory compromise, provided there is adequate ventilatory support. 4-Aminopyridine shows promising benefits in rapidly reversing the diaphragmatic blockade experimentally, but there are no studies of humans available [75].

Neuropathy secondary to reptile and insect toxins

Snakes

Snake envenomization after bites from cobras, kraits, coral snakes, pit vipers, and other snakes may produce clinical features related to neuromuscular junction (NMJ) dysfunction [78]. Commonly reported examination features include ptosis, bulbar and respiratory, and extremity weakness, all of which develop within 1 to 10 hours of exposure. Normal NMJ physiology may become disrupted at the presynaptic (α-bungarotoxin) or postsynaptic (β-bungarotoxin) nerve terminals [78]. Respiratory failure is the most serious and life-threatening consequence of snake envonimation, and aggressive respiratory support may be required. Isolated cases of distal sensory [79], sensorimotor [80], and pure motor [80] polyneuropathies are reported.

Ticks

A syndrome of rapidly progressive, pure motor weakness affecting limb, bulbar, respiratory, and ocular muscles occurs from exposure to certain tick species. Known as tick paralysis, the syndrome is caused by three tick varieties: *Dermacentor andersoni* (northwestern United States), *Dermacentor variabilis* (southeastern United States) [78], and *Ixodes holocyclus* (Australia) [81]. The toxin from *I. holocyclus* is shown to impair presynaptic release of acetylcholine [81], which also is suspected in North American species; thus, tick paralysis is most consistent with an NMJ disorder, rather than a peripheral polyneuropathy.

The clinical syndrome most commonly is observed in children under the age of 9 [82,83]. Symptoms of progressive, proximal greater-than-distal limb weakness develop approximately 3 to 7 days after attachment of the female tick [78,84]. The weakness steadily progresses unless the tick is removed. Dysarthria, dysphagia, and respiratory compromise requiring assistive ventilation develop with involvement of bulbar muscles. Facial weakness and weakness of extraocular muscles also may be seen [81,82,84]. Hypo- or areflexia is common, but sensation is spared. Electrodiagnostic studies reveal a consistent pattern of reduced motor amplitudes with normal to minimally slowed conduction velocities with normal sensory studies [81,83,84]. One report describes normal low and high frequency repetitive nerve stimulation [83]. CSF studies are unremarkable [83,84].

Removal of the tick results in rapid resolution of clinical weakness within 1 to 2 days [82,84], with recovery of motor amplitudes on electrodiagnostic testing [81,83,84]. Case reports from Australia note a slower clinical recovery than that seen in the United States, and mild worsening may be observed within even 24 to 48 hours after tick removal. Respiratory support was required for more than 1 week after tick removal in certain cases [81]. It is, therefore, suggested that antitoxin for *I. holocyclus* should be administered at the same time as tick removal to accelerate recovery [81].

The polyradiculoneuritis, cranial neuropathies, and GBS-like neuropathy associated with Lyme disease are other examples of neuropathic involvement related to tick exposure. As these are associated with the infectious organism, Borrelia burgdorferi, however, further descriptions of these entities are not provided in this article.

Neuropathy secondary to plant toxins

Buckthorn neuropathy

Tullidora toxin is present in the seeds of a shrub of the buckthorn family, *Karwinskia humboltiana*, found in southwestern Texas, New Mexico, California, and central and northern Mexico [85]. Ingestion of this toxin results in a subacute, progressive, symmetric motor polyneuropathy, similar to GBS [85–87]. Symptoms of motor weakness may not be noticed until a few weeks after ingestion, but once they begin, they may progress rapidly to quadriplegia with respiratory or bulbar paralysis within a few days. Spinal fluid typically is normal and displays no evidence of the albuminocytologic dissociation. Electrophysiologic testing on cats experimentally exposed to tullidora reveals diffuse motor conduction slowing, typical of a demyelinating polyneuropathy [87]. Initial reports support buckthorn neuropathy as a primary demyelinating disease, with Schwann cell enlargement and degeneration of the myelin sheath [85]. More recent electron microscopy studies, however, reveal widened periaxonal spaces and redistribution of cytoskeletal elements in the axoplasm, suggesting axonal loss with secondary demyelination [88]. Treatment generally is supportive and near complete functional recovery is expected if patients survive the initial insult.

Neurolathyrism

A pure motor spastic paraplegia can occur from prolonged ingestion of *Lathyrus sativus*, commonly referred to as the grass or chickling pea [89]. This plant is common to southern Europe and central Asia, and increased reliance on it as a food source in times of famine have led to large numbers of cases. Clinical signs usually are limited to upper motor neuron involvement. Lower motor neuron involvement is reported in 15% of patients [90], and a peripheral sensory polyneuropathy in 7% [91]. Electrophysiologic studies in symptomatic patients reveal primarily demyelinating abnormalities, including motor and sensory conduction slowing, prolonged distal motor latencies, and reduced motor unit recruitment on concentric needle

EMG [89,91]. Light and electron microscopy findings also support a demye-linating polyneuropathy, with irregular thickening, degeneration, and vesiculation of the myelin sheath in the paranodal regions [91]. Treatment is preventative, with discontinuation of further *Lathyrus* ingestion. Some patients notice mild improvement in spasticity for 1 to 3 months, although the neurologic illness typically is irreversible.

Ergotism

Ergot intoxication secondary to excessive ingestion of rye contaminated by the fungus, *Claviceps purpurea*, is linked to epidemics of limb ischemia and gangrene that occurred in the ninth to nineteenth centuries [92]. Modern cases of ergotism are rare but are reported in patients suffering from chronic migraines who use excessive doses of ergotamine tartrate. From this group, case reports of transient, isolated mononeuropathies, including bilateral peroneal and lateral popliteal neuropathies, are reported [92,93]. It is suggested the mononeuropathies are the result of nerve ischemia, possibly secondary to diffuse vasoconstriction; however, the limited clinical and electrophysiologic evidence does not provide convincing evidence to support this.

Summary

Many substances, organic and manufactured, may induce peripheral nerve damage when exposed to them. The expected clinical phenotype is of a distal, sensory or sensorimotor polyneuropathy, often painful, with axonal characteristics on electrodiagnostic and histopathologic analysis. Treatment is limited; often, the only effective management is supportive care and avoidance from or removal of the offending toxin. Fortunately, the majority of toxic neuropathies are self-limited and improves gradually after toxin elimination.

References

[1] Windebank AJ. Polyneuropathy due to nutritional deficiency and alcoholism. In: Dyck PJ, Thomas PK, editors. Peripheral neuropathy. 3rd edition. Philadelphia: WB Saunders; 1993. p. 1310–21.
[2] Behse F, Buchthal F. Alcoholic neuropathy: clinical, electrophysiologic, and biopsy findings. Ann Neurol 1977;2:95–110.
[3] Casey EB, Le Quesne PM. Electrophysiological evidence for a distal lesion in alcoholic neuropathy. J Neurol Neurosurg Psychiatry 1972;35:624–30.
[4] Blackstock E, Rushworth G, Gath D. Electrophysiologic studies in alcoholism. J Neurol Neurosurg Psychiatry 1972;35:326–34.
[5] Walsh JC, McLeod JG. Alcoholic neuropathy: an electrophysiological and histological study. J Neurol Sci 1970;10:457–69.

[6] D'Amour ML, Shahani BT, Young RR, et al. The importance of studying sural nerve conduction and late responses in the evaluation of alcoholic subjects. Neurology 1979;29: 1600–4.

[7] Mawdsley C, Mayer RF. Nerve conduction in alcoholic polyneuropathy. Brain 1965;88: 335–56.

[8] Shattuck GC. Relation of beriberi to polyneuritis from other causes. Am J Trop Med Hyg 1928;8:539–43.

[9] Victor M, Adams RD. On the etiology of the alcoholic neurologic diseases: with special references to the role of nutrition. Am J Clin Nutr 1961;9:379–97.

[10] North JD, Sinclair HM. Nutritional neuropathy: chronic thiamine deficiency in the rat. AMA Arch Pathol 1956;62:341–53.

[11] Fennelly J, Frank O, Baker H. Peripheral neuropathy of the alcoholic: I. Aetiological role of aneurin and other B-complex vitamins. BMJ 1964;2:1290–2.

[12] Layzer RB, Fishman RA, Schafer JA. Neuropathy following abuse of nitrous oxide. Neurology 1978;28:504–6.

[13] Marie RM, Le Biez E, Busson P, et al. Nitrous oxide anesthesia-associated myelopathy. Arch Neurol 2000;57:380–2.

[14] Ogundipe O, Pearson MW, Slater NG, et al. Sickle cell disease and nitrous oxide-induced neuropathy. Clin Lab Haematol 1999;21:409–12.

[15] Bosch EP, Smith BE. Disorders of peripheral nerves. In: Bradley WF, Daroff RB, Fenichel GM, et al, editors. Neurology in clinical practice. 3rd edition. Boston: Butterworth-Heinemann; 2000. p. 2119.

[16] Sesso RM, Iunes Y, Melo AC. Myeloneuropathy following nitrous oxide anaesthesia in a patient with macrocytic anaemia. Neuroradiology 1999;41:588–90.

[17] Stacy CB, Di Rocco A, Gould RJ. Methionine in the treatment of nitrous-oxide-induced neuropathy and myeloneuropathy. J Neurol 1992;239:401–3.

[18] Shafer SQ. Disorders of spinal cord, nerve, and muscle. Neurol Clin 1993;11:693–705.

[19] Challenor YB, Richter RW, Bruun B, et al. Nontraumatic plexitis and heroin addiction. JAMA 1973;225:958–61.

[20] Loizou LA, Boddie HG. Polyradiculneuropathy associated with heroin abuse. J Neurol Neurosurg Psychiatry 1978;41:855–7.

[21] Warner-Smith M, Darke S, Day C. Morbidity associated with non-fatal heroin overdose. Addiction 2002;97:963–7.

[22] Sinsawaiwong S, Phanthumchinda K. Pentazocine-induced fibrous myopathy and localized neuropathy. J Med Assoc Thai 1998;81:717–21.

[23] LeQuesne PM. Neuropathy due to drugs. In: Dyck PJ, Thomas PK, editors. Peripheral neuropathy. 3rd edition. Philadelphia: WB Saunders; 1993. p. 1571–81.

[24] Mukherjee SC, Rahman MM, Chowdhury UK, et al. Neuropathy in arsenic toxicity from groundwater arsenic contamination in West Begal, India. J Environ Sci Health [A] 2003; 38:165–83.

[25] Rusyniak DE, Furbee RB, Kirk MA. Thallium and arsenic poisoning in a small midwestern town. Ann Emerg Med 2002;39:307–11.

[26] Aminoff MJ. Effects of occupational toxins on the nervous system. In: Bradley WF, Daroff RB, Fenichel GM, Marsden CD, editors. Neurology in clinical practice. 3rd edition. Boston: Butterworth-Heinemann; 2000. p. 1511–9.

[27] Blom S, Lagerkvist B, Linderholm H. Arsenic exposure to smelter workers: clinical and neurophysiological studies. Scand J Work Environ Health 1985;11:265–9.

[28] Greenberg SA. Acute demyelinating polyneuropathy with arsenic ingestion. Muscle Nerve 1996;19:1611–3.

[29] Wax PM, Thornton CA. Recovery from severe arsenic-induced peripheral neuropathy with 2,3-dimercapto-1-propanesulphonic acid. J Toxicol Clin Toxicol 2000;38:777–80.

[30] Windebank AJ. Metal neuropathy. In: Dyck PJ, Thomas PK, editors. Peripheral neuropathy. 3rd edition. Philadelphia: WB Saunders; 1993. p. 1549–70.

[31] Rubens O, Logina I, Kravale I, et al. Peripheral neuropathy in chronic occupational inorganic lead exposure: a clinical and electrophysiological study. J Neurol Neurosurg Psychiatry 2001;71:200–4.

[32] Mitchell CS, Shear MS, Bolla KI, et al. Clinical evaluation of 58 organolead manufacturing workers. J Occup Environ Med 1996;38:372–8.

[33] Nielsen CJ, Nielsen VK, Kirkby H, et al. Absence of peripheral neuropathy in long-term lead-exposed subjects. Acta Neurol Scand 1982;65:241–7.

[34] Tromme I, Van Neste D, Dobbelaere F, et al. Skin signs in the diagnosis of thallium poisoning. Br J Dermatol 1998;138:321–5.

[35] Schaumberg HH, Berger AR. Human toxic neuropathy due to industrial agents. In: Dyck PJ, Thomas PK, editors. Peripheral neuropathy. 3rd edition. Philadelphia: WB Saunders; 1993. p. 1533–48.

[36] Gold BG, Voda J, Yu X, et al. The immunosuppressant FK506 elicits a neuronal heat shock response and protects against acrylamide neuropathy. Exp Neurol 2004;187:160–70.

[37] Pradat PF, Kennel P, Naimi-Sadaoui S, et al. Continuous delivery of neurotrophin 3 by gene therapy has a neuroprotective effect in experimental models of diabetic and acrylamide neuropathies. Hum Gene Ther 2001;12:2237–49.

[38] Belai A, Burnstock G. Acrylamide-induced neuropathic changes in rat enteric nerves: similarities with effects of streptozotocin-diabetes. J Auton Nerv Syst 1996;58:56–62.

[39] Huang CC, Chu CC, Wu TN, et al. Clinical course in patients with chronic carbon disulfide polyneuropathy. Clin Neurol Neurosurg 2002;104:115–20.

[40] Chu CC, Huang CC, Chu NS, et al. Carbon disulfide induced polyneuropathy: sural nerve pathology, electrophysiology, and clinical correlation. Acta Neurol Scand 1996;94:258–63.

[41] Goetz CG, Bolla KI, Rogers SM. Neurologic health outcomes and Agent Orange: Institute of Medicine report. Neurology 1994;44:801–9.

[42] Thomke F, Jung D, Besser R, et al. Increased risk of sensory neuropathy in workers with chloracne after exposure to 2, 3,7,8-polychlorinated dioxins and furans. Acta Neurol Scand 1999;100:1–5.

[43] Barbieri S, Pirovano C, Scarlato G, et al. Long-term effects of 2, 3,7,8-tetrachlorodibenzo-p-dioxin on the peripheral nervous system. Clinical and neurophysiological controlled study on subjects with chloracne from the Seveso area. Neuroepidemiology 1988;7:29–37.

[44] Grehl H, Grahmann F, Claus D, et al. Histologic evidence for a toxic polyneuropathy due to exposure to 2, 3,7,8-tetrachlorodibenzo-p-dioxin (TCDD) in rats. Acta Neurol Scand 1993; 88:354–7.

[45] Grahmann F, Claus D, Grehl H, et al. Electrophysiologic evidence for a toxic polyneuropathy in rats after exposure to 2, 3,7,8-tetrachlorodibenzo-p-dioxin (TCDD). J Neurol Sci 1993;115:71–5.

[46] Michalek JE, Akhtar FZ, Arezzo JC, et al. Serum dioxin and peripheral neuropathy in veterans of Operation Ranch Hand. Neurotoxicology 2001;22:479–90.

[47] Kim JS, Lim HS, Cho SI, et al. Impact of Agent Orange exposure among Korean Vietnam veterans. Ind Health 2003;41:149–57.

[48] Windebank AJ, Blexrud MD. Residual ethylene oxide in hollow fiber hemodialysis units is neurotoxic in vitro. Ann Neurol 1989;26:63–8.

[49] Brashear A, Unverzagt FW, Farber MO, et al. Ethylene oxide neurotoxicity: a cluster of 12 nurses with peripheral and central nervous system toxicity. Neurology 1996;46:992–8.

[50] Centers for Disease Control. n-Hexane-related peripheral neuropathy among automotive technicians–California, 1999–2000. MMWR 2001;50:1011–3.

[51] Pastore C, Izura V, Marhuenda D, et al. Partial conduction blocks in N-hexane neuropathy. Muscle Nerve 2002;26:132–5.

[52] Gluszcz-Zielinska A. [Occupational N-hexane neuropathy: clinical and neurophysiological investigation]. Med Pr 1999;50:31–6 [in Polish].

[53] Kuwabara S, Kai MR, Nagase H, et al. n-Hexane neuropathy caused by addictive inhalation: clinical and electrophysiological features. Eur Neurol 1999;41:163–7.

[54] Kuang S, Huang H, Liu H, et al. [A clinical analysis of 102 cases of chronic n-hexane intoxication]. Zhonghua Nei Ke Za Zhi 2001;40:329–31 [in Chinese].

[55] Pastore C, Marhuenda D, Marti J, et al. Early diagnosis of n-hexane-caused neuropathy. Muscle Nerve 1994;17:981–6.

[56] Chang AP, England JD, Garcia CA, et al. Focal conduction block in n-hexane polyneuropathy. Muscle Nerve 1998;21:964–9.

[57] Lifshitz M, Gavrilov V. Central nervous system toxicity and early peripheral neuropathy following dermal exposure to methyl bromide. J Toxicol Clin Toxicol 2000;38:799–801.

[58] De Haro L, Gastaut JL, Jouglard J, et al. Central and peripheral neurotoxic effects of chronic methyl bromide intoxication. J Toxicol Clin Toxicol 1997;35:29–34.

[59] Pearn J. Neurology of ciguatera. J Neurol Neurosurg Psychiatry 2001;70:4–8.

[60] Lawrence DN, Enriquez MB, Lumish RM, et al. Ciguatera fish poisoning in Miami. JAMA 1980;244:254–8.

[61] Butera R, Prockop LD, Buonocore M, et al. Mild ciguatera poisoning: case reports with neurophysiological evaluations. Muscle Nerve 2000;23:1598–603.

[62] Cameron J, Flowers AE, Capra MF. Electrophysiological studies on ciguatera poisoning in man (part II). J Neurol Sci 1991;101:93–7.

[63] Cameron J, Capra MF. The basis of the paradoxical disturbance of temperature perception in ciguatera poisoning. J Toxicol Clin Toxicol 1993;31:571–9.

[64] Hamblin PA, McLachlan EM, Lewis RJ. Sub-nanomolar concentrations of ciguatoxin-1 excite preganglionic terminals in guinea pig sympathetic ganglia. Naunyn Schmiedebergs Arch Pharmacol 1995;352:236–46.

[65] Allsop JL, Martini L, Lebris H, et al. Neurologic manifestations of ciguatera. 3 cases with a neurophysiologic study and examination of one nerve biopsy. Rev Neurol 1986;142:590–7.

[66] Lewis RJ, Jones A, Vernoux JP. HPLC/tandem electrospray mass spectrometry for the determination of Sub-ppb levels of Pacific and Caribbean ciguatoxins in crude extracts of fish. Anal Chem 1999;71:247–50.

[67] Purcell CE, Capra MF, Cameron J. Action of mannitol in ciguatoxin-intoxicated rats. Toxicon 1999;37:67–76.

[68] Trevett AJ, Mavo B, Warrell DA. Tetrodotoxic poisoning from ingestion of a porcupine fish (Diodon hystrix) in Papua New Guinea: nerve conduction studies. Am J Trop Med Hyg 1997; 56:30–2.

[69] Oda K, Araki K, Totoki T, et al. Nerve conduction study of human tetrodotoxication. Neurology 1989;39:743–5.

[70] Auerbach PS, Halstead BW. Hazardous aquatic life. In: Auerbach PS, Geehr E, editors. Management of wilderness and environmental allergies. 2nd edition. St. Louis: CV Mosby; 1989. p. 995–7.

[71] Doyle DD, Guo Y, Lustig SL, et al. Divalent cation competition with [3H] saxitoxin binding to tetrodotoxin-resistant and -sensitive sodium channels. A two-site structural model of ion/toxin interaction. J Gen Physiol 1993;101:153–82.

[72] Centers for Disease Control. Paralytic shellfish poisoning—Massachusetts and Alaska, 1990. MMWR 1991;40:157–61.

[73] Rodrigue DC, Etzel RA, Hall S, et al. Lethal paralytic shellfish poisoning in Guatemala. Am J Trop Med Hyg 1990;42:267–71.

[74] Gessner BD, Middaugh JP. Paralytic shellfish poisoning in Alaska: a 20-year retrospective analysis. Am J Epidemiol 1995;141:766–70.

[75] Chang FC, Spriggs DL, Benton BJ, et al. 4-aminopyridine reverses saxitoxin (STX)- and tetrodotoxin (TTX)-induced cardiorespiratory depression in chronically instrumented guinea pigs. Fundam Appl Toxicol 1997;38:75–88.

[76] De Carvalho M, Jacinto J, Ramos N, et al. Paralytic shellfish poisoning: clinical and electrophysiological observations. J Neurol 1998;245:551–4.

[77] Long RR, Sargent JC, Hammer K. Paralytic shellfish poisoning: a case report and serial electrophysiologic observations. Neurology 1990;40:1310–2.

[78] Harris JB, Goonetilleke A. Animal poisons and the nervous system: what the neurologist needs to know. J Neurol Neurosurg Psychiatry 2004;75(Suppl III):iii40–6.

[79] Seneviratne U, Dissanayake S. Neurological manifestations of snake bite in Sri Lanka. J Postgrad Med 2002;48:275–8.

[80] Kularatne SAM. Common krait (Bungarus caeruleus) bite in Anuradhapura, Sri Lanka: a prospective clinical study, 1996–98. Postgrad Med J 2002;78:276–80.

[81] Grattan-Smith PJ, Morris JG, Johnston HM, et al. Clinical and neurophysiological features of tick paralysis. Brain 1997;120:1975–87.

[82] Dworkin MS, Shoemaker PC, Anderson DE. Tick paralysis: 33 human cases in Washington state, 1946–1996. Clin Infect Dis 1999;29:1435–9.

[83] Venkataraman Vedanarayanan V, Evans OB, Subramony SH. Tick paralysis in children: electrophysiology and possibility of misdiagnosis. Neurology 2002;59:1088–90.

[84] Felz MW, Davis-Smith C, Swift TR. A 6-year old girl with tick paralysis. N Engl J Med 2000; 342:90–4.

[85] Calderon-Gonzalez R, Rizzi-Hernandez H. Buckthorn polyneuropathy. N Engl J Med 1967; 277:69–71.

[86] Aoki K, Munoz-Martinez EJ. Quantitative changes in myelin proteins in a peripheral neuropathy caused by tullidora. J Neurochem 1981;36:1–8.

[87] Hernandez-Cruz A, Munoz-Martinez EJ. Tullidora (Karwinskia Humboldtiana) toxin mainly affects fast conducting axons. Neuropathol Appl Neurobiol 1984;10:11–24.

[88] Heath JW, Ueda S, Bornstein MB, et al. Buckthorn neuropathy in vitro: evidence for a primary neuronal effect. J Neuropathol Exp Neurol 1982;41:204–20.

[89] Misra UK, Sharma VP. Peripheral and central conduction in neurolathyrism. J Neurol Neurosurg Psychiatry 1994;57:572–7.

[90] Cohn DF, Striefler M. Human neurolathyrism, a followup study of 200 patients. Arch Suisses Neurol Neurochir Psychiatrie 1981;128:151–6.

[91] Cohn DF, Streifler M, Dabush S, Messer G. Peripheral nerve changes in chronic neurolathyrism. Neurol India 1983;31:45–51.

[92] Merhoff GC, Porter JM. Ergot intoxication: historical review and description of unusual clinical manifestations. Ann Surg 1974;180:773–9.

[93] Perkin GD. Ischaemic lateral popliteal nerve palsy due to ergot intoxication. J Neurol Neurosurg Psychiatry 1974;37:1389–91.

ELSEVIER
SAUNDERS

Neurol Clin 23 (2005) 397–428

NEUROLOGIC
CLINICS

Toxic Myopathies

Ronan J. Walsh, MD[a],*, Anthony A. Amato, MD[b,c]

[a]Neuromuscular Division, Department of Neurology, Brigham and Women's Hospital,
Boston, MA, USA
[b]Neuromuscular Division, Department of Neurology, Clinical Neurophysiology Laboratory,
Brigham and Women's Hospital, Boston, MA, USA
[c]Harvard Medical School, Boston, MA, USA

Multiple drugs and toxins can cause myopathy [1–6]. Patients at risk for developing adverse reactions typically are those who have reduced abilities to metabolize or excrete the drug and its metabolites, as is the case in those who have liver and renal failure, infants and children, and elderly patients.

The exact incidence of toxic myopathies is unknown, but probably it is more common than is recognized. Early recognition is important, because they are potentially reversible on removal of the offending toxin, with greater likelihood of complete resolution the sooner this is achieved. Several general clinical features are useful in diagnosing a toxic myopathy correctly: lack of any other etiology for the myopathy; lack of any previous muscular symptoms; and resolution of the symptoms after withdrawal of the identified toxic agent. Drugs or toxins can produce mild symptoms of muscle pain and cramps or cause a severe weakness in which the patient may die as a result of widespread rhabdomyolysis and renal failure.

Muscle tissue is highly sensitive to drugs and toxins because of its high metabolic activity and multiple potential sites for foreign substances to disrupt the energy-producing pathways. Exogenous substances can have either a primary or secondary adverse affect on muscle tissue. Secondary effects of toxic medications may be due to compression, by causing the patient to become unconscious. The primary effect can be focal, as might occur from a drug being injected into a tissue, or generalized. Generalized toxic effect may result from the substance creating an electrolyte imbalance, inducing an immunologic response, or precipitating ischemia from a vascular

---

* Corresponding author. Neuromuscular Division, Department of Neurology, Brigham and Women's Hospital, 75 Francis Street, Tower 5D, Boston, MA 02115.
    E-mail address: rjwalsh@partners.org (R.J. Walsh).

reaction. Some drugs cause autophagic degeneration of the muscle tissue. Other toxic substances may affect protein synthesis adversely [7].

This review classifies the toxic myopathies according to their presumed pathogenic mechanisms (Table 1), focusing on drugs and toxins representative of major pathogenic processes affecting skeletal muscle, with the understanding that related substances have similar effects.

Necrotizing myopathies

Several drugs can cause a generalized necrotizing myopathy that can present as myalgias, weakness, myoglobinuria, or asymptomatic high creatine kinase (CK): hyper CK-emia. As is anticipated with any substance causing muscle necrosis, the electromyogram (EMG) may demonstrate increased insertional and spontaneous activity and small amplitude, short-duration, polyphasic, or "myopathic" motor unit action potentials (MUAP) [7].

Cholesterol-lowering drugs

Fibric acid derivatives

Clofibrate and gemfibrozil are branched-chain fatty acid esters used to treat hyperlipidemia. A toxic myopathy associated with these medications typically presents within 2 or 3 months after the drug is started but can be delayed up to 2 years [7–20]. Patients can develop generalized weakness, myalgias, cramps, and occasionally myoglobinuria. After stopping the medication, symptoms tend to resolve completely in several days to months. Patients who have renal insufficiency or those who are taking multiple fibric acid derivatives or 3-hydroxy-3-methylglutaryl coenzyme A (HMG-CoA) inhibitors are predisposed to developing a severe myopathy. Elevated serum CK levels usually are noted. Needle EMG may demonstrate fibrillation potentials, positive sharp waves, complex repetitive discharges, or myotonic discharges and myopathic MUAP in affected muscle groups but may be normal in individuals affected only mildly [7–9,19]. Muscle biopsies demonstrate scattered muscle fiber necrosis. The pathogenesis is unknown but is postulated to be destabilization of the lipophilic muscle membrane leading to muscle fiber degeneration [17].

3-hydroxy-3-methylglutaryl coenzyme A reductase inhibitors

HMG-CoA reductase is the rate-controlling enzyme in cholesterol synthesis. The three fermentation-derived statins—lovastatin, simvastatin, and provastatin—are shown to reduce the risk for mortality or major coronary events. Long-term efficacy and safety studies are lacking, however, for the synthetic statins—atorvostatin, fluvastatin, and cerivastatin [21].

All the major HMG-CoA reductase inhibitors—lovastatin [16,22–25], simvastatin [23,26–29], provastatin [23,30], atorvastatin [10,23,31], fluvastatin [23], and cerivastatin [21,23,32]—are associated with myopathy characterized by myalgias, proximal weakness, and, less commonly, myoglobinuria.

Serum CK can be elevated as much as 1000 times normal in patients who have severe toxic myopathy. The incidence of elevated serum CK or symptomatic myopathy generally is considered low, however. General reviews of statin myopathies cite a 2% to 7% incidence of myalgias [33] and 0.1% to 1.0% incidence of weakness or elevated CK [20,33,34] The National Heart, Lung, and Blood Institute advisory panel estimates the incidence of severe myopathy at approximately 0.08% each for lovastatin, simvastatin, and pravastatin [35]. The Food and Drug Administration estimates 0.15 deaths per million total statin prescriptions (not patients) resulting from rhabdomyolysis. Mortalities were found 16 to 80 times higher for cerivastatin than the other agents, however [36]. This led to the withdrawal of cerivastatin from the market. In the United States, of an estimated 700,000 users of cerivastatin, 31 had fatal rhabdomyolysis secondary to renal failure, and 385 patients developed nonfatal rhabdomyolysis [21]. Worldwide, an additional 21 deaths occurred. The concomitant use of fibric acids [10,17,24,25,37]—niacin [24], erythromycin [38], diltiazem [26,39–41], and cyclosporine [25]—increases the risk for toxic myopathy, as do renal insufficiency and liver disease.

Needle EMG usually demonstrates fibrillation potentials, positive sharp waves, myotonic discharges, and early recruitment of myopathic MUAP [7] in patients who have significant weakness. EMG of patients who have asymptomatic hyper-CK-emia, however, usually is normal.

Biopsies of severely affected muscles reveal muscle fiber necrosis with phagocytosis and small regenerating fibers (Fig. 1). Electron microscopy (EM) demonstrates the subsarcolemmal accumulation of autophagic lysosomes. Mild inflammatory infiltrate and membrane attack complex deposition on small blood vessels, reminiscent of dermatomyositis, is reported in one patient who had taken provastatin [30].

The pathogenesis of the myopathy secondary to HMG-CoA reductase inhibitors is unknown. Disruption of the cholesterol content in muscle membranes, predisposing the muscle fibers to rhabdomyolysis, has been postulated [14]. Other studies suggest that depletion of metabolites of geranylgeraniol is the primary cause of myotoxicity [42]. A third theory is that HMG-CoA reductase inhibitors decrease the levels of coenzyme Q, which could impair energy production [43].

Niacin

There are only a few reports of myopathy developing in patients treated with niacin [24,37]. In one report of three patients receiving niacin, myalgias and cramps in the legs were the predominant features [37]. Serum CK levels were elevated as much as tenfold. The symptoms improved and CK levels normalized after discontinuation of niacin. Neither EMG nor muscle biopsy results were reported. Rhabdomyolysis has been described in association with lovastatin and niacin [24]. The pathogenic mechanism of the myopathy likely is similar to that of the statins, as niacin can inhibit HMG-CoA reductase.

Table 1
Toxic myopathies

Pathogenic classification	Drug	Clinical features	Laboratory features	Histopathology
Necrotizing myopathy	Cholesterol-lowering agents Cyclosporine Labetolol Propofol Alcohol	Acute or insidious onset; proximal weakness; myalgias	Elevated serum CK; EMG: fibs, PSW, myotonia (statins, cyclosporine), myopathic MUAP	Many necrotic muscle fibers; no evidence of endomysial inflammatory cell infiltrate invading non-necrotic muscle fibers
Amphiphilic	Chloroquine Hydroxylchloroquine Aminodarone	Acute or insidious onset; proximal and distal weakness; myalgias; sensorimotor neuropathy; hypothyroid (amiodarone)	Elevated serum CK; EMG: fibs, PSW, myotonia (choroquine), myopathic MUAP; NCS: axonal sensorimotor neuropathy	Autophagic vacuoles and inclusions are apparent in some muscle fibers and in Schwann cells
Antimicrotubular	Colchicine Vincristine	Acute or insidious onset; proximal and distal weakness; myalgias; Sensorimotor neuropathy	Normal or elevated CK; EMG: fibs, PSW, myotonia (colchicine), myopathic MUAP; NCS: axonal sensorimotor neuropathy	Autophagic vacuoles and inclusions are evident in some muscle fibers; nerve biopsies demonstrate axonal degeneration
Mitochondrial myopathy	Zidovudine Other HIV-related antiretrovirals?	Acute or insidious onset; Proximal weakness; myalgias; rhabdomyolysis; painful sensory neuropathy	Normal or elevated CK; EMG: normal or myopathic; NCS: axonal sensory neuropathy/neuronopathy	Muscle biopsies reveal ragged red fibers, COX-negative fibers; also may see inflammatory cell infiltrates, cytoplasmic bodies, nemaline rods

Inflammatory myopathy	L-tryptophan D-penicillamine Cimetidine L-dopa Phenytoin Lamotrigine Interferon-α Hydroxyurea Imatinib	Acute or insidious onset; proximal weakness; myalgias	Elevated serum CK; EMG: fibs, PSW, myopathic MUAP	Perivascular, perimysial, or endomysial inflammatory cell infiltrates
Hypokalemic myopathy	Diuretics Laxatives Amphotericin Toluene abuse Licorice Corticosteroids Alcohol abuse	Acute proximal or generalized weakness; myalgias	Serum CK may be elevated; low serum potassium	May see scattered necrotic fibers and vacuoles
Unknown	Critical illness myopathy: corticosteroids; nondepolarizing neuromuscular blocking agents; sepsis	Acute generalized weakness including respiratory muscles	Serum CK can be normal or elevated; NCS: low amplitude CMAP with relatively normal SNAP; EMG: fibs, PSW, myopathic MUAP or no voluntary MUAP	Atrophy of muscle fibers, scattered necrotic fibers; absence of myosin thick filaments
	Omeprazole	Acute or insidious onset; proximal weakness; myalgias; sensorimotor neuropathy	Normal or slightly elevated serum CK EMG: myopathic MUAP; NCS: axonal sensorimotor neuropathy	Type II muscle fiber atrophy may be seen

(continued on next page)

Table 1 (*continued*)

Pathogenic classification	Drug	Clinical features	Laboratory features	Histopathology
	Isoretinoin	Acute or insidious onset; proximal weakness; myalgias	Normal or slightly elevated CK	Atrophy of fibers
	Finasteride		Serum CK is normal; EMG: myopathic MUAP	Variability in fiber size, type II fiber atrophy, increased internalized nuclei
	Emetine	Acute or insidious onset; proximal weakness; myalgias	Serum CKs mild to moderately elevated	Myofibrillar myopathy

Abbreviations: fibs, fibrillation potentials; NCS. nerve conduction studies; PSW, positive sharpwaves.

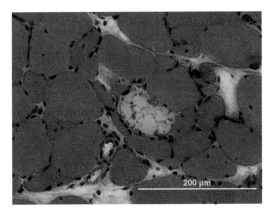

Fig. 1. Necrotizing myopathy. Muscle biopsy in a patient who had a statin myopathy revealed necrotic muscle fibers, variability in fiber size, and increased internalized nuclei (hematoxylin-eosin stain, original magnification ×10).

Immunophilins

Cyclosporine and tacrolimus

Cyclosporine and tacrolimus (ie, the immunophilins) are commonly used immunosuppressive agents, particularly for transplantation patients [44]. In patients taking cyclosporine, generalized myalgias and proximal muscle weakness develop within months after starting therapy [44–49]. There are a few reports of rhabdomyolysis with myoglobinuria in patients receiving cyclosporine concurrent with cholesterol lowering agents or colchicine [25,50–52]. Tacrolimus also is associated with severe rhabdomyolysis [53] and hypertrophic cardiomyopathy with congestive heart failure [54]. Improvement in myalgias, muscle strength, and cardiac function is seen with reduction or discontinuation of the offending agent. Routine nerve conduction studies are normal. Needle EMG demonstrates increased muscle membrane instability with fibrillation potentials, positive sharp waves, and myotonic potentials [46]. Small amplitude, short duration MUAP with early recruitment may be evident if patients have severe weakness. Serum CK usually is elevated. Muscle biopsies demonstrate necrosis, vacuoles, and type 2 muscle fiber atrophy.

The underlying pathogenesis of this myopathy and cardiomyopathy is not known. Similar to the cholesterol-lowering agents, the cyclophilins may destabilize the lipophilic muscle membrane. This may explain why the combination of cyclosporine and one of the more classic lipid-lowering agents (eg, fibric acid derivatives and statins) increases the risk for toxic myopathy.

Propofol

Propofol is an anesthetic agent used increasingly for sedating mechanically ventilated patients and treating status epilepticus. In children, several reports of rhabdomyolysis with myoglobinuria, metabolic acidosis, hypoxia, and myocardial arrest are associated with its use [55–57]. The reaction can be differentiated from malignant hyperthermia (MH) by the lack of persistent pyrexia and muscular rigidity. Misdiagnosed cases of acute quadriplegic myopathy (AQM) account for some of the other reported cases in the literature.

Serum CK levels are markedly elevated and myoglobinuria with renal failure may result. Massive muscle destruction can cause secondary hyperkalemia. Blood gases and serum chemistries demonstrate hypoxemia and severe metabolic acidosis. Muscle pathology has revealed necrosis of skeletal and cardiac muscle [55–57]. The patients who have AQM, who also received high-dose intravenous steroids, had prominent loss of thick filaments [58]. The mechanism of muscle toxicity is unknown. Discontinuation of propofol with supportive therapy for myoglobinuria, metabolic acidosis, hyperkalemia, and renal failure is the mainstay of treatment [7].

Labetolol

Labetolol is a commonly used α/β-blocker associated with rare reports of necrotizing myopathy [59,60]. Resulting proximal weakness or myalgias may present acutely or insidiously. Discontinuation of the medication results in improvement. Serum CK can be markedly elevated. Muscle biopsy may be normal [59] or reveal necrotic and regenerating fibers [60]. On EM, subsarcolemmal vacuoles were seen in one case [59]. The underlying pathogenesis is not known [7].

Amphiphilic drug myopathy

Amphiphilic drugs consist of a hydrophilic region and a hydrophobic region, which contain a primary or substituted positively charged amine group. It is these properties that account for a drug's ability to interact with the anionic phospholipids of cell membranes and organelles. This results in a neuromyopathy. The neuropathy frequently impairs function more than the myopathy [7].

Chloroquine

Chloroquine is a quinoline derivative used for treating malaria, sarcoidosis, systemic lupus erythematosis, scleroderma, and rheumatoid arthritis [6,61–65]. Chloroquine myopathy causes slowly progressive, painless, proximal weakness and atrophy, worse in the legs than the arms. Serum CK levels usually are elevated. Cardiomyopathy also can occur. A superimposed neuropathy leads to reduced sensation in some patients. Discontinuation of the medication results in resolution of the condition [7].

Mild slowing of motor and sensory nerve conduction velocities with mild to moderate reduction in the amplitudes is seen with the neuropathy [62,64]. Patients who have only the myopathy have normal motor and sensory studies [61]. Needle EMG reveals increased insertional activity with positive sharp waves and fibrillation potentials primarily in the proximal limb muscles [61,62,66]. Voluntary MUAP are predominantly polyphasic with decreased amplitude and duration [7].

Acid-phosphatase positive vacuoles are the most prominent abnormality on histopathology, present in as many as 50% of skeletal and cardiac muscle fibers [6,61–64]. Type 1 fibers are affected preferentially. The vacuoles on EM are noted to contain concentric lamellar myeloid debris and curvilinear structures. Nerve biopsies also contain autophagic vacuoles.

Pathogenesis is attributed to the drug's interaction with the lipid membrane. The drug-lipid complexes are resistant to digestion by lysosomal enzymes, which results in the formation of the autophagic vacuoles filled with myeloid debris.

Hydroxychloroquine

Hydroxychloroquine is related structurally to chloroquine and similarly produces a neuromyopathy [62]. With hydroxychloroquine the muscle weakness and histologic abnormalities usually are less severe. Vacuoles are typically absent on biopsy; despite this, EM generally demonstrates the pathologic accumulation of myeloid and curvilinear bodies [7].

Amiodarone

Amiodarone is an antiarrhythmic that also causes a neuromyopathy similar to chloroquine [65,67–70]. Patients develop severe proximal and distal weakness worse in the legs than the arms combined with distal sensory loss. Tremor and ataxia also are seen. Amiodarone also can result in hypothyroidism and an associated myopathy. Patients who have renal insufficiency may be more at risk for developing toxic neuromyopathy. CK levels are elevated. With discontinuation of the drug, muscle strength gradually improves.

Decreased amplitudes of CMAP and SNAP, particularly in the lower extremities, are evident on neurophysiologic testing [69]. On EMG, fibrillation potentials and positive sharp waves are evident in proximal and distal muscles. In proximal muscles, MUAP typically are polyphasic, short in duration, small in amplitude, and recruit early [7]. Distal muscles are more likely to have large-amplitude, long-duration polyphasic MUAP with decreased recruitment as a result of the associated neuropathy.

Autophagic vacuoles with myeloid inclusions are seen on muscle biopsies. In addition, neurogenic atrophy also can be appreciated, particularly in distal muscles. Besides myeloid debris, EM reveals myofibrillar disorganization. Myeloid inclusions also are evident on nerve biopsies. Pathogenesis is attributed to the drug interaction with the lipid membrane, similar to the other amphiphilic medications.

Antimicrotubular myopathies

Colchicine

Colchicine has been prescribed for gout for more than 200 years. It is weakly amphiphilic, but its therapeutic and toxic effect is considered secondary to inhibiting the polymerization of tubulin into microtubular structures [6,71]. Colchicine can cause a generalized peripheral neuropathy and myopathy. The neuromyopathy may develop after the long-term use of colchicine at customary doses or secondary to acute intoxication [4,72–74]. The neuromyopathy seems to develop more frequently in patients who have chronic renal failure. Progressive proximal muscle weakness develops over several months. One patient has been reported as having clinical myotonia [75]. The weakness resolves within 4 to 6 months after discontinuing the colchicine. Serum CK may be mildly elevated in asymptomatic patients or up to 50-fold in symptomatic patients. Nerve conduction studies commonly show a prolongation of the distal motor and sensory latencies in the upper and lower limbs [72–74]. Reduced compound muscle action potential (CMAP) and sensory nerve action potential (SNAP) amplitudes also may be noted. Needle EMG in the distal muscles demonstrates a reduced number of long-duration and high-amplitude MUAP firing at high rates, compatible with peripheral neuropathy. Alternatively, proximal limb and paraspinal muscles reveal early recruitment of MUAP, with short durations and low amplitudes, consistent with myopathy. Positive sharp waves, fibrillation potentials, and complex repetitive discharges are easily detectable in all muscle regions.

Muscle histology shows vacuolar myopathy with accumulation of lysosomes and autophagic vacuoles without necrosis (Fig. 2). The vacuoles react strongly with acid phosphatase. In addition, nerve biopsies can reveal evidence suggestive of a mild axonal neuropathy. The pathogenesis is believed to be the result of disruption of the microtubules arresting intracellular movement of lysosomes, resulting in the accumulation of autophagic vacuoles [72].

Vincristine

Vincristine is a potent chemotherapeutic agent that acts primarily by disrupting RNA and protein synthesis and the polymerization of tubulin into microtubules [6]. Its most important toxic effect, and the one that limits is use as a therapeutic agent, is severe peripheral axonal neuropathy. Much less common is the development of a proximal muscle weakness and myalgias [76]. Unfortunately, serum CK levels have not been reported in

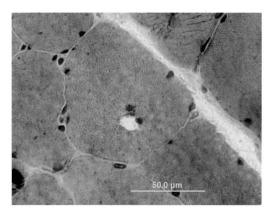

Fig. 2. Vacuolar myopathy. Muscle biopsy in a patient who had a neuromyopathy as a result of colchicine-demonstrated fibers with vacuoles (modified Gomori trichrome, original magnification ×10).

patients suspected of having a superimposed myopathy. Nerve conduction studies reveal an axonal peripheral neuropathy with signicantly reduced amplitudes of SNAPs and CMAPs [76]. Needle EMG of distally located muscles demonstrates positive sharp waves, fibrillation potentials, and neurogenic-appearing MUAP. EMG of proximal muscles, even in patients who have myalgias, reportedly are normal [76].

Muscle biopsies reveal mainly denervation atrophy and occasionally foci of segmental necrosis [76]. The pathogenic basis of the neuromyopathy presumably is similar to that of colchicine.

Drug-induced mitochondrial myopathy

Zidovudine (azidothymidine)

Skeletal muscle involvement in HIV infection includes inflammatory myopathy (polymyositis), microvasculitis, noninflammatory necrotizing myopathy, type 2 muscle fiber atrophy secondary to HIV-wasting syndrome, and a toxic myopathy secondary to azidothymidine (AZT) [77–88]. Clinically, AZT myopathy and the other myopathic disorders associated with HIV infection are indistinguishable, compounding the diagnostic difficulty. Indeed, muscle weakness may be multifactorial; an individual patient can have a HIV-associated myositis, nemaline rod myopathy, AZT-induced mitochondrial myopathy, and type 2 muscle fiber atrophy.

AZT myopathy presents with progressive proximal muscle weakness, myalgias, and fatigue, sometimes associated with elevated CK. These clinical features, however, do not help distinguish AZT myopathy from other HIV-related myopathies. A markedly elevated serum CK (eg, more than 5 times the upper limit of normal) is suggestive more of an HIV-associated myositis.

Muscle biopsies in AZT myopathy demonstrate ragged red fibers and cytochrome oxidase-negative fibers (Figs. 3A, B), whose number seems to correlate directly with the cumulative dose of AZT received by the patients [81,89]. In addition, necrotic fibers, cytoplasmic bodies, nemaline rods, and fibers with microvacuolation may be found on biopsy and coexist with the ragged red fibers [80,81,90]. EM confirms abnormalities of the mitochondria, myofilaments, and tubules. Significant endomysial inflammation and invasion of non-necrotic fibers may be lacking in pure AZT myopathy, in contrast to HIV-associated inflammatory myopathy.

Nerve conduction studies are normal, unless there is a concomitant peripheral neuropathy from the disease. Needle EMG examination demonstrates increase in needle insertional activity, with at times florid sustained runs of positive sharp waves and fibrillation potentials in some patients who have HIV-related myopathies and AZT myopathies [79,85,87]. Complex repetitive discharges occasionally are noted. Early recruitment of short

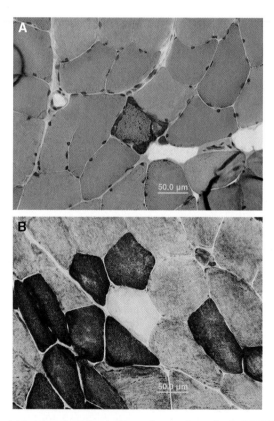

Fig. 3. Mitochondrial myopathy. Muscle biopsy in a patient who had HIV infection treated with zidovudine reveals ragged red fibers on (A) modified Gomori trichrome stain (original magnification ×10) and (B) cytochrome oxidase-negative fibers (original magnification ×10).

duration, small amplitude, polyphasic MUAP is seen, particularly in proximal muscles.

AZT acts as a false substitute for viral reverse transcriptase, but also for mitochondrial DNA polymerase, which probably accounts for the mitochondrial abnormalities present on muscle biopsy. Undoubtedly, AZT is implicated in the mitochondrial abnormalities evident on muscle biopsy. As discussed previously, however, the contribution of these mitochondrial abnormalities to the clinical muscle weakness remains controversial.

The percentage of patients who have myopathies that improve after AZT withdrawal is extremely variable, between 18% and 100% [79–81,83–85,91]. Discontinuation of AZT may be associated with a deleterious increase in HIV replication. It is advisable, therefore, to establish a histologic diagnosis before making a determination to discontinue AZT. The diagnosis still may not be clear, even after a muscle biopsy, as there may be signs of an inflammatory myopathy and mitochondrial abnormalities. Abundant abnormal spontaneous activity on EMG or markedly elevated serum CK levels favors an inflammatory myopathy rather than a mitochondrial myopathy. In such a case, a trial of intravenous immunoglobulin (IVIG) is recommended and, if this is ineffective, nonsteroidal anti-inflammatory medications or corticosteroids.

For those patients who have normal or only mildly elevated serum CK and normal or only slightly increased spontaneous activity on EMG, it may be impossible to distinguish AZT myopathy from other HIV-associated myopathies. A reasonable approach is to try a nonsteroidal anti-inflammatory drug with or without decreasing the dose of AZT [80]. If the patient does not improve in strength, discontinue AZT and use alternative newer antiretrovirals [92]. If there still is no objective improvement, perform a muscle biopsy and consider immunomodulating therapy (eg, IVIG) or corticosteroid treatment, if there is histologic evidence of an inflammatory myopathy. Patients can be rechallenged with AZT, particularly if there are no ragged red fibers on biopsy.

Other antiviral agents

According to some reports, the risk for mitochondrial myopathy with other nucleoside reverse transcriptase inhibitors, lamivudine (3TC), zalcitabine (ddC), and didanosine (ddI), is less than that of zidovudine (AZT) [93,94]. Mitochondrial toxicity does occur, however, with these medications, and hyperlactemia and hepatic steatosis do develop with these medications. Rare cases of rhabdomyolysis and myoglobinuria occur in patients taking other highly active antiretroviral therapy (HAART) medications, including tenofovir [95] and ritonavir [96]. The AIDS Clinical Trial Group randomized 2467 patients to receive one of four single or combination regimens with AZT, ddI, ddC, and their respective placebos [97]. Approximately 10% of patients had myalgias before treatment and 7% developed myalgia during treatment. No significant difference in the rate of myalgia or muscle weakness was seen between treatment arms. Five patients (0.5%) had elevated serum CK (>4 times normal) before treatment and 52 (5%) developed increased CK during treatment. In the AZT-ddC group, CK levels were significantly higher but this did not correlate with symptoms of myopathy. No comment was made on muscle biopsies; thus, it is unclear if the myopathies were secondary to mitochondrial toxicity or myositis.

Drug-induced inflammatory myopathy

L-tryptophan/eosinophilia-myalgia syndrome

There was a worldwide outbreak of this syndrome in the late 1980s and early 1990s traced to L-tryptophan pharmaceutical products manufactured by a single Japanese company [98–104]. Patients developed a subacute onset of generalized muscle pain and tenderness with variable degrees of weakness, skin changes, and a marked blood eosinophilia, with normal or elevated serum CK. Interestingly, the onset of symptoms can begin within a few weeks or there can be a latency of several years from the start of tryptophan ingestion. Associated symptoms included numbness, paresthesias, arthralgias, lymphadenopathy, dyspnea, abdominal pain, and mucocutaneous ulcers. Some patients developed a severe peripheral neuropathy simulating Guillain-Barré syndrome [99,105] or mononeuropathy multiplex [106]. Autoantibodies are absent and erythrocyte sedimentation rate usually is normal.

In muscle biopsies, the predominant pathologic change is perimysial and fascial inflammation [99]. The majority of inflammatory cells are CD8+ T cells and macrophages. Eosinophils and B cells account for less than 3% of the inflammatory cells. There is no deposition of membrane attack complex on blood vessels, unlike in dermatomyositis. Nerve biopsies also reveal inflammatory infiltrate, often perivascular in the epineurium, endoneurium, or perineurium accompanied by evidence of vasculopathy and angioneogenesis [99,101,106–108]. Significant axonal degeneration also has been appreciated.

The contaminants' pathologic role in the disorder is unknown but the eosinophilia suggests a form of allergic reaction. Discontinuation of L-tryptophan and treatment with high-dose corticosteroids usually is effective. Some patients experience relapses after withdrawal of steroids.

Toxic oil syndrome

Toxic oil syndrome is strikingly similar to the eosinophilia-myalgia syndrome associated with tryptophan [109]. This condition was restricted to an epidemic in Spain in 1981. The disorder was linked to the ingestion of illegally marked, denatured rapeseed oil used as a cooking substitute for olive oil. The toxic contaminant in the rapeseed oil, 3-phenylamino-

1,2-propanediol, chemically is similar to 3-(phenylamino) alanine, the adulterant in tryptophan that causes the eosinophilia-myalgia syndrome [110].

D-penicillamine

D-penicillamine is used for the treatment of Wilson's disease, rheumatoid arthritis, and other connective tissue disorders. D-penicillamine is associated with a 0.2% to 1.4% incidence of inflammatory myopathy [111–114]. Polymyositis and dermatomyositis are reported. The clinical, laboratory, histologic, and electrodiagnostic findings essentially are the same as those found in idiopathic forms of myositis. Cessation of the drug results in resolution of the symptoms. The medication may be restarted at a lower dosage without recurrence of the inflammatory myopathy.

Phenytoin

Hypersensitivity reactions to phenytoin characterized by fever, rash, and lymphadenopathy also can result in myalgias and muscle weakness with elevated serum CK [108]. Muscle biopsies demonstrate scattered necrotic and regenerating muscle fibers. The myopathy improves with discontinuation of the phenytoin and a short course of corticosteroids.

Procainamide

Proximal muscle weakness and myalgias are reported after procainamide administration [115,116]. Serum CK levels are elevated. EMG was reported as being consistent with a "patchy" myopathy (meaning the degree to which different muscles are involved can be variable, as is typical of inflammatory myopathy). Muscle biopsies demonstrate perivascular inflammation and rare necrotic muscle fibers. The pathogenesis may be related to lupus-like vasculitis, which can occur in patients treated with procainamide. The myopathy resolves after discontinuation of procainamide.

Interferon-α

Interferon-α is used in the treatment of viral hepatitis and certain malignancies (eg, chronic myelogenous leukemia [CML] and melanoma). A rare side effect of interferon-α is the occurrence of autoimmune disorders, including myasthenia gravis and myositis [117–119].

Imatinib mesylate

Imatinib mesylate (Gleevec) is a tyrosine kinase inhibitor used to treat patients who have CML. Imatinib inhibits the tyrosine kinase activity of the BCR-ABL oncoprotein in CML. Imatinib is tolerated well but myalgias occur in 21% to 52% of patients. The authors reported a patient who had

CML and who developed polymyositis while taking imatinib [120]. CML28 antibodies were detected in her serum. CML28 is identical to hRrp46p, a component of the human exosome, a multiprotein complex involved in processing RNA. Antibodies directed against hRrp46p and other components of the human exosome (eg, PM-Scl 100 and PM-Scl 75) are noted in patients who have polymyositis. The authors' patient's strength and serum CK normalized with discontinuation of the imatinib and a course of corticosteroids.

Tyrosine kinases are involved in signal transduction, cell growth, and differentiation. The mechanism by which imatinib therapy may cause myositis is unclear. The previous use of an immunomodulatory agent (eg, interferon-α), followed by imatinib leads to rapid apoptosis of leukemic cells. The subsequent release of a large bolus of leukemia antigens may have cross-reactivity with muscle antigens and generate an autoimmune response.

Other toxic myopathies

Steroid myopathy

A chronic excess of corticosteroid, from either endogenous (Cushing's syndrome) or exogenous (steroid medication administration) sources, results in proximal weakness and atrophy of the lower and upper limbs [121–125,155]. The distal extremities and oculobulbar and facial muscles are spared.

The incidence of exogenous corticosteroid myopathy is unknown. Women seem more prone to developing steroid-induced weakness than men, with a ratio of 2:1, but the reason is unclear. Prednisone doses of 30 mg/d or more (or equivalent doses of other corticosteroids) are associated with an increased risk for myopathy [125]. Fluorinated glucocorticoids (triamcinolone > betamethasone > dexamethasone) have a greater propensity for producing muscle weakness than the nonflourinated compounds [126]. Alternate-day dosing seems to reduce the risk for developing weakness. The muscle weakness may begin several weeks after the administration of steroids but more typically develops insidiously after chronic administration of oral high-dose steroids. In patients receiving high dosages of intravenous corticosteroids, with or without concomitant administration of neuromuscular blocking agents, an acute onset of severe generalized weakness can occur (acute quadriplegic myopathy, discussed later).

Serum CK is normal. Low serum potassium, as a result of glucocorticoid excess, may contribute to the weakness. Muscle biopsy reveals preferential atrophy of type 2 fibers, especially the fast twitch glycolytic-type 2B fibers (Fig. 4) [125,127,128]. There also may be a lesser degree of atrophy of type 1 muscle fibers. Necrosis or inflammation is not observed. Type 1 fibers commonly contain lipid droplets. On EM, mild mitochondrial abnormalities may be found.

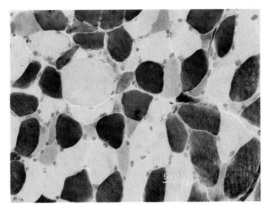

Fig. 4. Steroid myopathy. Muscle biopsy reveals preferential atrophy of type 2B fibers. On the ATPase stain at pH 4.5 the type 1 fibers are dark, type 2A are light, and type 2B stain intermediate (original magnification ×10).

The exact mechanism of corticosteroid myopathy is unknown. Corticosteroids bind to receptors on target cells and subsequently are internalized into the nuclei, where they regulate the transcription of specific genes. As a result, it is speculated that they decrease protein synthesis, increase protein degradation, alter carbohydrate metabolism, alter mitochondria, and reduce sarcolemmal excitability [129].

The recommended treatment of steroid myopathy is reduction in the dose, tapering to an alternate-day regimen, or switching to a nonflourinated steroid and encouraging exercise to prevent concomitant disuse atrophy [125,126,130].

A particular problem for neuromuscular physicians is the long-term use of high-dose steroids for treatment of immune-mediated neuromuscular disorders with associated weakness (eg, inflammatory myopathy, myasthenia gravis, and chronic inflammatory demyelinating polyneuropathy) [124,130,131]. The typical scenario occurs when, after an initial improvement, some patients experience a subsequent decline in muscle function. The cause of the relapse must then be determined (ie, disease exacerbation or steroid-induced weakness). If weakness occurs when the patient is taking chronic high doses of steroids, a steroid-induced myopathy perhaps is more likely. In contrast, if the weakness develops when the patient's steroids are tapered, relapse of the underlying disease process should be considered. An increasing serum CK in the case of an inflammatory myopathy points to an exacerbation of the myositis [130]. An EMG can be helpful as usually it is normal in steroid-induced myopathy as opposed to the prominent increase in spontaneous activity, myopathic MUAP, and early recruitment typically seen in inflammatory myopathies. In some cases, it may be impossible to state with certainty whether or not the new weakness is secondary to the steroid treatment or is related to a relapse of the underlying disease. The best approach in such cases is to taper the steroid medication and closely observe the patient. If improvement is observed, then the presumed cause of the worsened clinical condition is a result of the medication. Alternatively, if patients deteriorate, the weakness may be related to the underlying autoimmune disease and they may require increased doses of corticosteroids or other immunosuppressive agents.

Emetine

Emetine (Ipecac) hydrochloride has been used as an amebacide since the early part of the nineteenth century. It also is the major constituent of the emetic agent, ipecac. Patients who have eating disorders are reported to abuse ipecac. Overuse of emetine (500 to 600 mg per day for more than 10 days) can result in a profound, predominantly proximal myopathy and cardiomyopathy [132–134]. Symptoms are those of muscle pain, tenderness, and stiffness. Deep tendon reflexes usually are diminished, but the sensory examination is completely normal. Discontinuation of the medication leads to reversal of the myopathy. CK levels may be mildly to moderately elevated. The EMG examination may be normal or demonstrate increased insertional activity. Voluntary MUAPs are small amplitude with short duration and early recruitment.

Muscle histology in humans and animals who are given the medication reveals muscle atrophy of both fiber types: necrotic fibers, and small regenerating fibers. Scattered fibers contain cytoplasmic bodies. Changes in oxidative enzyme reactions result in "targetoid" or "moth-eaten" structures. On ultrastructural examination, there is evidence of myofibrillar degeneration in addition to compacted myofibrillar debris (cytoplasmic bodies). There are striking similarities between the histologic appearance of ipecac myopathy and that seen in myofibrillar myopathy (myofibrillar or desmin myopathy) [135,136].

Emetine inhibits protein synthesis. How this contributes to the associated myopathy is unclear, however. The myopathy improves with discontinuation of the emetine.

Acute quadriplegic myopathy (critical illness myopathy)

The possible causes for weakness in a patient in ICU include critical illness polyneuropathy [137], prolonged neuromuscular blockade [138,139], or acute quadraplegic myopathy. The terminology to descibe the myopathy varies and includes AQM, acute illness myopathy, critical illness myopathy, and myopathy associated with thick filament (myosin) [53,58,139–151]. In some cases, it is difficult to differentiate the myopathy from the neuropathy or from prolonged neuromuscular blockade. Not uncommonly, a combination of critical illness myopathy and neuropathy is seen. Critical illness neuropathy is reported more frequently than AQM in some series [152], whereas others find the myopathy more common [145,153,154]. In the largest series—88 patients who developed weakness while in an ICU—Lacomis et al found AQM was three times as common as critical illness polyneuropathy (42% versus 13%); prolonged neuromuscular blockade occurred in only one patient who also had AQM [145].

The first reported case of AQM occurred in a 24-year-old woman intubated for status asthmaticus with neuromuscular blockade and given high-dose intravenous corticosteroids [147]. Following the publication of this case there have been numerous reports of AQM developing in patients given high dose intravenous corticosteroids and/or nondepolarizing neuromuscular blockers [53,58,137,139–141,145,146,148–151,153,155–157]. Critically ill patients who have sepsis or multiorgan failure and who have not received either corticosteroids or nondepolarizing neuromuscular blocking agents, however, also are reported as having the disorder [142,143,150]. Transplant patients, who receive high doses of intravenous corticosteroids for prevention of rejection and neuromuscular blocking agents in the perioperative period, may be at increased risk for developing the disorder. In a prospective study of 100 consecutive adult patients undergoing liver transplantation, Campellone and colleagues report the development of AQM in seven patients [157].

Severe generalized muscle weakness develops over a period of several days in AQM. Ophthalmoplegia rarely is described as a complication [137,151]. Inability to wean off the ventilator leads to the diagnosis in many cases. Reflexes are diminished. Sensory examination usually is normal, although often it is difficult to assess in an intubated patient who has altered mental status. Deep tendon reflexes are decreased or absent. A mortality rate of 30% is reported in one large series secondary to multiple organ failure and sepsis rather than the myopathy [145]. In patients who survive, muscle strength recovers slowly over several months. Serum CK levels can be normal or moderately elevated in approximately 50% of patients.

The technique of direct muscle stimulation may be helpful in distinguishing AQM from critical illness myopathy, as described by Rich et al [149,153,158]. The amplitude of direct muscle–stimulated CMAP (dmCMAP) should be near normal despite a low or absent nerve stimulation–evoked CMAP (neCMAP) in critical illness polyneuropathy. In contrast, in myopathy, as the muscle membrane excitability is reduced, the neCMAP and dmCMAP should be very low. Theoretically, the ratio of neCMAP to dmCMAP should be close to 1:1 in a disorder of muscle membrane in-excitability and approach zero in a neuropathy or neuromuscular junction disorder. In reality, absent or reduced amplitudes of the dmCMAP with neCMAP/dmCMAP ratios greater than 0.9 were demonstrated in 11 patients who had critical illness myopathy, whereas neCMAP/dmCMAP ratios were 0.5 or less in patients who had severe neuropathy [149,153,158].

Muscle biopsies demonstrate type 2 muscle fiber atrophy with or without type 1 fiber atrophy [12,53,137,139,140,143–145,150,151] and a few reports describe muscle fiber necrosis [137,145,148,150,157]. Reactivity for myosin ATPase activity may be lost in type 1 fibers more than type 2 fibers. This corresponds to the loss of thick filaments (myosin) apparent ultrastructurally (Fig. 5) and on immunohistochemistry [12,53,139,141,142,144,145,150,157]. Actin, titin, and nebulin are spared or affected only at an advanced stage of the disease [150]. Some cases of AQM, however, do not demonstrate loss of myosin. Calpain expression is enhanced markedly in myosin-deficient AQM muscle biopsies [150].

A multifactorial etiology is likely, given the variable laboratory, histologic, and electrophysiologic features. Showalter and Engel suggest that calcium-activated proteases (calpains), which appear enhanced on muscle biopsies, may be responsible for degrading myosin [150]. Additionally, breakdown of muscle proteins, glycogen, and lipid may be related to cytokines released as a result of sepsis. Medical treatment (eg, antibiotics in sepsis and dialysis in renal failure) consists of supportive care and treating underlying systemic abnormalities. High-dose corticosteroids and non-depolarizing neuromuscular blockers should be stopped. Extensive physical therapy is required to prevent contractures and help regain muscle strength and functional abilities.

Omeprazole

Omeprazole is reported as the causative agent in several cases of neuromyopathy [144,159,160]. The predominant features are proximal weakness that primarily affects the lower extremities, paresthiasias, and a stocking distribution of sensory loss. Myalgias were reported in one patient [160]. Patients have diminished or absent deep tendon reflexes. Serum CK levels are normal or mildly elevated.

Nerve conduction studies reflect an axonal sensorimotor polyneuropathy with reduced amplitudes of SNAPs and CMAPs in the lower extremities.

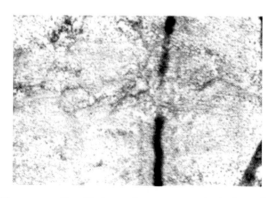

Fig. 5. Critical illness myopathy. Electron microscopy reveals the loss of the myosin thick filaments.

EMG was not mentioned in one case report, however [160]. Small polyphasic MUAPs on EMG were noted in a different patient, although nerve conduction studies were not performed [159].

Type 2 muscle fiber atrophy was the most prominent feature on muscle biopsies from two patients [159,160]. One patient had a superficial peroneal nerve biopsy, which demonstrated axonal degeneration [160]. The underlying pathogenesis for the neuromyopathy is unknown.

Muscle strength improved, sensory symptoms disappeared, and serum CK levels normalized after discontinuation of omeprazole. Symptoms recurred when omeprazole was restarted.

Drug-induced hypokalemic myopathy

Medications that cause hypokalemia include diuretics, laxatives, mineralocorticoids, amphotericin, lithium, and licorice [7]. Alcohol abuse and inhalation of toluene also are associated with hypokalemic myopathy (discussed later). Regardless of the etiology, the clinical, laboratory, histopathologic, and electrophysiologic features of hypokalemic myopathy are similar.

Malignant hyperthermia

MH is a mendelian autosomal dominant disorder precipitated by depolarizing muscle relaxants (eg, succinylcholine) and inhalational anesthetic agents (eg, halothane) [161]. It is characterized by severe muscle rigidity, myoglobinuria, fever, tachycardia, cyanosis, and cardiac arrhythmias. The incidence varies from 0.5% to 0.0005% in patients exposed to general anesthesia [161]. At least 50% of patients clinically manifesting the disorder have had previously uneventful anesthesia [162]. MH can manifest during surgery or in the postoperative period. Exercise, ingestion of caffeine, and stress rarely trigger attacks of MH [163].

Interictally serum CK can be normal or mildly elevated in patients susceptible to MH. During attacks of MH, serum CK levels are elevated markedly. Myoglobinuria and hyerkalemia can develop. Lactic acidosis, hypoxia, and hypercarbia are evident.

Neurophysiology usually is normal interictally unless the patient has a predisposing myopathic disorder (eg, muscular dystrophy). Therefore, routine nerve conductions studies and EMG are not helpful in distinguishing who may be at risk for developing MH.

The in vitro muscle contracture test is used to diagnose individuals susceptible to MH [161]. Strips of muscle are stimulated at 0.1 to 0.2 Hz for 1 to 5 seconds and tension is measured by a strain-gauge. Varying concentrations of halothane and caffeine are applied and the resultant tension produced by muscle stimulation is recorded. Compared with those without malignant hyperthermia much lower concentrations of caffeine and halothane produce muscle contractions in patients who have MH than those required in normal muscle tissue [7].

Nonspecific histopathologic features seen on muscle biopsy after an attack of MH include fiber size variability, increased internal nuclei, moth-eaten fibers, and necrotic fibers. MH is believed to arise secondary to excessive calcium release by the ryanodine receptor, a calcium channel in the sarcoplasmic reticulum. The ryanodine receptor bridges the gap between the sarcoplasmic reticulum and the T tubule. The excessive intracytoplasmic calcium leads to increased muscle contraction, increased use of oxygen and ATP, and overproduction of heat. In humans, nonsense and in-frame mutations in the RYR1 gene also are associated with central core myopathy and the moderate form of multi-minicore myopathy. The mechanism by which various anesthetic agents and depolarizing muscle relaxants trigger the exaggerated release of calcium from the sarcoplasmic reticulum via the ryanodine receptor is not known, however.

Mutations in the ryanodine receptor gene account for only a minority of patients who have MH. Other genetic loci associated with susceptibility to MH have been identified. The CACNL1A3 gene encoding the α1-subunit of the human skeletal muscle dihydropyridine-sensitive L-type voltage-dependent calcium channel (VDCC) represents the MHS2 locus and is responsible for the disease in a large French family. The mutation is localized in a very different part of the α1-subunit of the human skeletal muscle VDCC, compared with previously reported mutations found in patients who had hypokalemic periodic paralysis. Thus, the MHS2 gene seems to be allelic to potassium-sensitive periodic paralysis, paramyotonia congenita, and related disorders. Patients who are compound heterozygotes with a mutation in the ryanodine receptor and a mutation in the α subunit of the VDCC also are reported. MHS3 is linked to chromosome 7q21-q22 (in the region of a gene encoding subunit calcium channel CACNA2) [164]. A close association is formed at the skeletal muscle triadic junctions between the ryanodine receptor and the L-type VDCC, and the two channel complexes seem to function together in excitation-contraction coupling. Chromosome 3q13.1 is linked to MHS4 but the gene has yet to be identified [165]. MHS5 is caused by mutations in the dihydropteridine receptor gene on chromosome 1q31 (allelic to hypokalemic periodic paralysis) [166]. Linkage to chromosome 5p is demonstrated in other families (MHS6) [167]. In addition to these disorders, it is well known that patients who have dystrophinopathies are susceptible to developing MH [168]. Thus, various myopathic disorders affecting the structural proteins of the muscle membrane or ion channels can cause MH.

The best treatment is prevention; patients at risk for MH should not be given known triggering anesthetic agents. MH is a medical emergency requiring several therapeutic steps [161]. Initially, the anesthetic agent is discontinued while 100% oxygen is delivered. Dantrolene should be administered at a dose of 2 to 3 mg/kg every 5 minutes for a total of 10 mg/kg. The stomach, bladder, and lower gastrointestinal tract are lavaged with iced saline solution and cooling blankets are applied.

Correction of acidosis and hyperkalemia is instituted with sodium bicarbonate, hyperventilation, dextrose, insulin, and occasionally calcium chloride. Urinary output is maintained with hydration, furosemide or mannitol. The patient must be monitored and treated for cardiac arrhythmias.

Myopathies resulting from drug abuse

Alcoholic myopathy

Neuropathy is associated more commonly with chronic alcohol abuse than myopathy [71]. Despite this, however, five types of muscle disorders are recognized with respect to the toxic effects of alcohol: (1) acute necrotizing myopathy, (2) acute hypokalemic myopathy, (3) chronic alcoholic myopathy, (4) asymptomatic alcoholic myopathy, and (5) alcoholic cardiomyopathy [1,6,7,71].

Acute necrotizing myopathy usually develops in patients consuming excessive alchohol for some time. The clinical features are acute muscle pain, tenderness to palpation, cramping, swelling, weakness and markedly elevated CK after or during a recent, particularly intense binge. There is marked variability in the number, location, and degree of muscle involvement. Myoglobinuria and acute renal failure can develop in some patients. Muscle cramps resolve over the course of several days. The remainder of the symptoms often last several weeks.

Muscle histology reveals widespread muscle fiber necrosis. Marked intracellular edema is present with separation of myofibrils. Tubular aggregates have been noted. Ultrastructurally, there is disorganization of the sarcomere structure and degeneration of mitochondria. Supportive medical care and nutritional supplementation (many patients are malnourished) are the mainstay of treatment.

Acute hypokalemic myopathy, which is alcohol induced, manifests as acute generalized weakness similar to other forms of hypokalemic myopathy. It can be differentiated from acute necrotizing myopathy by the absence of muscle cramping, pain, swelling, and tenderness. Muscle weakness evolves over 1 or 2 days. CK levels are markedly elevated. Potassium level is low, ranging between 1.4 and 2.1 meq/L. If muscle biopsy is performed within the acute time frame, it demonstrates vacuolar changes. The clinical symptoms and histologic abnormalities resolve quickly once the hypokalemia is treated adequately.

Chronic alcoholic myopathy presents with an insidious onset of primarily lower limb proximal limb girdle weakness. The degree of weakness may vary. A random pattern of muscle fiber atrophy, necrosis, and regeneration can be seen on muscle biopsy. It is unclear if the disorder is caused by a toxic influence of alcohol on muscle (a true "myopathy") or if the weakness arises from malnutrition or a toxic peripheral neuropathy.

An asymptomatic alcoholic myopathy has been suggested to explain elevated serum CK levels found coincidentally in alcoholics evaluated for unrelated conditions. These patients do not complain of weakness and their physical examination does not reveal striking evidence of a myopathic disorder. Muscle biopsy histology is unknown for this class of patients and the true nature of this presumed form of alcoholic myopathy is questionable. The etiology of the elevated serum CK may be related to subclinical necrotizing myopathy, hypokalemia, or muscle trauma [7].

Some patients presenting with acute muscle weakness (acute necrotizing myopathy or hypokalemic myopathy) and alcohol abuse have normal or only mildly abnormal sensory and motor studies. EMG examination of the proximal muscles demostrates increased insertional activity, and short-duration, low-amplitude MUAPs firing at high rates with minimal force production [169–174]. These patients seem to have a primary myopathic process with little evidence of a peripheral neuropathy. Treated with medical support and correction of any electrolyte disturbances, the membrane instability resolves and there is little in the way of residual MUAP abnormalities.

The frequent occurrence of a sensorimotor peripheral neuropathy in patients who have a history of chronic excess alcohol abuse [173,175–179,180] can lead to diagnostic confusion with respect to the presence or absence of a myopathic process, clinically and on electrophysiologic testing.

The mechanism by which alcohol causes these myopathies is not known. Alcohol's metabolism may lead to the accumulation of toxic metabolites (eg, acetaldehyde) or free radicals, which may be toxic to lipid membranes [71]. Alcohol also may have a direct toxic effect on various ion channels. There is speculation by some investigators that chronic alcohol abuse impairs glycolysis and glycogenolysis [181,182]. Detailed biochemical studies, however, do not confirm defects in oxidative metabolism [183]. Further work is required to elucidate fully the pathogenic role of alcohol in myopathies.

Myopathies secondary to illicit drugs

Muscle fiber necrosis has been reported with use of illicit drugs and controlled narcotics (heroin, meperidine, cocaine, pentazocine, piritramide, amphetamines, and so forth) [1,6,7,184–187]. There are several mechanisms of muscle injury, including direct muscle trauma (eg, needle injury), rhabdomyolysis secondary to pressure and ischemic necrosis related to prolonged loss of consciousness, ischemia resulting from vasoconstriction, rhabdomyolysis caused by generalized status epilepticus, and the direct toxic effects of the drugs (or adulterants) on muscle tissue. Serum CK levels are markedly elevated. Nerve conduction studies are normal. Needle EMG examination reveals fibrillation potentials and positive sharp waves. MUAP with short durations and small amplitude are recruited early with minimal contraction. Muscle biopsies demonstrate widespread necrosis.

Inhalation of volatile agents (eg, toluene) also causes generalized muscle weakness and, occasionally, myoglobinuria. Toluene causes distal renal tubular acidosis with associated severe hypokalemia, hypophosphatemia, and mild hypocalcemia. Muscle strength returns after correction of the electrolyte abnormalities and abstaining from inhaling volatile agents [7].

References

[1] Argov Z. Drug-induced neuromuscular disorders in man. 5th edition. Edinburgh (Scotland): Churchill-Livingstone; 1988.
[2] Baker PC. Drug-induced and toxic myopathies. Semin Neurol 1983;3:265–73.
[3] Griggs RC, Mendell JR, Miller RG. Myopathies of systemic disease. Philadelphia: FA Davis; 1995.
[4] Kuncl RW, George EB. Toxic neuropathies and myopathies. Curr Opin Neurol 1993;6: 695–704.
[5] Lane RJ, Mastaglia FL. Drug-induced myopathies in man. Lancet 1978;2:562–6.
[6] Mastaglia FL. Toxic myopathies, vol. 18. Amsterdam: Elsevier Science; 1992.
[7] Amato AA, Dumitru D. Acquired myopathies. In: Dumitru D, Amato AA, Zwarts MJ, editors. Electrodiagnostic medicine. 2nd edition. Philadelphia: Hanley & Belfus; 2002. p. 1265–432.
[8] Abourizk N, Khalil BA, Bahuth N, et al. Clofibrate-induced muscular syndrome. Report of a case with clinical, electromyographic and pathologic observations. J Neurol Sci 1979; 42:1–9.
[9] Denizot M, Fabre J, Pometta D, et al. Clofibrate, nephrotic syndrome, and histological changes in muscle. Lancet 1973;1:1326.
[10] Duell PB, Connor WE, Illingworth DR. Rhabdomyolysis after taking atorvastatin with gemfibrozil. Am J Cardiol 1998;81:368–9.
[11] Gabriel R, Pearce JM. Clofibrate-induced myopathy and neuropathy. Lancet 1976;2: 906.
[12] Kwiecinski H. Myotonia induced with clofibrate in rats. J Neurol 1978;219:107–16.
[13] Langer T, Levy RI. Acute muscular syndrome associated with administration of clofibrate. N Engl J Med 1968;279:856–8.
[14] London SF, Gross KF, Ringel SP. Cholesterol-lowering agent myopathy (CLAM). Neurology 1991;41:1159–60.
[15] MacLennan DH, Phillips MS. Malignant hyperthermia. Science 1992;256:789–94.
[16] Marais GE, Larson KK. Rhabdomyolysis and acute renal failure induced by combination lovastatin and gemfibrozil therapy. Ann Intern Med 1990;112:228–30.
[17] Pierce LR, Wysowski DK, Gross TP. Myopathy and rhabdomyolysis associated with lovastatin-gemfibrozil combination therapy. JAMA 1990;264:71–5.
[18] Pierides AM, Alvarez-Ude F, Kerr DN. Clofibrate-induced muscle damage in patients with chronic renal failure. Lancet 1975;2:1279–82.
[19] Rush P, Baron M, Kapusta M. Clofibrate myopathy: a case report and a review of the literature. Semin Arthritis Rheumatol 1986;15:226–9.
[20] Shepherd J. Fibrates and statins in the treatment of hyperlipidaemia: an appraisal of their efficacy and safety. Eur Heart J 1995;16:5–13.
[21] Furberg CD, Pitt B. Commentary: withdrawal of cervistatin from the world market. Curr Control Trials Cardiovasc Med 2001;2:205–7.
[22] Corpier CL, Jones PH, Suki WN, et al. Rhabdomyolysis and renal injury with lovastatin use. Report of two cases in cardiac transplant recipients. JAMA 1988;260:239–41.

[23] Jones P, Kafonek S, Laurora I, Hunninghake D. Comparative dose efficacy study of atorvastatin versus simvastatin, pravastatin, lovastatin, and fluvastatin in patients with hypercholesterolemia (the CURVES study). Am J Cardiol 1998;81:582–7.

[24] Reaven P, Witztum JL. Lovastatin, nicotinic acid, and rhabdomyolysis. Ann Intern Med 1988;109:597–8.

[25] Tobert JA. Efficacy and long-term adverse effect pattern of lovastatin. Am J Cardiol 1988; 62:28J–34J.

[26] Galper JB. Increased incidence of myositis in patients treated with high-dose simvastatin. Am J Cardiol 1998;81:259.

[27] Deslypere JP, Vermeulen A. Rhabdomyolysis and simvastatin. Ann Intern Med 1991;114: 342.

[28] Davidson MH, Stein EA, Dujovne CA, et al. The efficacy and six-week tolerability of simvastatin 80 and 160 mg/day. Am J Cardiol 1997;79:38–42.

[29] Berland Y, Vacher Coponat H, Durand C, et al. Rhabdomyolysis with simvastatin use. Nephron 1991;57:365–6.

[30] Schalke BB, Schmidt B, Toyka K, et al. Pravastatin-associated inflammatory myopathy. N Engl J Med 1992;327:649–50.

[31] Bakker-Arkema RG, Best J, Fayyad R, et al. A brief review paper of the efficacy and safety of atorvastatin in early clinical trials. Atherosclerosis 1997;131:17–23.

[32] von Keutz E, Schluter G. Preclinical safety evaluation of cerivastatin, a novel HMG-CoA reductase inhibitor. Am J Cardiol 1998;82:11J–7J.

[33] Hodel C. Myopathy and rhabdomyolysis with lipid-lowering drugs. Toxicol Lett 2002;128: 159–68.

[34] Hamilton-Craig I. Statin-associated myopathy. Med J Aust 2001;175:486–9.

[35] Pasternak RC, Smith SC Jr, Bairey-Merz CN, et al. ACC/AHA/NHLBI clinical advisory on the use and safety of statins. J Am Coll Cardiol 2002;40:567–72.

[36] Staffa JA, Chang J, Green L. Cerivastatin and reports of fatal rhabdomyolysis. N Engl J Med 2002;346:539–40.

[37] Litin SC, Anderson CF. Nicotinic acid-associated myopathy: a report of three cases. Am J Med 1989;86:481–3.

[38] Ayanian JZ, Fuchs CS, Stone RM. Lovastatin and rhabdomyolysis. Ann Intern Med 1988; 109:682–3.

[39] Mousa O, Brater DC, Sunblad KJ, et al. The interaction of diltiazem with simvastatin. Clin Pharmacol Ther 2000;67:267–74.

[40] Kanathur N, Mathai MG, Byrd RP Jr, et al. Simvastatin-diltiazem drug interaction resulting in rhabdomyolysis and hepatitis. Tenn Med 2001;94:339–41.

[41] Lewin JJ 3rd, Nappi JM, Taylor MH. Rhabdomyolysis with concurrent atorvastatin and diltiazem. Ann Pharmacother 2002;36:1546–9.

[42] Flint OP, Masters BA, Gregg RE, et al. Inhibition of cholesterol synthesis by squalene synthase inhibitors does not induce myotoxicity in vitro. Toxicol Appl Pharmacol 1997; 145:91–8.

[43] Folkers K, Langsjoen P, Willis R, et al. Lovastatin decreases coenzyme Q levels in humans. Proc Natl Acad Sci USA 1990;8:8931–4.

[44] Amato AA, Barohn RJ. Neurological complications of transplantations. In: Harati Y, Rolack LA, editors. Practical neuroimmunology. Boston: Butterworth-Heineman; 1997. p. 341–75.

[45] Arellano F, Krup P. Muscular disorders associated with cyclosporine [letter]. Lancet 1991; 337:915.

[46] Costigan DA. Acquired myotonia, weakness and vacuolar myopathy secondary to cyclosporine [abstract]. Muscle Nerve 1989;12:761.

[47] Goy JJ, Stauffer JC, Deruaz JP, et al. Myopathy as possible side-effect of cyclosporin. Lancet 1989;1:1446–7.

[48] Grezard O, Lebranchu Y, Birmele B, et al. Cyclosporin-induced muscular toxicity. Lancet 1990;335:177.

[49] Noppen M, Velkeniers B, Dierckx R, et al. Cyclosporine and myopathy. Ann Intern Med 1987;107:945–6.

[50] Norman DJ, Illingworth DR, Munson J, et al. Myolysis and acute renal failure in a heart-transplant recipient receiving lovastatin. N Engl J Med 1988;318:46–7.

[51] Rieger EH, Halasz NA, Wahlstrom HE. Colchicine neuromyopathy after renal transplantation. Transplantation 1990;49:1196–8.

[52] Volin L, Jarventie G, Ruutu T. Fatal rhabdomyolysis as a complication of bone marrow transplantation. Bone Marrow Transplant 1990;6:59–60.

[53] Hirano M, Ott BR, Raps EC, et al. Acute quadriplegic myopathy: a complication of treatment with steroids, nondepolarizing blocking agents, or both. Neurology 1992;42:2082–7.

[54] Atkison P, Joubert G, Barron A, et al. Hypertrophic cardiomyopathy associated with tacrolimus in paediatric transplant patients. Lancet 1995;345:894–6.

[55] Hanna JP, Ramundo ML. Rhabdomyolysis and hypoxia associated with prolonged propofol infusion in children. Neurology 1998;50:301–3.

[56] Parke TJ, Stevens JE, Rice AS, et al. Metabolic acidosis and fatal myocardial failure after propofol infusion in children: five case reports. BMJ 1992;305:613–6.

[57] Strickland RA, Murray MJ. Fatal metabolic acidosis in a pediatric patient receiving an infusion of propofol in the intensive care unit: is there a relationship? Crit Care Med 1995;23:405–9.

[58] Hanson P, Dive A, Brucher JM, et al. Acute corticosteroid myopathy in intensive care patients. Muscle Nerve 1997;20:1371–80.

[59] Teicher A, Rosenthal T, Kissin E. Labetalol-induced toxic myopathy. Br Med J (Clin Res Ed) 1981;282:1824–5.

[60] Willis JK, Tilton AH, Harkin JC, et al. Reversible myopathy due to labetalol. Pediatr Neurol 1990;6:275–6.

[61] Eadie MJ, Ferrier TM. Chloroquine myopathy. J Neurol Neurosurg Psychiatry 1966;29:331–7.

[62] Estes ML, Ewing-Wilson D, Chou SM, et al. Chloroquine neuromyotoxicity. Clinical and pathologic perspective. Am J Med 1987;82:447–55.

[63] Mastaglia FL. Adverse effects of drugs on muscle. Drugs 1982;24:304–21.

[64] Mastaglia FL, Papadimitriou JM, Dawkins RL, et al. Vacuolar myopathy associated with chloroquine, lupus erythematosus and thymoma. Report of a case with unusual mitochondrial changes and lipid accumulation in muscle. J Neurol Sci 1977;34:315–328.

[65] Costa-Jussa FR, Jacobs JM. The pathology of amiodarone neurotoxicity. I. Experimental studies with reference to changes in other tissues. Brain 1985;108(Pt 3):735–52.

[66] Masanes F, Barrientos A, Cebrian M, et al. Clinical, histological and molecular reversibility of zidovudine myopathy. J Neurol Sci 1998;159:226–8.

[67] Alderson K, Griffin JW, Cornblath DR, et al. Neuromuscular complications of amiodarone therapy. Neurology 1987;37(Suppl):355.

[68] Jacobs JM, Costa-Jussa FR. The pathology of amiodarone neurotoxicity. II. Peripheral neuropathy in man. Brain 1985;108(Pt 3):753–69.

[69] Meier C, Kauer B, Muller U, Ludin HP. Neuromyopathy during chronic amiodarone treatment. A case report. J Neurol 1979;220:231–9.

[70] Fernando Roth R, Itabashi H, Louie J, et al. Amiodarone toxicity: myopathy and neuropathy. Am Heart J 1990;119:1223–5.

[71] Victor M, Sieb JP. Myopathies due to drugs, toxins, and nutritional deficiency. 2nd edition. New York: McGraw Hill; 1994.

[72] Kuncl RW, Cornblath DR, Avila O, Duncan G. Electrodiagnosis of human colchicine myoneuropathy. Muscle Nerve 1989;12:360–4.

[73] Kuncl RW, Duncan G, Watson D, et al. Colchicine myopathy and neuropathy. N Engl J Med 1987;316:1562–8.

[74] Riggs JE, Schochet SS Jr, Gutmann L, et al. Chronic human colchicine neuropathy and myopathy. Arch Neurol 1986;43:521–3.

[75] Rutkove SB, De Girolami U, Preston DC, et al. Myotonia in colchicine myoneuropathy. Muscle Nerve 1996;19:870–5.

[76] Bradley WG, Lassman LP, Pearce GW, et al. The neuromyopathy of vincristine in man. Clinical, electrophysiological and pathological studies. J Neurol Sci 1970;10:107–31.

[77] Bailey RO, Turok DI, Jaufmann BP, et al. Myositis and acquired immunodeficiency syndrome. Hum Pathol 1987;18:749–51.

[78] Bessen LJ, Greene JB, Louie E, et al. Severe polymyositis-like syndrome associated with zidovudine therapy of AIDS and ARC. N Engl J Med 1988;318:708.

[79] Chalmers AC, Greco CM, Miller RG. Prognosis in AZT myopathy. Neurology 1991;41: 1181–4.

[80] Dalakas MC, Illa I, Pezeshkpour GH, et al. Mitochondrial myopathy caused by long-term zidovudine therapy. N Engl J Med 1990;322:1098–105.

[81] Grau JM, Masanes F, Pedrol E, et al. Human immunodeficiency virus type 1 infection and myopathy: clinical relevance of zidovudine therapy. Ann Neurol 1993;34:206–11.

[82] Reyes MG, Casanova J, Varricchio F, et al. Zidovudine myopathy. Neurology 1992;42: 1252.

[83] Manji H, Harrison MJ, Round JM, et al. Muscle disease, HIV and zidovudine: the spectrum of muscle disease in HIV-infected individuals treated with zidovudine. J Neurol 1993;240:479–88.

[84] Peters BS, Winer J, Landon DN, et al. Mitochondrial myopathy associated with chronic zidovudine therapy in AIDS. Q J Med 1993;86:5–15.

[85] Simpson DM, Bender AN. Human immunodeficiency virus-associated myopathy: analysis of 11 patients. Ann Neurol 1988;24:79–84.

[86] Simpson DM, Bender AN, Farraye J, et al. Human immunodeficiency virus wasting syndrome may represent a treatable myopathy. Neurology 1990;40(3 Pt 1):535–8.

[87] Simpson DM, Citak KA, Godfrey E, et al. Myopathies associated with human immunodeficiency virus and zidovudine: can their effects be distinguished? Neurology 1993;43:971–6.

[88] Till M, MacDonell KB. Myopathy with human immunodeficiency virus type 1 (HIV-1) infection: HIV-1 or zidovudine? Ann Intern Med 1990;113:492–4.

[89] Mhiri C, Baudrimont M, Bonne G, et al. Zidovudine myopathy: a distinctive disorder associated with mitochondrial dysfunction. Ann Neurol 1991;29:606–14.

[90] McComas AJ, Sica RE, McNabb AR, et al. Evidence for reversible motoneurone dysfunction in thyrotoxicosis. J Neurol Neurosurg Psychiatry 1974;37:548–58.

[91] Simpson DM, Slasor P, Dafni U, et al. Analysis of myopathy in a placebo-controlled zidovudine trial. Muscle Nerve 1997;20:382–5.

[92] Jay CA, Hench K, Ropka M. Improvement of AZT myopathy after change to dideoxyinsine (ddI) or dideoxycytosine (ddC) [abstract]. Neurology 1993;43(Suppl 2): A373–4.

[93] Benbrik E, Chariot P, Bonavaud S, et al. Cellular and mitochondrial toxicity of zidovudine (AZT), didanosine (ddI) and zalcitabine (ddC) on cultured human muscle cells. J Neurol Sci 1997;149:19–25.

[94] Pedrol E, Masanes F, Fernandez-Sola J, et al. Lack of muscle toxicity with didanosine (ddI). Clinical and experimental studies. J Neurol Sci 1996;138:42–8.

[95] Callens S, De Roo A, Colebunders R. Fanconi-like syndrome and rhabdomyolysis in a person with HIV infection on highly active antiretroviral treatment including tenofovir. J Infect 2003;47:262–3.

[96] Mah Ming JB, Gill MJ. Drug-induced rhabdomyolysis after concomitant use of clarithromycin atorvastatin, lopinavir/ritanovir in a patient with HIV. AIDS Patient Care STDS 2003;17:207–10.

[97] Simpson DM, Katzenstein DA, Hughes MD, et al. Neuromuscular function in HIV infection: analysis of a placebo-controlled combination antiretroviral trial. AIDS Clinical Group 175/801 Study Team. AIDS 1998;12:2425–32.

[98] Sieb JP, Gillessen T. Iatrogenic and toxic myopathies. Muscle Nerve 2003;27:142–56.

[99] Smith BE, Dyck PJ. Peripheral neuropathy in the eosinophilia-myalgia syndrome associated with L-tryptophan ingestion. Neurology 1990;40:1035–40.

[100] Sakimoto K. The cause of the eosinophilia-myalgia syndrome associated with tryptophan use. N Engl J Med 1990;323:992–3.

[101] Sagman DL, Melamed JC. L-tryptophan-induced eosinophilia-myalgia syndrome and myopathy. Neurology 1990;40:1629–30.

[102] Hertzman PA, Blevins WL, Mayer J, et al. Association of the eosinophilia-myalgia syndrome with the ingestion of tryptophan. N Engl J Med 1990;322:869–73.

[103] Donofrio PD, Stanton C, Miller VS, et al. Demyelinating polyneuropathy in eosinophilia-myalgia syndrome. Muscle Nerve 1992;15:796–805.

[104] Belongia EA, Hedberg CW, Gleich GJ, et al. An investigation of the cause of the eosinophilia-myalgia syndrome associated with tryptophan use. N Engl J Med 1990;323: 357–65.

[105] Heiman-Patterson TD, Bird SJ, Parry GJ, et al. Peripheral neuropathy associated with eosinophilia-myalgia syndrome. Ann Neurol 1990;28:522–8.

[106] Selwa JF, Feldman EL, Blaivas M. Mononeuropathy multiplex in tryptophan-associated eosinophilia-myalgia syndrome. Neurology 1990;40:1632–3.

[107] Turi GK, Solitare GB, James N, et al. Eosinophilia-myalgia syndrome (L-tryptophan-associated neuromyopathy). Neurology 1990;40:1793–6.

[108] Harney J, Glasberg MR. Myopathy and hypersensitivity to phenytoin. Neurology 1983;33: 790–1.

[109] Kilbourne EM, Rigau-Perez JG, Heath CW Jr, et al. Clinical epidemiology of toxic-oil syndrome. Manifestations of a new illness. N Engl J Med 1983;309:1408–14.

[110] Mayeno AN, Belongia EA, Lin F, et al. 3-(Phenylamino)alanine, a novel aniline-derived amino acid associated with the eosinophilia-myalgia syndrome: a link to the toxic oil syndrome? Mayo Clin Proc 1992;67:1134–9.

[111] Dawkins RL, Zilko PJ, Carrano J, et al. Immunobiology of D-penicillamine. J Rheumatol Suppl 1981;7:56–61.

[112] Hall JT, Fallahi S, Koopman WJ. Penicillamine-induced myositis: observations and unique features in two patients and review of the literature. Am J Med 1984;77:719.

[113] Takahashi K, Ogita T, Okudaira H, et al. D-penicillamine-induced polymyositis in patients with rheumatoid arthritis. Arthritis Rheum 1986;29:560–4.

[114] Taneja V, Mehra N, Singh YN. HLA-D region genes and susceptibility to D-penicillamine-induced polymyositis. Arthritis Rheum 1990;33:1445–7.

[115] Fontiveros ES, Cumming WJ, Hudgson P. Procainamide-induced myositis. J Neurol Sci 1980;45:143–7.

[116] Lewis CA, Boheimer N, Rose P, et al. Myopathy after short term administration of procainamide. Br Med J (Clin Res Ed) 1986;292:593–4.

[117] Cirigliano G, Della Rossa A, Tavoni A, et al. Polymyositis occurring during alpha-interferon treatment for malignant melanoma: a case report and review of the literature. Rheumatol Int 1999;19:65–7.

[118] Dietrich LL, Bridges AJ, Albertini MR. Dermatomyositis after interferon alpha treatment. Med Oncol 2000;17:64–9.

[119] Hengstman GJ, Vogels OJ, ter Laak HJ, et al. Myositis during long-term interferon-alpha treatment. Neurology 2000;54:2186.

[120] Srinivasan J, Wu C, Amato AA. Inflammatory myopathy associated with imitinab therapy. J Clin Neuromusc Dis 2004;5:119–21.

[121] Coomes EN. The rate of recovery of reversible myopathies and the effects of anabolic agents in steroid myopathy. Neurology 1965;15:523–30.

[122] Engel AG. Metabolic and endocrine myopathies. 5th edition. Edinburgh (Scotland): Churchill-Livingstone; 1988.

[123] Golding DN, Murray SM, et al. Corticosteroid myopathy. Ann Phys Med 1961;6:171–7.

[124] Williams RS. Triamcinolone myopathy. Lancet 1959;1:698–701.

[125] Kissel JT, Mendell JR. The endocrine myopathies. In: Rowland LP, DiMauro S, editors. Handbook of clinical neurology, vol. 18. Amsterdam (the Netherlands): Elsevier Science Publishers; 1992. p. 527–51.

[126] Faludi G, Gotlieb J, Meyers J. Factors influencing the development of steroid-induced myopathies. Ann N Y Acad Sci 1966;138:62–72.

[127] Hudgson P, Kendall-Taylor P. Endocrine myopathies. In: Mastaglia FL, Walton JN, editors. Skeletal muscle pathology. Edinburgh (Scotland): Churchill Livingstone; 1992. p. 493–509.

[128] Pleasure DE, Walsh GO, Engel WK. Atrophy of skeletal muscle in patients with Cushing's syndrome. Arch Neurol 1970;22:118–25.

[129] Kaminski HJ, Ruff RL. Endocrine myopathies (hyper- and hypofunction of adrenal, thyroid, pituitary, and parathyroid glands and iatrogenic corticosteroid myopathy). In: Engel AG, Franzini-Armstrong C, editors. Myology. 2nd edition. New York: McGraw-Hill; 1994. p. 1726–53.

[130] Amato AA, Barohn RJ. Idiopathic inflammatory myopathies. Neurol Clin 1997;15: 615–48.

[131] Maclean K, Schurr PH. Reversible amyotrophy complicating treatment with fludrocortisone. Lancet 1959;1:701–3.

[132] Bennett HS, Spiro AJ, Pollack MA, et al. Ipecac-induced myopathy simulating dermatomyositis. Neurology 1982;32:91–4.

[133] Mateer JE, Farrell BJ, Chou SS, et al. Reversible ipecac myopathy. Arch Neurol 1985;42: 188–90.

[134] Palmer EP, Guay AT. Reversible myopathy secondary to abuse of ipecac in patients with major eating disorders. N Engl J Med 1985;313:1457–9.

[135] Amato AA, Jackson CE, Lampkin S, et al. Myofibrillar myopathy: no evidence of apoptosis by TUNEL. Neurology 1999;52:861–3.

[136] Amato AA, Kagan-Hallet K, Jackson CE, et al. The wide spectrum of myofibrillar myopathy suggests a multifactorial etiology and pathogenesis. Neurology 1998;51: 1646–55.

[137] Zochodne DW, Ramsay DA, Saly V, et al. Acute necrotizing myopathy of intensive care: electrophysiological studies. Muscle Nerve 1994;17:285–92.

[138] Barohn RJ, Jackson CE, Rogers SJ, et al. Prolonged paralysis due to nondepolarizing neuromuscular blocking agents and corticosteroids. Muscle Nerve 1994;17:647–54.

[139] Gooch JL. AAEM case report #29: prolonged paralysis after neuromuscular blockade. Muscle Nerve 1995;18:937–42.

[140] al-Lozi MT, Pestronk A, Yee WC, Flaris N, et al. Rapidly evolving myopathy with myosin-deficient muscle fibers. Ann Neurol 1994;35:273–9.

[141] Danon MJ, Carpenter S. Myopathy with thick filament (myosin) loss following prolonged paralysis with vecuronium during steroid treatment. Muscle Nerve 1991;14: 1131–9.

[142] Deconinck N, Van Parijs V, Beckers-Bleukx G, et al. Critical illness myopathy unrelated to corticosteroids or neuromuscular blocking agents. Neuromuscul Disord 1998;8:186–92.

[143] Gutmann L, Blumenthal D, Schochet SS. Acute type II myofiber atrophy in critical illness. Neurology 1996;46:819–21.

[144] Lacomis D, Giuliani MJ, Van Cott A, et al. Acute myopathy of intensive care: clinical, electromyographic, and pathological aspects. Ann Neurol 1996;40:645–54.

[145] Lacomis D, Petrella JT, Giuliani MJ. Causes of neuromuscular weakness in the intensive care unit: a study of ninety-two patients. Muscle Nerve 1998;21:610–7.

[146] Lacomis D, Smith TW, Chad DA. Acute myopathy and neuropathy in status asthmaticus: case report and literature review. Muscle Nerve 1993;16:84–90.

[147] MacFarlane IA, Rosenthal FD. Severe myopathy after status asthmaticus. Lancet 1977; 2:615.

[148] Ramsay DA, Zochodne DW, Robertson DM, et al. A syndrome of acute severe muscle necrosis in intensive care unit patients. J Neuropathol Exp Neurol 1993;52:387–98.

[149] Rich MM, Teener JW, Raps EC, et al. Muscle is electrically inexcitable in acute quadriplegic myopathy. Neurology 1996;46:731–6.

[150] Showalter CJ, Engel AG. Acute quadriplegic myopathy: analysis of myosin isoforms and evidence for calpain-mediated proteolysis. Muscle Nerve 1997;20:316–22.

[151] Sitwell LD, Weinshenker BG, Monpetit V, et al. Complete ophthalmoplegia as a complication of acute corticosteroid- and pancuronium-associated myopathy. Neurology 1991;41:921–2.

[152] Witt NJ, Zochodne DW, Bolton CF, et al. Peripheral nerve function in sepsis and multiple organ failure. Chest 1991;99:176–84.

[153] Rich MM, Bird SJ, Raps EC, et al. Direct muscle stimulation in acute quadriplegic myopathy. Muscle Nerve 1997;20:665–73.

[154] Latronico N, Fenzi F, Recupero D, et al. Critical illness myopathy and neuropathy. Lancet 1996;347:1579–82.

[155] Road J, Mackie G, Jiang TX, et al. Reversible paralysis with status asthmaticus, steroids, and pancuronium: clinical electrophysiological correlates. Muscle Nerve 1997;20: 1587–90.

[156] Landrigan PJ. Illness in Gulf War veterans. Causes and consequences. JAMA 1997;277: 259–61.

[157] Campellone JV, Lacomis D, Kramer DJ, et al. Acute myopathy after liver transplantation. Neurology 1998;50:46–53.

[158] Rich MM, Pinter MJ, Kraner SD, et al. Loss of electrical excitability in an animal model of acute quadriplegic myopathy. Ann Neurol 1998;43:171–9.

[159] Garrot FJ, Lacambrac D, Del Sert T, et al. Subacute myopathy during omeprazole therapy [letter]. Lancet 1994;340:672.

[160] Faucheux JM, Tournebize P, Viguier A, et al. Neuromyopathy secondary to omeprazole treatment. Muscle Nerve 1998;21:261–2.

[161] Bertorini TE. Myoglobinuria, malignant hyperthermia, neuroleptic malignant syndrome and serotonin syndrome. Neurol Clin 1997;15:649–71.

[162] Griggs RC, Mendell JR, Miller RG. Myopathies of systemic disease. Evaluation and treatment of myopathies. Philadelphia: FA Davis; 1995. p. 355–85.

[163] Nelson TE, Flewellen EH. Current concepts. The malignant hyperthermia syndrome. N Engl J Med 1983;309:416–8.

[164] Iles DE, Lehmann-Horn F, Scherer SW, et al. Localization of the gene encoding the alpha 2/delta-subunits of the L-type voltage-dependent calcium channel to chromosome 7q and analysis of the segregation of flanking markers in malignant hyperthermia susceptible families. Hum Mol Genet 1994;3:969–75.

[165] Sudbrak R, Procaccio V, Klausnitzer M, et al. Mapping of a further malignant hyperthermia susceptibility locus to chromosome 3q13.1. Am J Hum Genet 1995;56: 684–91.

[166] Monnier N, Procaccio V, Stieglitz P, et al. Malignant-hyperthermia susceptibility is associated with a mutation of the alpha 1-subunit of the human dihydropyridine-sensitive L-type voltage-dependent calcium-channel receptor in skeletal muscle. Am J Hum Genet 1997;60:1316–25.

[167] Robinson RL, Monnier N, Wolz W, et al. A genome wide search for susceptibility loci in three European malignant hyperthermia pedigrees. Hum Mol Genet 1997;6:953–61.

[168] Sethna NF, Rockoff MA, Worthen HM, et al. Anesthesia-related complications in children with Duchenne muscular dystrophy. Anesthesiology 1988;68:462–5.

[169] Hibi S, Misawa A, Tamai M, et al. Severe rhabdomyolysis associated with tacrolimus. Lancet 1995;346:702.

[170] Ekbom K, Hed R, Kirstein L, et al. Muscular affections in chronic alcoholism. Arch Neurol 1964;10:449–58.

[171] Mayer RF, Garcia-Mullin R, Eckholdt JW. Acute "alcoholic" myopathy. Neurology 1968; 18:275.

[172] Oh SJ. Chronic alcoholic myopathy: an entity difficult to diagnose. South Med J 1972;65: 449–52.

[173] Perkoff GT. Alcoholic myopathy. Annu Rev Med 1971;22:125–32.

[174] Rubenstein AE, Wainapel SF. Acute hypokalemic myopathy in alcoholism. A clinical entity. Arch Neurol 1977;34:553–5.

[175] Faris AA, Reyes MG. Reappraisal of alcoholic myopathy. Clinical and biopsy study on chronic alcoholics without muscle weakness or wasting. J Neurol Neurosurg Psychiatry 1971;34:86–92.

[176] Faris AA, Reyes MG, Abrams BM. Subclinical alcoholic myopathy: electromyographic and biopsy study. Trans Am Neurol Assoc 1967;92:102–6.

[177] Norman MG, Temple AR, Murphy JV. Infantile quadriceps-femoris contracture resulting from intramuscular injections. N Engl J Med 1970;282:964–6.

[178] Oh SJ. Alcoholic myopathy, a critical review. Ala J Med Sci 1972;9:79–95.

[179] Rossouw JE, Keeton RG, Hewlett RH. Chronic proximal muscular weakness in alcoholics. S Afr Med J 1976;50:2095–8.

[180] Worden RE. Pattern of muscle and nerve pathology in alcoholism. Ann N Y Acad Sci 1976; 273:351–9.

[181] Trounce I, Byrne E, Dennett X. Biochemical and morphological studies of skeletal muscle in experimental chronic alcoholic myopathy. Acta Neurol Scand 1990;82:386–91.

[182] Bollaert PE, Robin-Lherbier B, Escanye JM, et al. Phosphorus nuclear magnetic resonance evidence of abnormal skeletal muscle metabolism in chronic alcoholics. Neurology 1989;39: 821–4.

[183] Cardellach F, Galofre J, Grau JM, et al. Oxidative metabolism in muscle mitochondria from patients with chronic alcoholism. Ann Neurol 1992;31:515–8.

[184] Cogen FC, Rigg G, Simmons JL, et al. Phencyclidine-associated acute rhabdomyolysis. Ann Intern Med 1978;88:210–2.

[185] Richter RW, Pearson J, Bruun B, et al. Neurological complications of addiction to heroin. Bull N Y Acad Med 1973;49:3–21.

[186] Richter RW, Challenor YB, Pearson J, et al. Acute myoglobinuria associated with heroin addiction. JAMA 1971;216:1172–6.

[187] Van den Bergh PY, Guettat L, Vande Berg BC, et al. Focal myopathy associated with chronic intramuscular injection of piritramide. Muscle Nerve 1997;20:1598–600.

ELSEVIER
SAUNDERS

NEUROLOGIC
CLINICS

Neurol Clin 23 (2005) 429–459

Toxin-Induced Movement Disorders

Eric J. Pappert, MD

Division of Neurology, Department of Medicine, University of Texas, Health Science Center,
2379 NE Loop 410, Suite 12, San Antonio, TX 78217, USA

The term *movement disorder* includes a vast array of conditions exemplified by abnormalities of volitional motor control or by the presence of excessive involuntary movements. Typically, disorders of the spinal cord, motor neuron, peripheral nerve, muscle, or impairment of the execution of learned sequences of movement are excluded from this group of disorders. Movement disorders have traditionally been divided into two classes: hypokinetic and hyperkinetic. Hypokinetic disorders are characterized by a delay in the initiation of movement, and when the movement occurs, it is slow and low in amplitude. Hyperkinetic disorders, characterized by spontaneous, involuntary movements, include dystonia, chorea, myoclonus, tic, and tremor. Often, however, hypokinetic and hyperkinetic components are present in the same disorder.

Movement disorders occur as part of idiopathic or genetic diseases, but may also present in the setting of metabolic, vascular, infectious, and endocrinologic abnormalities. The use of certain classes of prescription drugs, including antipsychotics, selective serotonin reuptake inhibitors, and antiepileptics, may also result in certain abnormalities of movement. Comprehensive reviews of this subject have previously been published [1–3] and are not considered further. Movement disorders have also occurred following exposure to neurotoxins (Table 1). These compounds have been classified as heavy metals, gases, pesticides, organic solvents, and other chemicals. Although the neurologic manifestations of poisoning by certain toxins have been attributed to cellular hypoxia due to mitochondrial dysfunction or to the generation of free radicals, some agents are relatively selective in their toxicity to lenticular or striatal neurons and produce signs and symptoms related to these structures [4,5]. This article reviews the movement disorders that may occur following exposure to various environmental and industrial toxins.

E-mail address: pappert@uthscsa.edu

Table 1
Toxin-induced movement disorders in humans

Toxin	Parkinsonism	Dystonia	Chorea	Myoclonus	Tics	Tremor
Aluminum	No	No	No	Yes	No	Yes
Amphetamine	No	Possible	Yes	Yes	Yes	No
Bismuth	No	No	No	Yes	No	No
Butane	No	Yes	No	Yes	No	No
Carbon disulfide	Yes	No	No	No	No	Yes
Carbon monoxide	Yes	Yes	Yes	No	Yes	Yes
Carbon tetrachloride	Yes	No	No	No	No	No
Chlordecone	No	No	No	Yes	No	Yes
Cocaine	No	Possible	Yes	No	Yes	No
Cyanide	Yes	No	No	No	No	Yes
Cycad seed	Yes	No	No	No	No	Yes
Dichloroethane	No	No	No	Yes	No	No
Dioxin	No	Yes	No	No	No	Yes
Ethyl alcohol	Yes	Yes	Yes	No	No	Yes
Gasoline	No	No	Yes	No	No	No
Glue	No	No	Yes	No	No	No
Manganese	Yes	No	No	Yes	No	Yes
Mercury	Possible	No	No	Yes	No	Yes
Methyl alcohol	Yes	Yes	No	No	No	No
Methyl bromide	No	No	No	Yes	No	Yes
Methyl chloride	No	No	No	Yes	No	No
Methyl ethyl ketone	No	No	No	Yes	No	Yes
MPTP	Yes	Yes	Yes	No	No	Yes
n-Hexane	Yes	No	No	No	No	No
3-Nitropropionic acid	No	Yes	Yes	No	No	No
Tetanus toxin	No	No	No	Yes	No	Yes
Tetraethyl lead	No	No	Yes	Yes	No	Yes
Toluene	No	No	No	Yes	No	Yes

Parkinsonism

Parkinsonism is the clinical condition in which an individual has signs that include combinations of bradykinesia, resting tremor, rigidity, and postural instability. The prototypic parkinsonian syndrome is idiopathic Parkinson's disease (PD) in which a specific and localized degeneration of dopaminergic cells in the substantia nigra occurs [6]. Other non-PD parkinsonian syndromes may have nigrostriatal system damage, but this degeneration occurs in the context of wider, diffuse, or multifocal anatomic alterations, and the parkinsonism is only one of several accompanying neurologic signs. Drug-induced parkinsonism, seen with patients who ingest antidopaminergic drugs (specifically neuroleptics or reserpine), can be reversible, but is clinically indistinguishable from PD [7]. Parkinsonism may also be induced by a variety of toxins that inhibit oxidative processes or mitochondrial respiration, including manganese, carbon monoxide, cyanide, and carbon disulfide. Although the possibility exists that contact with a toxicant may contribute to the cause of PD, at present, parkinsonism appears to be an uncommon consequence of occupational or environmental toxin exposure. Neurotoxin-based models, however, have been important in exploring the pathogenesis of sporadic PD.

1-Methyl-4-phenyl-1,2,3,6-tetrahydropyridine

The model produced by the neurotoxin 1-methyl-4-phenyl-1,2,3,6-tetrahydropyridine (MPTP), an inhibitor of complex I of the mitochondrial respiratory chain, has had a competitive advantage over other models because MPTP causes intoxication in humans. It induces a syndrome virtually identical to PD [8]. The discovery of this toxin occurred following the development of parkinsonism (in addicts) caused by drugs contaminated with MPTP [9]. This finding led to the subsequent development of mouse and primate models of PD using this neurotoxin [10–12]. The major metabolite of MPTP is 1-methyl-4-phenylpyridinium ion, and its production is mediated by monoamine oxidase [13–15]. This biotransformation can be blocked by pretreatment with agents that inhibit monoamine oxidase type B [15]. In most nonhuman primates, MPTP causes rigidity, akinesia, postural instability, and a predominately posturokinetic tremor [10]. These symptoms are successfully treated with levodopa and dopamine agonists. Investigators evaluated the exposure of nearly 400 intravenous drug users to the neurotoxin [16], with most remaining asymptomatic [17]. Acute effects were reported in 7 symptomatic index cases with moderate to severe parkinsonism who experienced injection-site burning, disorientation, a dream-like sensation, visual aberrations, metallic taste, muscle jerks, and variable twisting postures [8]. Within 2 weeks of MPTP exposure, these individuals developed a rapidly progressive parkinsonian syndrome with uniformly moderate to severe bradykinesia, rigidity, instability, dysarthria, hypomimia, flexed posture, micrographia, and freezing [8]. In addition to the more severe cases of MPTP-induced parkinsonism, milder symptoms may be present. Although not unvarying, many severely affected subjects developed limited upgaze, seborrhea, dystonia, and tremor. A detailed study of the tremor in 4 patients revealed that movement exhibited all the characteristics of a parkinsonian rest tremor, in that it was asymmetric, distal in location, dampened by movement, and exhibited an alternating agonist and antagonist contraction rate of 4.5 and 5.0 Hz, respectively [18,19]. Although MPTP-induced parkinsonism responded dramatically to levodopa, within weeks to months, typical motor fluctuations and dyskinesias occurred [20]. Over time, worsening of symptoms occurred in patients with moderate to severe MPTP-induced parkinsonism. In some of the originally asymptomatic or mildly affected individuals, symptoms typical for PD materialized [16,21].

Using fluorodopa F^{18} and high-resolution photon emission tomography (PET), Snow et al [22] scanned 9 humans exposed to MPTP to determine whether there is a caudate-putamen gradient in humans with minimal to severe parkinsonism induced by MPTP, as is seen in idiopathic PD. Compared with 10 patients with PD and 6 normal subjects, the MPTP group had an equal degree of reduction of dopaminergic function in the caudate and putamen, in contrast to the greater putaminal loss in PD [22]. The pathology induced by MPTP includes the selective loss of dopaminergic neurons in brain areas similar to idiopathic PD, yet the injury is less diffuse and primarily confined to the substantia nigra. In a detailed neuropathologic study of MPTP-induced parkinsonism, brain tissue from subjects with survival times of 3 to 16 years after exposure revealed moderate to severe depletion of pigmented nerve cells in the substantia nigra in each case [23]. Lewy bodies were not present. Two thirds of the individuals demonstrated gliosis and clustering of microglia around nerve cells, with one patient having additional large amounts of extraneuronal melanin present. Although the mechanisms by which this occurs is unclear, the investigators suggested that these findings indicate active, ongoing nerve cell loss and that a time-limited insult to the nigrostriatal system potentially may set in motion a self-perpetuating process of neurodegeneration [24].

Manganese

Manganese is an essential trace metal, and toxicity from this agent has been described since the early 1800s. Previously, cases typically followed excessive occupational exposure through mining manganese ore [25]. Industrial exposure and rare instances of manganese intoxication during total parenteral nutrition and from fungicide have also been reported [26,27]. Manganese is absorbed through the gastrointestinal system and lungs and easily crosses the blood-brain barrier, most likely through carrier-mediated transport [28]. Manganese increases free radical formation, inhibits antioxidant function, and may enhance auto-oxidation of dopamine by a higher-valence manganese ion. It may additionally reduce energy production as a mitochondrial toxin and possibly increase glutamate's neurotoxic effects [29–31]. Three clinical syndrome stages are generally recognized in manganese-related neurotoxicity: (1) behavioral changes, (2) parkinsonism, and (3) dystonia with severe gait disturbances [32]. Extrapyramidal symptoms including masked facies, salivation, micrographia, bradykinesia, and rigidity predominate, regardless of whether manganese contact occurs through mining or industrial exposure [33–37]. Patients may have variable degrees of rigidity and bradykinesia, with one symptom relatively more prominent than the other. Although uncommon, tremor may occasionally be severe and "flapping" in nature. Dystonia of differing severities may occur in combination when the parkinsonism is severe, resembling the clinical picture seen in Wilson's disease [32–36]. When walking, patients may take small steps on the balls of their feet. Their heels are elevated and rotated outward, associated with an extended posture and flexed arms. This is known as a "cock walk." Other abnormal examination findings may include hyper-reflexia, dysmetria, emotional lability, and mild dementia [35,36]. Miners exposed to manganese dust by inhalation may experience so-called "manganese madness" as a prodrome to the development of the movement disorder. Fatigue, headache, insomnia, illusions, hallucinations, irritability, and aggressiveness characterize this "madness." This constellation of symptoms is generally absent in those exposed to industrial manganese [35,36]. A comparison of the clinical features of 15 career welders with two control groups with PD demonstrated no differences in the clinical manifestations, with the exception that the age of disease onset was younger in the welding group with parkinsonism [37]. The syndrome may resolve if further exposure is prevented at an early stage; however, it usually follows a progressive course, even when patients are removed from the environment of high manganese content [38]. Early studies of levodopa therapy in patients with manganese-induced parkinsonism have reported anywhere from dramatic improvement of rigidity, bradykinesia, and balance to no change in clinical signs [35,37,39–41]. Recently, Koller et al [42] reported a small, long-term, double-blind controlled study of high-dose levodopa treatment of patients with manganese-induced parkinsonism. No effect of levodopa was observed on either clinical rating scale or on objective measures. Neuroimaging studies in nonhuman primates and patients with manganese intoxication have revealed high signal intensities confined to the striatum, globus pallidus, and substantia nigra pars reticulata on T1-weighted MRIs. Despite continued neurologic dysfunction, these imaging findings resolve after manganese withdrawal [43–45]. Several reports of fluorodopa F^{18} PET studies in cases of manganese intoxication in nonhuman primates and humans have been normal [46,47]. Pathologic studies in humans and animals clearly demonstrate that manganese toxicity is associated with damage to basal ganglia structures [48–50]. The globus pallidus and substantia nigra pars reticulata are predominately involved. Damage to the caudate nucleus, putamen, subthalamic nucleus, and substantia nigra pars compacta occurs to a lesser degree with variable involvement of the substantia nigra pars compacta [51].

Solvents

It is well known that exposure to solvents in an occupational setting may lead to central nervous system damage and parkinsonism. The most important solvents in this respect are methanol, carbon disulfide, and n-hexane. Poisoning with methyl alcohol (methanol, CH_3OH), a common solvent and chemical intermediate, most commonly occurs from its ingestion as a substitute for, or adulterant of, ethyl alcohol. Although methanol itself is not toxic, its oxidative metabolism leads to the formation of formaldehyde and formic acid [52]. These chemicals achieve high concentrations within the putamen and are believed to have selective toxicity to this region [53]. Acute intoxication may resemble ethyl alcohol inebriation but quickly evolves into delirium, coma, or death from the systemic effects of metabolic acidosis or brain edema. Survivors of intoxication may experience several types of central nervous system abnormalities including blindness, pseudobulbar speech, and cognitive impairment [54,55]. Movement disorders are generally uncommon sequelae following methanol poisoning [56–58]; however, permanent parkinsonian motor impairment has been described for some long-term survivors of methanol poisoning [59,60]. Brain CT and MRI studies in survivors have revealed cystic resorption of the putamen [61,62]. Increased dopamine β-hydroxylase and decreased methionine-enkephalin cerebrospinal fluid levels in a survivor may suggest that methanol toxicity results in alterations of the central noradrenergic activity and the opioid system [63]. Pathologic studies in individuals with methanol intoxication have demonstrated bilateral necrosis of the putamen, optic atrophy, and diffuse lesions in the cerebral cortex, gray matter nuclei, and anterior horn [61,64].

Carbon disulfide is a colorless, highly volatile solvent used in the production of viscose rayon and cellophane and is a fumigant to counter grain infestations. Industrial intoxication of workers may occur through inhalation or cutaneous absorption [65]. Carbon disulfide is rapidly accumulated in the brain and may cause manic behavior, including sleep disruption, hypersexuality, mood fluctuations, nightmares, hallucinations, and paranoia [66,67]. These effects are followed by depression, dysmetria, memory dysfunction, sensorimotor peripheral and cranial neuropathy, and parkinsonism [68]. Parkinsonism was seen in up to 30% of persons intoxicated with carbon disulfide prior to the adoption of modern safety regulations [67,68]. Although acute intoxications are uncommon, chronic low-grade exposure remains problematic [69–71]. In one study of 21 grain workers who had chronic exposure to carbon disulfide, most self-reporting individuals had abnormalities of movement including cogwheel rigidity (80%), bradykinesia (71%), posturoaction tremor (52%), and resting tremor (48%) [72]. Neuroimaging studies in this population may be normal or show central demyelination [72]. The few available human and primate pathologic studies demonstrate diffuse neuronal loss and demyelination, with focal necrosis of globus pallidus and substantia nigra [73,74]. Although the specific mechanism of neurotoxicity is unknown, carbon disulfide may produce its adverse effects through the inhibition of cytochrome oxidase or the formation of dithiocarbamate metabolites and subsequent chelation of metal ions [65,75].

n-Hexane is metabolized to 2,5-hexanedion and, with chronic exposure, may induce peripheral nerve injury and parkinsonism [76,77]. Distinct from the pattern of abnormalities seen in PD, PET studies in these individuals demonstrate regional striatal abnormalities of the nigrostriatal dopaminergic system and of glucose metabolism [78]. Pathologic examination and immunohistochemical analysis of the brain in individuals who expired following n-hexane exposure revealed neuronal loss in the periaqueductal gray, pedunculopontine nucleus, and locus ceruleus; severe dopaminergic neuronal loss with gliosis in the substantia nigra; and near complete loss of striatal tyrosine hydroxylase immunostaining [79].

Finally, rare cases of parkinsonism associated with chronic inhalation of carbon tetrachloride have also been reported [80].

Cyanide

Cyanide blocks trivalent iron in the cellular respiration enzymes and inactivates cytochrome oxidase and other oxidative enzymes. These actions result in cessation of cell respiration and respiratory arrest [81]. Cyanide exhibits a particular affinity for structures with a high oxygen requirement and therefore leads to hemorrhagic necrosis. Poisoning with this agent can occur acutely by volitional ingestion as a result of a suicide attempt and is generally lethal when more than 3 mg/kg of body weight are consumed [82]. Survival after cyanide intoxication is exceptional [83]. Dizziness, headaches, vertigo, agitation, seizures, coma, and death usually occur within seconds to minutes after acute ingestion [84]. Chronic intoxication through inhalation or dermal absorption may also take place by way of occupational exposure in the mining or metal industries. A variety of neurologic signs and symptoms may occur in this setting, including dementia, parkinsonism, and delayed dystonia with parkinsonism [4,85,86]. Early MRI studies following survival of cyanide intoxication may be unremarkable, yet typical bilateral areas of hyperintensity in the lentiform nuclei and the caudate nuclei are usually seen [83,87–89]. With marked contrast enhancement, additional discrete, bilateral hyperintense alterations high in the frontoparietal region can also be seen, suggestive of pseudolaminar necrosis. Later, areas of hemorrhagic necrosis with hyperintense signal changes are seen in the striatum and globus pallidus [90]. A 6-fluorodopa PET study in a patient who survived cyanide ingestion but later developed parkinsonism revealed bilateral decreased uptake in the basal ganglia, providing evidence of functional impairment of dopaminergic nigrostriatal neurons related to direct toxicity of cyanide or to the effects of secondary cerebral hypoxia [88]. A pathologic report in an 18-year-old man who died 19 months after having survived a suicide attempt with cyanide and developing parkinsonism, revealed major destructive changes in the globus pallidus and putamen, with sparing of the melanin-containing zone of substantia nigra [4].

Carbon monoxide

Carbon monoxide is a clear, odorless gas and its inhalation has been the mechanism of attempted suicides since ancient times [91]. More recently, occupational poisonings have occurred when gasoline engines are used in poorly ventilated settings or through the use of methylene chloride for paint stripping [92,93]. Chronic low-dose inhalation as may occur in firefighters may be associated with delayed cognitive symptoms and could increase the risk of the development of parkinsonism in later life [94–96]. Exposure may also occur when coal or charcoal is used for cooking or as a source of household heating [97] or in artificially self-contained environments [98]. Carbon monoxide has a much greater affinity for hemoglobin oxygen-sites compared with oxygen, and after entering the blood stream, it binds with the ferrous ion complex of protoporphyrin IX, prohibiting oxygen binding [99]. This action results in a functional anoxia with subsequent tissue damage. Carbon monoxide additionally inhibits ATP production by binding to mitochondrial cytochrome oxidase, further potentiating the anoxic injury [99]. Acute intoxication is fatal in 2% to 25% of exposed individuals, and up to 40% of survivors suffer neurologic sequelae [93, 100,101]. Individuals with acute carbon monoxide poisoning may have vague symptoms that are inadvertently related to a viral syndrome. These symptoms include headache, dizziness, and visual aberrations, which may quickly evolve to loss of consciousness, seizures, coma, cardiac arrest, and death [91,93]. Survivors can remain in a persistent vegetative state, but nearly 70% recover [102]. Although the mental status may improve within days to weeks, additional central nervous system sequelae including personality alternations and memory dysfunction may occur that may eventually progress to profound apathy and mutism [93,103]. Parkinsonian signs may be seen in up to 80% of cases with prominent masked facies, decreased arm swing, rigidity, shuffling gait, postural reflex impairment, urinary incontinence, and occasional rest or intention tremor [5,97,104]. This clinical presentation is typically delayed in presentation from 2 to 26 weeks and may be progressive and associated with other movement disorders including dystonia and choreathetosis. This neurologic deterioration may continue, remain static, or subsequently improve [103,105]. Levodopa and anticholinergic drugs are generally ineffective [5]. MRI may disclose diffuse high-intensity white matter signals and bilateral pallidal necrosis [106]. Pathologically, when death occurs acutely from carbon monoxide poisoning, the findings mirror those seen with other forms of asphyxiation, including cerebral swelling, capillary congestion, and petechial hemorrhages [107]. White matter changes and internal pallidal necrosis and hemorrhage in the anterior and superior sections are the primary pathologic changes [102,107,108].

Cycad seed toxicity

A neurologic syndrome referred to as "amyotrophic lateral sclerosis and parkinsonism-dementia complex of Guam" (ALS/PDC), particularly prevalent in the Guamanian Chamorro population, has been related to the ingestion of a neurotoxin. First recognized early in the last century [109–112], various etiologic theories of this disorder have been proposed.

The use of the seeds of a cycad, *Cycas rumphii*, drew suspicion because they were already known by the Chamorro people to be toxic [113]. β-Methylamino-L-alanine (BMAA) [114] is produced by cyanobacteria of the genus *Nostoc*, which are root symbionts of cycads [115], and monkeys fed large doses of this toxin had an acute and reversible neurologic disorder that included parkinsonism [116,117]. The doses of BMAA received by these animals were well beyond those that would be ingested by humans in a typical diet, casting doubt on the association of this toxin and the human disorder. More recently, it has been suggested that the doses of cycad toxin ingested by the Chamorro population may have been enhanced indirectly by consuming not only the flour of the cycad but also flying foxes [118] that are eaten by the indigenous island people on ceremonial gatherings [119,120]. These animals ingest large quantities of the seeds of *C rumphii*, and biomagnification could result when the toxins accumulate (or are chemically modified) in the tissues of this mammal [121]. Cox et al [115] demonstrated that bound BMAA, in addition to free BMAA, can bioaccumulate from cyanobacterial symbionts in the root tissues of *C micronesica* throughout the food chain. BMAA is then consumed by Chamorro people in their traditional diets. These investigators demonstrated BMAA within brain tissues of Chamorro patients who died of ALS/PDC in Guam [115]. Bound to protein, BMAA functions as an endogenous neurotoxic reservoir, slowly releasing neurotoxin directly into the cerebral tissues through protein metabolism [122]. The results of other studies propose that the delivery of the neurotoxin inside the brain may produce varied dysfunction [123]. These possibilities include the alteration or truncation of neuroproteins, the formation of dimers that covalently bind metal ions, and the capture and release of metal ions by BMAA complexes that may interfere with the proper function of *N*-methyl-D-aspartate and α-amino-3-hydroxy-5-methyl-4-isoxazolepropionic acid receptors (or BMAA may act as a chronic agonist at these same receptors) [124–126]. This last possibility can effectively convert a single ingestion of BMAA into a prolonged, constant low-level exposure of this neurotoxin within brain tissues, resulting in neuronal death through excitotoxicity [122].

The incidence of PDC now greatly exceeds ALS and typically includes both parkinsonism and dementia. The mean age at onset of PDC has increased in successive studies to 68 years in men and women [127], and PDC is twice as common in men than in women [128]. Patients with PDC typically present with parkinsonism that is similar to idiopathic PD, including increased muscle tone and bradykinesia; however, their involvement is generally more symmetric [128]. Masked facies, decreased blink rate, and hypophonic speech are frequent. The gait is abnormal with slow, short steps with an overall apraxic pattern. Although a posturoaction tremor is more common, rest tremor occurs in nearly one third of patients [128]. Parkinsonism is generally followed by cognitive decline within a few years, yet in about 30% of patients [129,130], dementia precedes the motoric symptoms. Treatment with dopaminergic agents results in some improvement of parkinsonism in patients with PDC, although to a much less dramatic degree than with idiopathic PD [131,132].

Alcohol

Many movement disorders are associated with alcohol intake and withdrawal, including parkinsonism [133–136]. Chronic alcoholics of both sexes who have little or no indication of hepatic dysfunction have been reported to demonstrate transient parkinsonism. These individuals are observed to have the typical features of masked facies, bradykinesia, stooped posture, coarse rest tremor, rigidity, and a shuffling gait [135,136]. These classic features are at times associated with a prominent glabellar reflex and extraocular eye movement abnormalities. This parkinsonian syndrome may occur repeatedly during periods of alcohol withdrawal, along with other characteristic signs of confusion, posturoaction tremor, and ataxia. Neuroimaging studies are generally nonspecific in these individuals [134,137]. Although the exact pathophysiology of this phenomenon is unknown, it most likely represents a reversible aberration of nigrostriatal dopaminergic transmission, suggested by long-term follow-up studies that have failed to reveal any sustained movement disorder in individuals with past parkinsonism during alcohol withdrawal [138].

Dystonia

Dystonia is a slow muscle contortion that causes an abnormal, sustained body posture, frequently with a twisting character. This movement disorder is primarily seen in its idiopathic form, typically generalized in distribution in childhood, and usually focal or segmental in adults. In addition to idiopathic forms, certain metabolic derangements, structural disorders, drug use, and toxins may have dystonia as a consequence. As an example, patients who recover following cyanide intoxication may experience the occurrence of dystonia [87]. The dystonia following such intoxication is usually delayed in onset and progressive in character. It may present in isolation but is usually found in combination with varying degrees of parkinsonism and, in one report, eye-lid apraxia [86,139]. The movement abnormality generally stabilizes over time and then may gradually improve or eventually resolve. Dopaminergic therapy has been beneficial in some patients [140,141]. Neuroimaging studies in these individuals show diffuse atrophy and hypodensities on CT images and T2 hyperintensities on MRI scans in the bilateral putamen and external globus pallidus, correlating with postmortem findings [139].

As described earlier, long-term survivors of methanol poisoning typically have permanent parkinsonism, but cases of dystonia have also been described [142,143]. LeWitt and Martin [143] reported a 30-year-old chronic schizophrenic man who survived methanol intoxication but developed a persistent, predominately dystonic disorder. Generalized dystonic posturing with prominent involvement of the hands was present. The speech was dysphonic, with mild paucity of movements and an intermittent posturoaction tremor of the upper extremities. Although rigidity was felt on examination, a cogwheeling character was absent. After arising slowly, the patient's posture was erect. He walked with an unusual toe-walking, shuffling quality in the absence of hesitation, difficulty turning, or impairment of balance. Although there was no response to anticholinergics, isolated improvement in the rigidity occurred with dopaminergic therapy [143]. In a separate report, a 40-year-old alcoholic woman who survived an attempted suicide by ingesting methanol experienced typical visual abnormalities, but a year later had the additional onset of difficulty speaking and chewing [142]. Her examination revealed mild dysarthria, a shuffling gait, reduced arm swing, and minimal bradykinesia. Although she was able to open and close her mouth volitionally, when eating or drinking, an involuntary jaw closure significantly impaired these activities. The movements did not improve with oral pharmacologic therapy using anticholinergics, dopaminergics, or injections of botulinum toxin into the masseters and temporalis muscles [142]. In this same case, neuroimaging studies revealed symmetric low densities in the putamen and head of the caudate nuclei. Electrophysiologic investigations studying the blink reflex and silent period of the masseter muscle demonstrated facilitation of R2, an associated R3 component, an enhanced recovery-cycle curve of R2 responses, and bilaterally absent masseter muscle silent periods [142]. The investigators speculated that these findings may have resulted from basal ganglia dysfunction leading to hypoactive inhibitory control on the pontomedullary interneuronal net regulating these polysynaptic circuits.

3-Nitropropionic acid is a widely distributed plant and fungal neurotoxin that irreversibly inhibits succinate dehydrogenase, an enzyme contained within the Krebs cycle and complex II in the mitochondrial electron transport chain [144]. This toxin induces inhibition of energy metabolism, resulting in damage to the basal ganglia, hippocampus, spinal tracts, and peripheral nerves in animals. Reports of an acute, noninflammatory encephalopathy in mainly young individuals following ingestion of mildewed sugarcane containing the arthrinium-produced 3-nitropropionic acid mycotoxin were first reported in the early 1970s from Northern China [145]. Severe intoxications typically result in a short prodrome consisting of nausea, vomiting, and anorexia, followed by frequent seizures and coma within a day of exposure [146]. Status epilepticus, opisthotonic posturing, and decerebrate rigidity occurred in up to one half of the cases. Dystonia was seen in patients within 2 months of intoxication and included grimacing, spasms of the extremities, and torticollis, with overlying athetosis and choreiform movements of the hands and fingers. No parkinsonism has been observed in any dystonic patient. The movements were permanent but nonprogressive and typically not amenable to pharmacologic treatment. CT in these individuals demonstrated diffuse atrophy and bilateral lenticular nuclei and globus pallidal hypodensities with occasional involvement of the caudate nuclei [146]. A neuropathologic study was carried out in rats intoxicated with 3-nitropropionic acid and anthrinium cultures [147]. Consistent bilateral caudate-putamen and globus pallidus necrosis was found in the animals with both poisonings in accordance with the bilateral lenticular hypodensities found by CT scanning in patients of mildewed sugarcane poisoning with delayed dystonia [147].

Finally, Klawans [148] reported a group of railroad workers who were exposed to dioxin during cleaning up of a chemical spillage and followed medically for 6 years. Fatigue and muscle aching were the initial neurologic complaints. Detailed neurologic examination demonstrated dystonic writer's cramp and/or other action dystonias of the hands in nearly half of the subjects. The dystonia was generally mild and occurred within the first 2 to 3 years of the toxic exposure. Postural and intention tremor was also displayed in two hirds of the individuals.

Chorea, choreoathetosis, and ballismus

Chorea is a rapid, unpredictable body movement that generally spreads from one muscle group to another. When twisted movements accompany the rapid jerk, the term *choreoathetosis* is used; in contrast, ballismus involves large-amplitude and proximal, rather than distal, movements of the same character. The neuroanatomic areas of interest for chorea, choreoathetosis, and ballismus include the striatum, subthalamic nucleus, and anterior thalamus [149,150]. Substances that adversely affect the normal chemistry of these structures are associated with the production of chorea and include amphetamine, cocaine, and alcohol. The association of amphetamine use and the occurrence of chorea may relate to its central dopaminergic activity [151,152]. This effect may be further enhanced when amphetamine abuse occurs in the setting of oral birth control use, which increases striatal postsynaptic dopaminergic sensitivity [153]. Among other complex effects, cocaine is known to bind dopamine, norepinephrine, and serotonin reuptake sites, preventing removal of these neurotransmitters from the synaptic clefts [154,155]. Cocaine blocks dopamine reuptake acutely, producing a rapid rise in the availability of dopamine in the synaptic cleft [156]. With chronic exposure, a complex series of alterations occur in an attempt to surmount the dopaminergic overstimulation [157–159]. Amphetamine-related choreiform movements are usually generalized and involve the extremities, head, and neck. In acute intoxications, the movements are not present in isolation but are associated with other signs that include dry mucous membranes, delirium, psychosis, and rarely, rhabdomyolysis [160–162]. The movements occurring in cocaine abusers are likely under-reported because they are typically self-limited and not life threatening.

Some cultural subgroups have even incorporated language to describe the choreic movements associated with cocaine use, including "crack dancing" and "boca torcida," which translated means "twisted mouth" [163]. Daras et al [163] described seven individuals whose addiction resulted in the nearly daily use of cocaine for a period of 8 months to 5 years who presented with choreoathetotic movements. The movements involved the extremities in all seven patients, whereas two also had eye blinking or lip smacking. The onset of the movements was nearly immediate after cocaine use in half of the patients but delayed by a few hours in the remaining individuals. The movements lasted from 2 days to less than a week, with gradual disappearance following minimal if any treatment. In a separate study, chronic amphetamine- and cocaine-dependent abusers as a group were also shown to have a significantly increased abnormal involuntary movement scale score compared with age-matched normal controls, an occurrence most marked in younger subjects [164].

Potentially related to functional dopamine receptor supersensivity, transient choreic dyskinesias have been reported in alcohol abusers, most commonly in younger female alcoholics [133,165]. These movements are typically seen 1 to 2 weeks after the cessation of alcohol but may also occur during periods of heavy binging [133,166–168]. Jerky, choreic movements and sinuous, writhing movements are present and appear most prominently in the lingual-oral region, causing twisting and pursing of the lips and mouth, with overlying tongue protrusions and facial grimacing. Movements in the lower extremities are rare. As the movements uniformly dissipate spontaneously over time, pharmacologic treatment is not required. Hepatic function studies in these patients are not typically elevated, in contrast to patients with portosystemic shunts in acquired heptolenticular degeneration from severe alcoholic liver disease who may have chronic or persistent choreiform movements [169]. Other substances of abuse, including the inhalation of glue and gasoline fumes, have been associated with the occurrence of chorea [170–172].

Whether in conjunction with other movement disorders or in isolation, transitory chorea of the extremities, face, and neck can occur as a delayed phenomenon following the resolution of a carbon monoxide–induced coma. The movements generally occur one week or more into recovery and last less than 6 months [173,174]. The chorea occurs in association with other neurologic deficits including dysarthria and memory disturbances. CT and MRI studies have revealed symmetric bilateral lesions in the infarction in the head of the caudate nucleus, putamen, and globus pallidus [174,175].

Myoclonus

Myoclonus is less well characterized than the other movement disorders. The term is used to describe brief, lightning-like involuntary jerks sufficient in amplitude to move joints. These movements may be focal or generalized, rhythmic or arrhythmic. The abnormal movement may be an active muscle contraction, termed *positive myoclonus*, or a sudden lapse of muscle contraction, termed *asterixis* or *negative myoclonus*. Myoclonus may present as part of a complex neurologic syndrome related to a variety of medications or intoxicants. Typically, the myoclonic jerks in these settings are generalized or multifocal, asymmetric, nonrhythmic, and commonly stimulus sensitive or induced by voluntary movement. Generally, the myoclonic jerking occurs in association with encephalopathy, altered mental status, or even coma in these syndromes. Other neurologic signs, including ataxia, headache, and seizures, may be present with certain intoxications. Several toxins produce encephalopathies in which myoclonus can be a prominent feature. These include intoxications with bismuth, aluminum, methyl bromide, cooking oil that contains anilines, and tetraethyl lead.

Bismuth

In 1974, two independent researchers published nearly simultaneous reports of a total of 11 patients with myoclonic encephalopathy following oral bismuth subgallate or bismuth subnitrate administration, often used to improve stool consistency and odor following colostomy [176,177]. Thereafter, multiple other similar cases were reported in Europe, the United States, and Australia [178–184]. These patients often had an initial presentation with depressed mood, apathy, and irritability as a prodrome, rapidly followed by mental status changes, hallucinations, myoclonus, ataxia, and dysarthria. Severe intoxications resulted in convulsions, coma, and death. The myoclonus was either multifocal or generalized and occurred spontaneously or was provoked by action or sensory stimulation. The symptoms in this disorder generally resolved with the discontinuation of the therapy, but utilization of chelation therapy with dimercaprol was necessary in the severe cases.

Aluminum

Although occupational exposure to industrial aluminum typically does not induce nervous system disorders in patients with normal renal function, there have been isolated reports of individuals with apparent aluminum neurotoxicity. These patients were exposed to aluminum during the smelting process or through inhalation of aluminum dust. Focal epilepsy, hyperreflexia, seizures, tremor, incoordination, ataxia, coma, and death have been observed in such individuals. Controversy exists as to whether these symptoms resulted from exposure to aluminum alone or other associated chemicals [185–187]. Acute or chronic aluminum toxicity, however, has clearly been established to occur in uremic patients. Acute neurotoxicity with plasma levels of greater than 500 mg/mL generally manifests as generalized tonic-clonic seizures and is associated with agitation, confusion, myoclonic jerking, coma, and death [188]. This constellation of symptoms may appear within days of deferoxamine chelation therapy that results in displacement of sequestered aluminum from bone or following after extended periods of treatment with aluminum compounds and citrate. During the 1970s, initial reports of maintenance dialysis patients developing the insidious onset of mental deterioration, speech disturbance, apraxia, and myoclonus were first published [189]. The sudden onset of hesitant, nonfluent speech with both dysphasic and dysarthric components is the earliest and most characteristic sign of this disorder [190]. Cognitive abnormalities appear more gradually, with poor concentration, inattention, and delirium with occasional psychosis. Mutism and a global dementia may be seen after 6 months of symptoms [189,190]. In some patients, seizures were also present and typically heralded an inexorable progressive decline resulting in death. The average duration of illness of these more seriously ill patients was less than 7 months. Routine biochemical studies were unremarkable, and osteodystrophy was not a prominent feature [189]. Usually antedating the neurologic syndrome, serial EEGs showed progressive slowing of the background rhythm, with the later development of a high-voltage spike-wave pattern intermixed with abundant slow activity [190]. All standard neuroimaging studies of these patients were normal. Postmortem evaluations of the brain demonstrated mild spongiform pathology in the cerebral cortex, with other nonspecific changes [191]. Treatment was generally ineffective, but ventriculo-peritoneal shunting produced transient neurologic improvement in one patient [190]. Epidemiologic investigations showed high aluminum levels in city water during the period of the outbreak [189]. In a prospective study attempting to assess whether other, less severe, neuropsychologic abnormalities were also associated with aluminum, Sprague et al [192] evaluated patients receiving chronic dialysis. Quantitative measures of asterixis, myoclonus, motor strength, and sensation were used to evaluate motor function, and measures of dementia, memory, language, and depression were used to evaluate cognitive function. Patients with elevated aluminum levels had an increase in the number of neurologic abnormalities observed and an increase in severity of myoclonus, asterixis, and lower extremity weakness [192]. These patients also showed a significant impairment in memory, but no abnormalities were noted on tests of dementia, depression, or language. No significant correlation between sex, age, presence of diabetes, mode of dialysis, years of chronic renal failure, years of dialysis, or years of aluminum ingestion correlated with any neurologic or neurobehavioral measurement or serum aluminum level [192].

Mercury

The major physical forms of mercury to which humans are exposed are mercury vapor emitted from natural and dental amalgam sources and methylmercury compounds found in seafood and freshwater fish [193]. The effects of severe exposure to mercury vapor include a triad of symptoms, including erethism, tremor, and gingivitis. Methylmercury primarily affects nervous system tissue, causing ataxia and visual aberrations. Although relatively uncommon, sporadic cases of acute inorganic mercurial poisoning occur and may be associated with tremor and intention myoclonus [194], as described in the original publication of the "Mad Hatter syndrome" [195]. Roullet et al [196] described a 58-year-old laboratory-glassware manufac- turer who was referred for a nearly 2-year history of coarse "tremor" of the upper extremities. After examination, severe intention and action myoclo- nus was found in association with mild memory impairment. Mercury levels were high in blood and urine, resulting from inhalation of mercury vapor. With dimercaprol treatment, minimal unilateral intention tremor remained. Epidemic intoxications still occur with organic mercury substances and may also cause similar symptoms including generalized or action-induced myoclonus with overlying tremor, ataxia, and encephalopathy [197].

Manganese

As discussed in an earlier section, metal manganese may produce varied movement disorders but is primarily associated with parkinsonism in association with a posturoaction tremor and dystonia. More recently, Ono et al [198] reported a single case of a 17-year-old male welder exposed to manganese who presented with myoclonic jerks mainly in the right upper and lower extremities. There was no associated parkinsonism or tremor. Laboratory studies revealed elevated levels of manganese in the blood and hair and MRI demonstrated high-intensity signals in the globus pallidus on T1-weighted images. The movements and imaging abnormalities were abated after the institution of chelation therapy.

Methyl bromide, methyl chloride, methyl ethyl ketone, and toluene

Methyl bromide is widely used as a fumigant for pest and pathogen control in food supplies, warehouses, barges, buildings, and furniture. The primary route for exposure is inhalation, and because of its frequent use around humans and human-related activities, fatal accidents have occurred. The US Clean Air Act mandates a complete phase-out of the import and manufacture of methyl bromide by January 2005 [199]. Methyl bromide is acutely very toxic [200]. With chronic exposure, central nervous system toxicity predominates, but the symptoms may be masked by the severity of acute effects [200]. Symptoms of acute exposure include mucosal irritation, malaise, nausea, vomiting, headache, dizziness, and breathing difficulties. With continued exposure, these symptoms (after a variable latent period) are followed by visual disturbances, speech abnormalities, peripheral neuropathy, incoordination, myoclonus, seizures, psychosis, and at times, death [201,202]. The myoclonus may be spontaneous or induced by somatosensory stimulation or voluntary movements and is multifocal and sometimes generalized. Although the seizures are typically unresponsive to diazepam, clonazepam, and diphenylhydantoin, they were suppressed by induction of a thiopental coma [203]. The myoclonus may be variably responsive to the multiple-drug treatment of 5-hydroxytryptophan, γ-aminobutyric acid, and clonazepam [204]. Prior subchronic exposure and high serum bromide concentrations were likely to be factors contributing to the severity of symptoms. A direct correlation between serum bromide concentrations and the severity of neurologic symptoms could not be demonstrated [203]. Electrophysiologic studies have revealed giant and asymmetric somatosensory evoked potentials in a patient with predominantly unilateral, spontaneous, and intention myoclonus after 3 days of voluntary methyl bromide intoxication, suggesting that myoclonus could be related to an abnormal reactivity of somatomotor and somatosensory cortices to the afferent volleys triggered by voluntary movements [204]. Back-averaging studies have shown a biphasic EEG spike of maximal amplitude at the central region contralateral to the corresponding myoclonic jerk, preceding it by a short interval, whereas long latency reflexes were enhanced [205]. These electrophysiologic findings suggest that the myoclonus in this setting is of the cortical reflex category. Postmortem anatomic studies have revealed mainly necrosis of both inferior colliculi, with gliosis in the upper brain stem reticular formation and moderate changes in the dentate and pontine nuclei [201]. The mechanism of toxicity for methyl bromide is currently unknown, although its alkylating properties and the potential for inducing reactive intermediates through metabolic transformations are theorized to be possible mechanisms [206].

Methyl chloride is a methylating agent used in the production of tetramethyl lead, butyl rubber, and polystyrene foams. The principal route of intoxication is by inhalation or absorption through the skin. It is rapidly absorbed by the blood, with some investigators attributing its toxicity to enzyme-catalyzed methylation [207]. It is a potent central nervous system depressant and may be associated with headache, dizziness, confusion, speech abnormalities, diplopia, and incoordination [208,209]. Seizures and stimulus-sensitive myoclonus may also occur [210,211]. Pharmacodynamic studies have shown the compound to be rapidly absorbed by the blood, with most researchers attributing the toxicity to an enzyme-catalyzed methylation reaction in the body.

Methyl ethyl ketone and toluene are volatile hydrocarbon solvents used in the manufacture of resins, rubber, glue, adhesives, lacquer, paint, and paint removers. Welch et al [212] reported a case of a 38 year-old laborer who experienced acute methyl ethyl ketone and toluene intoxication during each of two spray paintings in an enclosed, unventilated garage. Nausea, headaches, dizziness, and respiratory difficulty developed acutely with impaired concentration, memory loss, dysarthria, ataxia, and an intention tremor occurring over the next few days. MRI of the brain and EEG were normal. Isolated exposure to methyl ethyl ketone may also produce neurologic symptoms including dizziness, posturoaction tremor, gait ataxia, and reversible, multifocal myoclonus [213]. EEGs in this case have shown a normal background activity with overlying bursts or theta waves and generalized spikes. Although transient in nature, the myoclonus and tremor is dramatically improved with ethyl alcohol administration. Chronic, low-grade exposure of methyl ethyl ketone has been associated with the occurrence of polyneuropathy in humans [214]. Chronic, isolated toluene intoxication has been associated with stimulus-sensitive spinal myoclonus in addition to upper-extremity tremor and memory disturbances. Electrophysiologic studies failed to reveal a C-reflex or giant somatosensory evoked potentials, and EEGs showed no spikes [215].

Other intoxications

Commonly available gasoline may be abused by inhalation in an attempt to obtain a euphoric effect. Related to the presence of tetraethyl lead, this substance may cause an acute encephalopathy associated with irritability, visual hallucinations, incoordination, and myoclonus [171,172,216]. Goldings and Stewart [171] reported a case of a 15-year old boy who presented with the acute onset of confusion, insomnia, headache, and shaking, followed by hallucinations, formication, an action tremor, myoclonus, chorea, and ataxia. The diagnosis was confirmed with the establishment of the abuse and plasma lead levels in the toxic range. Chelation therapy reversed the clinical symptoms. In a retrospective study of 25 patients (aged 5–27 years) admitted to a tertiary referral hospital system in Australia with chronic gasoline intoxication, Goodheart and Dunne [172] reported a high prevalence of seizures and 40% death rate. All had an altered mental status and nearly half had a movement disorder consisting of myoclonus (9) or chorea (8) in addition to ataxia (13). High blood lead levels on presentation were highly correlated with a poor prognosis. A nearly uniformly disappointing outcome occurred in the 18 patients who received treatment with agents to reduce the lead load.

Dichloroethane is commonly used in the dry cleaning industry. A single case report of an accidental ingestion of an ointment containing this substance resulted in symptoms consisting of two phases [217]. Initially, the individual presented with somnolence, seizures, and myoclonus, followed by permanent mental dysfunction, dysarthria, and ataxia. These neurologic symptoms were accompanied by acute renal and hepatic failure and anemia. Butane and butane-containing products are readily available around the household and can be abused or be accidentally inhaled. Butane has been associated with a myoclonic encephalopathy [218]. One case of presumed inadvertent butane inhalation was reported by Peatfield and Boothman [219] following the use of an oven cleaner by a previously healthy woman.

After a lengthy cleaning using this product, the individual developed gastrointestinal symptoms followed by involuntary, irregular, predominately myoclonic movements of the chest, neck, and upper abdomen that occurred spontaneously but also were triggered by auditory stimuli. In addition, the movements had an overlying dystonic component. EEG studies were unrevealing. The movements resolved after 2 days of valproic acid administration.

Tetanus toxin affects the central and peripheral nervous system by depressing motor neuron inhibitory interneuronal synapses and by damaging interneurons and motor neurons [220]. As a result, the inhibitory terminals of the spinal interneurons release a reduced amount of glycine and γ-aminobutyric acid and block postsynaptic inhibition of motor neurons [221]. Warren et al [222] recently published a report of a 60 year-old man who presented with stiffness and painful spasms of his right upper extremity, face, and neck 1 week after sustaining an abrasion. These symptoms were followed by dysphagia and respiratory failure resulting in intubation and treatment with tetanus immune globulin. While recuperating, the patient demonstrated generalized, stimulus-sensitive myoclonus elicited by sudden, unexpected sounds and taps to the torso and face. Consisting of eye blinks and neck and trunk flexion with abduction and flexion of the arms, the responses did not habituate. The myoclonus was associated with a coarse upper-extremity tremor, generalized muscle stiffness, and twitches. The remaining examination was unremarkable other than brisk tendon reflexes, excluding ankle jerks. The abnormal movements rapidly improved with the administration of clonazepam and baclofen. The clinical examination findings and the results of electrophysiologic studies that revealed bilateral rostro-caudal activation of axial and limb muscles after stimulation of single peripheral nerves suggest that tetanus intoxication results in myoclonus of brainstem origin [222].

Tics

Tics are stereotypical, nonrhythmic, brief movements or sounds that are not usually constantly present but occur out of a background of normal motor activity. Simple motor tics consist of sudden, brief, abrupt, isolated movements, whereas complex motor tics are more complicated and often include coordinated movements. Simple vocal tics consist of inarticulate noises and single sounds, whereas complex vocal tics have linguistic meaning and may include full or truncated words. Although most patients with tics have this movement disorder as part of Gilles de la Tourette's syndrome (GTS), secondary tic disorders caused by prescription medications, trauma, encephalitis, and other neurodegenerative conditions have been reported. Rare cases of toxin-induced tics have been described, including those related to cocaine and carbon monoxide exposure.

Pascual-Leone and Dhuna [223] reported 4 patients with cocaine-induced multifocal tics, of whom two had a severe exacerbation of symptoms previously diagnosed as GTS. One of these 2 patients with GTS experienced the exacerbation following an initial exposure to cocaine. The second individual was a habitual cocaine snorter and had a worsening of tics after smoking "crack" for the first time. The remaining 2 non-GTS patients were also habitual cocaine abusers who experienced new-onset tics following a high-dose binge of cocaine. In a separate retrospective review of 411 patients with tic disorders who presented between 1988 and 1998 to the movement disorders clinic at Columbia-Presbyterian Medical Center, 22 individuals were identified who presented after the age of 21 [224]. One of these patients developed the tic disorder during an extended 2-year daily intranasal cocaine binge. Initially, the patient noticed transient facial movements that occurred during acute intoxication and typically subsided as the drug's effects waned. Over time, the movements persisted, with the eventual development of complex tics including stereotypical head turning and shoulder movements. The patient had no past history of childhood tics, cranial trauma, encephalitis, or exposure to psychiatric medications. Others have reported the onset of tics after the resolution of coma following exposure to carbon monoxide [225,226]. These patients developed stereo-typical movements of the head, shoulder, or face, at times accompanied by vocalizations and coprolalia. Neuroimaging studies with CT and MRI revealed bilateral globus pallidus lesions. One case was successfully treated with clonazepam [225].

Other tremors

Tremors are defined as rhythmic to-and-fro oscillations and are named for the body position in which they are most prominent: rest, when the tremor is maximal at repose, as seen in parkinsonism; postural, when the tremor develops as a patient maintains a position; and kinetic, when the tremor develops as a patient carries out a movement. In addition, rhythmic to-and-from movements that only occur in association with a particular type of activity have been described. These task-specific tremors include primary writing tremor, vocal tremor, and orthostatic tremor. Although most instances of posturoaction tremor are related to sporadic or familial essential tremor or an exaggeration of the physiologic tremor, the association of toxins and tremor has long been known. As has been discussed in previous sections, tremor may occur in association with other types of movement abnormalities following exposure to mercury [227], lead [171,227,228], manganese, dioxin [148], methyl bromide [229], methyl ethyl ketone and toluene [212], and carbon disulfide [72]. Exposure to the polycyclic chlorinated hydrocarbon insecticide, chlordecone (Kepone), also has resulted in the occurrence of tremor. Chlordecone can be absorbed through oral, respiratory, and dermal routes, the last thought to be the most significant [230]. In the mid-1970s, over half of 133 persons who had worked at a pesticide plant that produced Kepone developed a previously un-recognized clinical disorder characterized by weight loss, pleuritic and joint pain, oligospermia, nervousness, tremor, and opsoclonus [231]. Clinical manifestations abated following treatment with cholestyramine, which reduced blood levels of chlordecone [232,233]. The site of action and pathophysiologic effects of chlordecone on the central nervous system are unknown. Finally, although not causing tremor specifically in humans, some toxins such as oxotremorine, harmaline, and DDT have been used to produce experimental animal models of tremor for research purposes [234,235].

Summary

Toxins can be cited as a cause of several movement disorders, but this association is rare and the resultant syndromes usually include additional signs that are not typical for the idiopathic movement disorders. Most instances of confirmed toxin-induced movement disorders show lesions on CT and MRI scans of cortical or subcortical structures. A common underlying element in these toxin-induced syndromes is the development of lesions primarily in the pallidum and striatum. Because many toxins result in lesions affecting these structures, a selective vulnerability to hypoxic or metabolic insults has long been postulated. The susceptibility of these structures may relate to a number of factors, including the pattern of oxidative metabolism, heavy metal concentration, vascular perfusion, and neuronal innervation. Finally, in addition to causing disability, certain neurotoxins have led to a better understanding of human disease through the development of research models. As an example, the MPTP model has not only provided an animal model to study therapeutic strategies in PD but has also contributed important insights into the mechanisms of neuronal degeneration

References

[1] Pappert EJ. Neuroleptic-induced movement disorders acute and subacute syndromes. In: Vinken PJ, Bruyn GW, editors. Handbook of clinical neurology: intoxications of the nervous system. Part II. Amsterdam: Elsevier; 1994. p. 273–310.

[2] Tanner CM. Drug-induced movement disorders (tardive dyskinesia and dopa-induced dyskinesia). In: Vinken PJ, Bryn GW, Klawans HL, editors. Handbook of clinical neurology: extrapyramidal disorders. Amsterdam: Elsevier; 1986. p. 185–204.

[3] Lang AE, Weiner WJ. Drug-induced movement disorders. Mt. Kisco (NY): Futura Publishing Co.; 1992.

[4] Uitti RJ, Rajput AH, Ashenhurst EM, et al. Cyanide-induced parkinsonism: a clinico-pathologic study. Neurology 1985;35:921–5.

[5] Klawans HL, Stein RW, Tanner CM, et al. A pure parkinsonian syndrome following acute carbon monoxide intoxication. Arch Neurol 1982;39:302–4.

[6] Bernheimer H, Birkmayer W, Hornykiewicz O, et al. Brain dopamine and the syndrome of Parkinson and Huntington. Clinical, morphological and neurochemical correlations. J Neurol Sci 1973;20:415–55.

[7] Goetz CG, Klawans HL, Tanner CM. Movement disorders induced by neurolpetic drugs. In: Shah RS, editor. Neurolpetic drugs. New York: Plenum Publishing; 1986. p. 302–30.

[8] Ballard PA, Tetrud JW, Langston JW. Permanent parkinsonism in humans due to 1-methyl-4-phenyl-1,2,3,6-tetrahydropyridine (MPTP): seven cases. Neurology 1985;35: 949–56.

[9] Langston JW, Ballard PA Jr. Parkinson's disease in a chemist working with 1-methyl-4-phenyl-1, 2,5,6- tetrahydropyridine. N Engl J Med 1983;309:310.

[10] Burns RS, Chiueh CC, Markey SP, et al. A primate model of parkinsonism: selective destruction of dopaminergic neurons in the pars compacta of the substantia nigra by N-methyl-r-phenyl-1,2,3,6-tetranydropyridine. Proc Natl Acad Sci USA 1983;80:4546–50.

[11] Langston JW, Forno LS, Rebert CS, et al. Selective nigral toxicity after systemic administration of 1-methyl-4-phenyl-1,2,3,6-tetrahydropyridine (MPTP) in the squirrel monkey. Brain Res 1984;292:390–4.

[12] Bloem BR, Irwin I, Buruma OJ, et al. The MPTP model: versatile contributions to the treatment of idiopathic Parkinson's disease. J Neurol Sci 1990;97:273–93.

[13] Langston JW, Irwin I, Langston EB, et al. 1-Methyl-4-phenyl-pyridinium ion (MPP+): identification of a metabolite of MPTP, a toxin selective to the substantia nigra. Neurosci Lett 1984;48:87–92.

[14] Markey SP, Johannessen JN, Chiueh CC, et al. Intraneuronal generation of a pyridinium metabolite may cause drug-induced parkinsonism. Nature 1984;311:464–7.

[15] Chiba K, Trevor AJ, Castagnoli N Jr. Metabolism of the neurotoxic tertiary amine, MPTP, by brain monoamine oxidase. Biochem Biophys Res Commun 1984;120:575–8.

[16] Ruttenber AJ, Garbe PL, Kalter HD, et al. Meperidine analog exposure in California narcotics abusers: initial epidemiologic findings. In: Markey SP, Cstagnoli N Jr, Trevor AJ, et al, editors. MPTP: a neurotoxin producing a parkinsonian syndrome. New York: Academic Press; 1986. p. 339–53.

[17] Calne DB, Langston JW, Martin WRW, et al. Positron emission tomography after MPTP: observations relating to the cause of Parkinson's disease. Nature 1985;317:246–8.

[18] Tetrud JW, Langston JW, Redmond DE Jr, et al. MPTP-induced tremor in human and non-human primates. Neurology 1986;36:308.

[19] Tetrud JW, Langston JW. Tremor in MPTP-induced parkinsonism. Neurology 1992;42: 407–10.

[20] Langston JW, Ballard PA. Parkinsonism induced by 1-methyl-4-phenyl-1,2,3,6-tetra-hydropyridine (MPTP): implications for treatment and the pathogenesis of Parkinson's disease. Can J Neurol Sci 1984;11:160–5.

[21] Langston JW. MPTP-induced parkinsonism: how good a model is it? In: Fahn S, Marsen CD, Teychenne P, et al, editors. Recent advances in Parkinson's disease. New York: Raven Press; 1986. p. 119–26.

[22] Snow BJ, Vingerhoets FJ, Langston JW, et al. Pattern of dopaminergic loss in the striatum of humans with MPTP induced parkinsonism. J Neurol Neurosurg Psychiatry 2000;68: 313–6.

[23] Langston JW, Forno LS, Tetrud J, et al. Evidence of active nerve cell degeneration in the substantia nigra of humans years after 1-methyl-4-phenyl-1,2,3,6-tetrahydropyridine exposure. Ann Neurol 1999;46:598–605.

[24] Forno LS, Langston JW, DeLanney LE, et al. An electron microscopic study of MPTP-induced inclusion bodies in an old monkey. Brain Res 1988;448:150–7.

[25] Crouper J. Sur les effets du peroxide de manganese. J Chim Med Pharm Toxicol 1837;3: 223–5.

[26] Nagatomo S, Umehara F, Hanada K, et al. Manganese intoxication during total parenteral nutrition: report of two cases and review of the literature. J Neurol Sci 1999;162: 102–5.

[27] Meco G, Bonifati V, Vanacore N, et al. Parkinsonism after chronic exposure to the fungicide maneb (manganese ethylene-bis-dithiocarbamate). Scand J Work Environ Health 1994;20:301–5.

[28] Aschner M, Aschner JL. Manganese neurotoxicity: cellular effects and blood-brain barrier transport. Neurosci Beh Rev 1991;15:333–40.

[29] Donaldson J, Labaella FS, Gesser D. Enhanced autoxidation of dopamine as a possible basis of mangaese neurotoxicity. Neurotoxicology 1981;2:53–64.

[30] Donaldson J. The pathophysiology of trace metal: neurotrasmitter interaction in the CNS. Trends Pharmacol Sci 1981;1:75–7.

[31] Graham DG. Catecholamine toxicity: a proposal for the molecular pathogenesis of manganese neurotoxicity and Parkinson's disease. Neurotoxicology 1984;5:83–96.

[32] Pal PK, Samii A, Calne DB. Manganese neurotoxicity: a review of clinical features, imaging and pathology. Neurotoxicology 1999;20:227–38.

[33] Mena I, Marin O, Fuenzalida S, et al. Chronic manganese poisoning: clinical picture and manganese turnover. Neurology 1967;17:128–36.

[34] Huang CC, Chu NS, Lu CS, et al. Chronic manganese intoxication. Arch Neurol 1989;46: 1104–6.

[35] Cook DG, Fahn S, Brait KA. Chronic manganese intoxication. Arch Neurol 1974;30: 59–64.

[36] Barbeau A. Manganese and extrapyramidal disorders. Neurotoxicology 1984;5:13–36.

[37] Racette BA, McGee-Minnich L, Moerlein SM, et al. Welding-related parkinsonism: clinical features, treatment, and pathophysiology. Neurology 2001;56:8–13.

[38] Huang CC, Chu NS, Lu CS, et al. Long-term progression in chronic manganism. Neurology 1998;50:698–700.

[39] Mena I, Court J, Fuenzalida S, et al. Modification of chronic manganese poisoning: treatment with L-dopa and 5-OH tryptophane. N Engl J Med 1970;282:5–10.

[40] Rosenstock HA, Simons DG, Meyer JS. Chronic manganism: neurologic and laboratory studies during treatment with levodopa. JAMA 1971;217:1354–8.

[41] Lu CS, Huang CC, Chu NS, et al. Levodopa failure in chronic manganism. Neurology 1994;44:1600–2.

[42] Koller WC, Lyons KE, Truly W. Effect of levodopa treatment for parkinsonism in welders: a double-blind study. Neurology 2004;62:730–3.

[43] Eriksson H, Tedroff J, Thuomas KA, et al. Manganese induced brain lesions in *Macaca fascicularis* as revealed by positron emission tomography and magnetic resonance imaging. Arch Toxicol 1992;66:403–7.

[44] Nelson K, Gulnick J, Korn T, et al. Manganese encephalopathy: utility of early magnetic resonance imaging. Br J Ind Med 1993;50:510–3.

[45] Newland MC, Ceckler TL, Kordower JH, et al. Visualizing manganese in the primate basal ganglia with magnetic resonance imaging. Exp Neurol 1989;106:251–8.

[46] Shinotoh H, Snow BJ, Hewitt KA, et al. MRI and PET studies of manganese-intoxicated monkeys. Neurology 1995;45:1199–204.

[47] Wolters EC, Huang CC, Clark C, et al. Positron emission tomography in manganese intoxication. Ann Neurol 1989;26:647–51.

[48] Pentschew A, Ebner FF, Kovatch RM. Experimental manganese encephalopathy in monkeys: a preliminary report. J Neuropathol Exp Neurol 1963;22:488–99.

[49] Eriksson H, Magiste K, Plantin LO, et al. Effects of manganese oxide on monkeys as revealed by a combined neurochemical, histological and neurophysiological evaluation. Arch Toxicol 1987;61:46–52.

[50] Shukla GS, Chandra SV. Species variation in manganese induced changes in brain biogenic amines. Toxicol Lett 1979;3:249–53.

[51] Neff NH, Barrett RE, Costa E. Selective depletion of caudate nucleus dopamine and serotonin during chronic manganese dioxide administration to squirrel monkeys. Experientia 1969;25:1140–1.

[52] Ritchie JM. The aliphatic alcohols. In: Goodman LS, Gilman A, editors. The pharmacological basis of therapeutics. London: Macmillan; 1970. p. 135–50.

[53] Symon L, Pasztor E, Dorsch NWC. Physiological responses of local areas of the cerebral circulation in experimental primates determined by the method of hydrogen clearance. Stroke 1973;4:632–4.

[54] Branch A, Tonning DJ. Acute methyl alchol poisoning. Observations in some thirty cases. Can J Public Health 1945;36:147–51.

[55] Schneck SA. Methanol. In: Vinken PJ, Bruyn GW, editors. Handbook of clinical neurology, vol 36. Amsterdam: Elsevier; 1979. p. 351–60.

[56] Bennett IL, Cary FH, Mitchell GL, et al. Acute methyl alcohol poisoning: a review based on experiences in an outbreak of 323 cases. Medicine 1953;32:431–63.

[57] Kenney AH, Mellinkoff SM. Methyl alcohol poisoning. Ann Intern Med 1951;34:331–8.

[58] Borhaus EC. Methyl alcohol poisoning: a clinical and pathological study of 11 fatal cases. Illinois Med J 1930;57:260–3.

[59] Riegel H, Wolf G. Schwere neurologische Ausfalle als Folge einer Methylalkoholvergif-tung. Fortschr Neurol Psychiatr 1966;34:346–51.

[60] Guggenheim MA, Couch JR, Weinberg W. Motor dysfunction as a permanent com-plication of methanol ingestion. Arch Neurol 1971;24:550–4.

[61] McLean DR, Jacobs H, Mielke BW. Methanol poisoning: a clinical and pathological study. Ann Neurol 1980;8:161–7.

[62] Aquilonius SM, Aksmark H, Enokson P. Computerized tomography in severe methanol intoxication. BMJ 1978;1:929–30.

[63] Verslegers W, Van den Kerchove M, Crols R, et al. Methanol intoxication. Parkinsonism and decreased Met-enkephalin levels due to putaminal necrosis. Acta Neurol Belg 1988;88: 163–71.

[64] Potts AM, Praglin J, Farkas J, et al. Studies on the visual toxicity of methanol. Am J Ophthalmol 1953;40:76–83.

[65] Seppalainen AM, Haltia M. Carbon disulfide. In: Spencer PS, Schaumberg HH, editors. Experimental and clinical neurotoxicology. Baltimore: Williams & Wilkins; 1980. p. 356–73.

[66] Negro F. Les syndromes parkinsoniens par intoxication sulfide-carbonee. Rev Neurol 1930;49:518–22.

[67] Ranaletti A. Die berufliche Schwefelkohlenstoffvergiftung in Italien: Klink und Exper-imente. Arch Gwerbepathol Gewerbehyg 1931;2:664–75.

[68] Quarelli G. Les syndrome strio-pallidal dans l'intoxication chronique par sulfure de carbon (Syndrome de Quarelli). Presse Med 1937;1:533–5.

[69] Aaserud O, Gjerstad L, Nakstad P, et al. Neurological examination, computerized tomography, cerebral blood flow and neuropsychological examination in workers with long-term exposure to carbon disulfide. Toxicology 1988;49:277–82.

[70] Aaserud O, Hommeren OJ, Tvedt B, et al. Carbon disulfide exposure and neurotoxic sequelae among viscose rayon workers. Am J Ind Med 1990;18:25–37.

[71] Vigliani EC. Carbon disulphide poisoning in viscose rayon factories. Br J Ind Med 1954;11: 235–44.

[72] Peters HA, Levine RL, Matthews CG, et al. Extrapyramidal and other neurologic manifestations associated with carbon disulfide fumigant exposure. Arch Neurol 1988;45: 537–40.

[73] Alpers BJ, Lewy FH. Changes in the nervous system following carbon disulfide poisoning in animals and in man. Arch Neurol Psychiatry 1940;44:725–6.

[74] Richter R. Degeneration of the basal ganglia in monkeys from chronic carbon disulfide poisoning. J Neuropathol Exp Neurol 1945;4:324–53.

[75] Bus JS. The relationship of carbon disulfide metabolism to development of toxicity. Neurotoxicology 1985;4:73–80.

[76] Spencer PS, Couri D, Schaumburg HH. n-Hexane and methyl n-butyl ketone. In: Spencer PS, Schaumberg HH, editors. Experimental and clinical neurotoxicology. Baltimore: Williams & Wilkins; 1980. p. 456–75.

[77] Vanacore N, Gasparini M, Brusa L, et al. A possible association between exposure to n-hexane and parkinsonism. Neurol Sci 2000;21:49–52.

[78] Pezzoli G, Antonini A, Barbieri S, et al. n-Hexane-induced parkinsonism: pathogenetic hypotheses. Mov Disord 1995;10:279–82.

[79] Pezzoli G, Strada O, Silani V, et al. Clinical and pathological features in hydrocarbon-induced parkinsonism. Ann Neurol 1996;40:922–5.

[80] Melamed E, Lavy S. Parkinsonism associated with chronic inhalation of carbon tetrachloride. Lancet 1977;7(1):1015.

[81] Henschler D. Wichtige Gifte und Vergiftungen. In: Forth W, Henschler D, Rummel W, editors. Allgemeine und spezielle pharmakologie und toxikologie. 5th edition. Wissenschaftsverlag: Mannheim; 1987. p. 751–2.

[82] Moeschlin S. Klinik und Therapie der Vergiftungen. 6th edition. Stuttgart: Georg Thieme Verlag; 1980. p. 252–6.

[83] Feldman JM, Feldman MD. Sequelae of attempted suicide by cyanide ingestion: a case report. Int J Psychiatr Med 1990;20:173–9.

[84] Borron SW, Baud FJ. Acute cyanide poisoning: clinical spectrum, diagnosis, and treatment. Arh Hig Rada Toksikol 1996;47:307–22.

[85] Lopez-Ibor J. Neurologische Erscheinungen infolge van Blausaureintoxikationen. Arch Psychiatr Nervenkr 1943;116:18–25.

[86] Grandas F, Artieda J, Obeso JA. Clinical and CT scan findings in a case of cyanide intoxication. Mov Disord 1989;4:188–93.

[87] Rosenow F, Herholz K, Lanfermann H, et al. Neurological sequelae of cyanide intoxication: the patterns of clinical, magnetic resonance imaging and positron emission tomography findings. Ann Neurol 1995;38:825–8.

[88] Rosenberg NL, Myers JA, Martin WR. Cyanide-induced parkinsonism: clinical, MRI, and 6-fluorodopa PET studies. Neurology 1989;39:142–4.

[89] Messing B, Storch B. Computer tomography and magnetic resonance imaging in cyanide poisoning. Eur Arch Psychiatry Neurol Sci 1988;237:139–43.

[90] Rachinger J, Fellner FA, Stieglbauer K, et al. MR changes after acute cyanide intoxication. Am J Neurorad 2002;23:1398–401.

[91] Koumbourlis AC, Skoutakis VA. Carbon monoxide poisoning: diagnosis and treatment. Clin Toxicol Consult 1982;4:51–69.

[92] Norkool DM, Kirkpatrick JN. Treatment of acute carbon monoxide poisoning with hyperbaric oxygen: a review of 115 cases. Ann Emerg Med 1985;14:1168–71.

[93] Smith JS, Brandon S. Morbidity from acute carbon monoxide poisoning at three year follow-up. BMJ 1973;1:318–21.

[94] Myers RAM, Shyder SK, Emhoff TA. Subacute sequelae of carbon monoxide poisoning at three year follow-up. Ann Emerg Med 1985;14:1163–7.

[95] Fennell EB, Booth MP, Moberg PJ, et al. Neuropsychological evaluation of 1 case of acute simultaneous exposure to moderate levels of carbon monoxide [abstract]. Neurology 1991;41(Suppl):237.

[96] Minerbo GM, Jankovic J. Prevalence of Parkinson's disease among firefighters [abstract]. Neurology 1990;40(Suppl):348.

[97] Choi IS. Delayed neurologic sequelae of carbon monoxide toxicity. Arch Neurol 1983;40: 433–5.

[98] Lassinger BK, Kwak C, Walford RL, et al. Atypical parkinsonism and motor neuron syndrome in a Biosphere 2 participant: a possible complication of chronic hypoxia and carbon monoxide toxicity? Mov Dis 2004;19:465–9.

[99] Spencer PS, Butterfield PG. Environmental agents and Parkinson's disease. In: Ellenberg JH, Koller WC, Langston JW, editors. Etiology of Parkinson's disease. New York: Marcel Dekker; 1995. p. 319–65.

[100] Shillito JH, Drinker CK, Shaughnessy TJ. The problem of nervous and mental sequelae in carbon monoxide poisoning. JAMA 1936;106:669–74.

[101] Richardson JC, Chambers RA, Heywood PM. Encephalopathies of anoxia and hypoglycemia. Arch Neurol 1959;1:178–82.

[102] Garland H, Pearce J. Neurological complications of carbon monoxide poisoning. Q J Med 1967;36:445–55.

[103] Lee MS, Marsden CD. Neurological sequelae following carbon monoxide poisoning: clinical course and outcome according to the clinical types and brain computed tomography scan findings. Mov Disord 1994;9:550–8.

[104] Choi IS. Parkinsonism after carbon monoxide poisoning. Eur Neurol 2002;48:30–3.

[105] Ginsberg MD. Delayed neurological deterioration following hypoxia. Adv Neurol 1979;26: 21–43.

[106] Shon YH, Jeong Y, Kim HS, et al. The brain lesion responsible for parkinsonism after carbon monoxide poisoning. Arch Neurol 2000;57:1214–8.

[107] Jellinger K. Exogenous lesions of the pallidum. In: Vinken PJ, Bryn GW, Klawans HL, editors. Handbook of clinical neurology. New York: Elsevier; 1986. p. 465–91.

[108] Kobayahsi K, Isaki K, Fukutani Y, et al. CT findings of the interval form of carbon monoxide poisoning compared with neuropathological findings. Eur Neurol 1984;23:34–43.

[109] Zimmerman HM. Monthly report to medical officer in command, US Navy Medical Research Unit No. 2, 1945:221.

[110] Arnold A, Edgren DC, Palladino VS. Amyotrophic lateral sclerosis: fifty cases observed on Guam. J Nerv Ment Dis 1953;117:135–9.

[111] Koener DR. Amyotrophic lateral sclerosis on Guam: a clinical study and review of the literature. Ann Intern Med 1952;37:1204–20.

[112] Kurland LT, Mulder DW. Epidemiologic investigations of amyotrophic lateral sclerosis. I. Preliminary report on geographic distribution, with special reference to the Mariana Islands, including clinical and pathologic observations. Neurology 1954;5:355–78; and 6:438–48.

[113] Norstag KJ, Nichols TJ. The Biology of cycads. Ithaca (NY): Cornell University Press; 1997.

[114] Vega A, Bell EA. α-Amino-β-methylaminoproprionic acid, a new amino acid from seeds of Cycas circinalis. Phytochemistry 1967;6:759–62.

[115] Cox PA, Banack SA, Murch SJ. Biomagnification of cyanobacterial neurotoxins and neurodegenerative disease among the Chamorro people of Guam. Proc Natl Acad Sci USA 2003;100:13380–3.

[116] Spencer PS, Nunn PB, Hugon J, et al. Motorneurone disease on Guam: possible role of a food neurotoxin. Lancet 1986;1:965.

[117] Spencer PS, Nunn PB, Hugon J, et al. Guam amyotrophic lateral sclerosis-parkinsonism-dementia linked to a plant excitant neurotoxin. Science 1987;237:517–22.

[118] Cox PA, Sacks OW. Cycad neurotoxins, consumption of flying foxes, and ALS-PDC disease in Guam. Neurology 2002;58:956–9.

[119] Mickelburgh SP, Hutson AM, Racey PA. Old World fruit bats: an action plan for their conservation. Gland, Switzerland: IUCN; 1992.

[120] Zhang ZX, Anderson DW, Mantel N, et al. Motor-neuron disease in Guam: geographic and familial occurrence, 1956–85. Acta Neurol Scand 1996;94:51–79.

[121] Wiles GJ, Fujita MS. Food plants and economic importance of flying foxes on Pacific Islands. Biol Rep 1992;90:24–35.

[122] Murch SJ, Cox PA, Banack SA. A mechanism for slow release of biomagnified cyanobacterial neurotoxins and neurodegenerative disease in Guam. Proc Natl Acad Sci USA 2004;101:12228–31.

[123] Hursthouse MB, Motevalli M, O'Brien P, et al. X-ray crystal structure of a copper (II) complex of neurotoxic amino acid, DL-α-amino-β-methylaminoproprionic acid. J Chem Soc Dalton Trans 1990;1985–7.

[124] Nunn PB, O'Brien P, Pettit LD, et al. Complexes of zinc, copper, and nickel with the nonprotein amino acid L-alpha-amino-beta-methylaminopropionic acid: a naturally occurring neurotoxin. J Inorg Biochem 1989;37:175–83.

[125] Weiss JH, Sensi SL. Zn (2+): a novel ionic mediator of neural injury in brain disease. Trends Neurosci 2000;23:365–71.

[126] Carriedo SG, Yin ZH, Weiss JH. Motor neurons are selectively vulnerable to AMPA/ kainate receptor-mediated injury in vitro. J Neurosci 1996;16:4069–79.

[127] Hirano A, Kurland LT, Krooth RS, et al. Parkinsonism-dementia complex, an endemic disease on the island of Guam. I. Clinical features. Brain 1961;84:642–61.

[128] Galasko D, Salmon DP, Craig U-K, et al. Clinical features and changing patterns of neurodegenerative disorders on Guam, 1997–2000. Neurology 2002;58:90–7.

[129] Elizan TS, Hirano A, Abrams BM, et al. Amyotrophic lateral sclerosis and parkinsonism-dementia complex of Guam. Neurological re-evaluation. Arch Neurol 1966;14:356–68.

[130] Chen KM, Chase TN. Parkinsonism-dementia complex. In: Vinken PJ, Bryn GM, Klawans HL, editors. Handbook of clinical neurology, vol. 49. Extrapyramidal disorders. New York: Elsevier Science; 1986. p. 167–83.

[131] Doi H, Chen KM, Chase TN, et al. Effect of L-dopa on clinical duration and quality of life in PDC of Guam. Clin Neurol (Japan) 1983;23:935–42.

[132] Holden EM, Brody JA, Chase TN. Parkinsonism-dementia of Guam: treatment with levodopa and L-alpha-methyldopahydrazine. Neurology 1974;24:263–5.

[133] Neiman J, Lang AE, Fornazzari L, et al. Movement disorders in alcoholism: a review. Neurology 1990;40:741–6.

[134] Carlen PL, Lee MA, Jacob M, et al. Parkinsonism provoked by alcoholism. Ann Neurol 1981;9:84–6.

[135] Lang AE, Marsden CD, OBeso JA, et al. Alcohol and Parkinson disease. Ann Neurol 1982; 12:254–6.

[136] Shen WW. Extrapyramidal symptoms associated with alcohol withdrawal. Biol Psychiatry 1984;19:1037–43.

[137] Carlen PL, Wilkinson DA, Wortzman G, et al. Cerebral atrophy and functional deficits in alcoholics without clinically apparent liver disease. Neurology 1981;31:377–85.

[138] Shandling M, Carlen PL, Lang AE. Parkinsonism in alcohol withdrawal: a follow-up study. Mov Dis 1990;5:36–9.

[139] Carella F, Grassi MP, Savoiardo M, et al. Dystonic-parkinsonian syndrome after cyanide poisoning: clinical and MRI findings. J Neurol Neurosurg Psychiatry 1988;51:1345–8.

[140] Borgohain R, Singh AK, Radhakrishna H, et al. Delayed onset generalised dystonia after cyanide poisoning. Clin Neurol Neurosurg 1995;97:213–5.

[141] Valenzuela R, Court J, Godoy J. Delayed cyanide induced dystonia. J Neurol Neurosurg Psychiatry 1992;55:198–9.

[142] Quartarone A, Girlanda P, Vita G, et al. Oromandibular dystonia in a patient with bilateral putaminal necrosis after methanol poisoning: an electrophysiological study. Eur Neurol 2000;44:127–8.

[143] LeWitt PA, Martin SD. Dystonia and hypokinesis with putaminal necrosis after methanol intoxication. Clin Neuropharmacol 1988;11:161–7.

[144] Gould DH, Gustine DL. Basal ganglia degeneration, myelin alteration, and enzyme inhibition induced in mice by the plant toxin 3-nitropropionic acid. Neuropathol Appl Neurobiol 1982;8:377–93.

[145] Liu XJ. Investigation of the etiology of mildewed sugarcane poisoning. A review. Chung Hua Yu Fang I Hsueh Tsa Chih 1986;20:306–8.

[146] He F, Zhang S, Qian F, et al. Delayed dystonia with striatal CT lucencies induced by a mycotoxin (3-nitropropionic acid). Neurology 1995;45:2178–83.

[147] Fu Y, He F, Zhang S, et al. Consistent striatal damage in rats induced by 3-nitropropionic acid and cultures of arthrinium fungus. Neurotoxicol Teratol 1995;17:413–8.

[148] Klawans HL. Dystonia and tremor following exposure to 2,3,7-tetrachlorodibenzo-p-dioxin. Mov Disord 1987;2:255.

[149] Diersen G, Bergman LL, Gioino G, et al. Hemiballismus following surgery for Parkinson disease. Arch Neurol Psychiat 1961;5:627–37.

[150] Hughes B. Involuntary movements following stereotactic operations. J Neurol Neurosurg Psychiat 1965;28:291–303.

[151] Klawans HL, Weiner WJ. The effect of d-amphetamine on choreiform movement disorders. Neurology 1974;24:312–8.

[152] Kanazawa I, Kimura M, Murata M, et al. Choreic movements in the macaque monkey induced by kainic acid lesions of the striatum combined with l-dopa. Pharmacological, biochemical, and physiological studies on neural mechanisms. Brain 1990;113:509–35.

[153] Leys D, Bourgeois P, Destee A, Petit H. [Acute choreic syndrome and psychotic state induced by an amphetaminic drug.] Rev Neurol (Paris) 1985;141:499–500.

[154] Johanson C-E, Fischman MW. The pharmacology of cocaine as related to its abuse. Pharmacol Rev 1989;41:3–52.

[155] Ritz MC, Lamb RJ, Goldberg SR, et al. Cocaine receptors on dopamine transporters are related to self-administration of cocaine. Science 1987;237:1214–22.

[156] Dackis CA, Gold MS. New concepts in cocaine addiction: the dopamine depletion hypothesis. Neurosci Biobehav Rev 1985;9:469–77.

[157] Trulson ME, Babb S, Joe JC, et al. Chronic cocaine administration depletes tyrosine hydroxylase immunoreactivity in the rat nigral striatal system: quantitative light microscopic studies. Exp Neurol 1986;94:744–56.

[158] Volkow ND, Fowler JS, Wolf AP, et al. Effects of chronic cocaine abuse on postsynaptic dopamine receptors. Am Psychiatry 1990;147:719–24.

[159] Peris J, Boyson SJ, Cass WA, et al. Persistence of neurochemical changes in dopamine systems after repeated cocaine administration. J Pharmacol Exp Ther 1990;253:38–44.

[160] Sperling LS, Horowitz JL. Methamphetamine-induced choreoathetosis and rhabdomyolysis. Ann Intern Med 1994;121:986.

[161] Rhee KJ, Albertson TE, Douglas JC. Choreoathetoid disorder associated with amphetamine-like drugs. Am J Emerg Med 1988;6:131–3.

[162] Lundh H, Tunving K. An extrapyramidal choreiform syndrome caused by amphetamine addiction. J Neurol Neurosurg Psychiatry 1981;44:728–30.

[163] Daras M, Koppel BS, Atos-Radzion E. Cocaine-induced choreoathetoid movements ('crack dancing'). Neurology 1994;44:751–2.

[164] Bartzokis G, Beckson M, Wirshing DA, et al. Choreoathetoid movements in cocaine dependence. Biol Psychiatry 1999;45:1630–5.

[165] Balldin J, Alling C, Gottfries CG, et al. Changes in dopamine receptor sensitivity in humans after heavy alcohol intake. Psychopharmacology (Berlin) 1985;86:142–6.

[166] Mullin PJ, Kershaw PW, Bolt JMW. Choreoathetotic movement disorder in alcoholism. BMJ 1970;4:278–81.

[167] Fornazzari L, Carlen PL. Transient choreiform dyskinesias during alcohol withdrawal. Can J Neurol Sci 1982;9:89–90.

[168] Curry KH. Choreoathetosis and alcohol withdrawal. Med J Aust 1985;143:265–6.

[169] Toghill PJ, Johnston AW, Smith JF. Choreoathetosis in portosystemic encephalopathy. J Neurol Neursurg Psychiatry 1967;30:358–63.

[170] Bartolucci G, Pellettier JR. Glue sniffing and movement disorder. J Neurol Neurosurg Psychiatry 1984;47(11):1259.

[171] Goldings AS, Stewart RM. Organic lead encephalopathy: behavioral change and movement disorder following gasoline inhalation. J Clin Psychiatry 1982;43:70–2.

[172] Goodheart RS, Dunne JW. Petrol sniffer's encephalopathy. A study of 25 patients. Med J Aust 1994;160:178–81.

[173] Meucci G, Rossi G, Mazzoni M. A case of transient choreoathetosis with amnesic syndrome after acute monoxide poisoning. Ital J Neurol Sci 1989;10:513–7.

[174] Davous P, Rondot P, Marion MH, et al. Severe chorea after acute carbon monoxide poisoning. J Neurol Neurosurg Psychiatry 1986;49:206–8.

[175] Schwartz A, Hennerici M, Wegener OH. Delayed choreoathetosis following acute carbon monoxide poisoning. Neurology 1990;40:741–6.

[176] Burns R, Thomas DW, Barron VJ. Reversible encephalopathy possibly associated with bismuth subgallate ingestion. BMJ 1974;1:220–3.

[177] Buge A, Rancurel G, Poisson M, et al. [Myoclonic encephalopathies induced by bismuth salts. 6 cases observed during long-term oral treatment.] Nouv Presse Med 1974;3: 2315–20.

[178] Emile J, De Bray JM, Bernat M, et al. [Scapular and vertebral osteopathies during acute myoclonic bismuth encephalopathies. Apropos of 8 cases.] Ann Med Interne (Paris) 1979; 130:75–80.

[179] Liessens JL, Monstrey J, Vanden Eeckhout E, et al. Bismuth encephalopathy. A clinical and anatomo-pathological report of one case. Acta Neurol Belg 1978;78:301–9.

[180] Loseke N, Retif J, Coune A, et al. [Myoclonic bismuth-induced encephalopathy. Case report (author's translation).] Acta Gastroenterol Belg 1978;41:72–80.

[181] Hillemand P, Palliere M, Laquais B, et al. [Bismuth treatment and blood bismuth levels.] Sem Hop 1977;53:1663–9.

[182] Supino-Viterbo V, Sicard C, Risvegliato M, et al. Toxic encephalopathy due to ingestion of bismuth salts: clinical and EEG studies of 45 patients. J Neurol Neurosurg Psychiatry 1977; 40:748–52.

[183] Buge A, Rancurel G, Dechy H. [Bismuth myoclonic encephalopathies. Their course and lasting or definitive late complications.] Rev Neurol (Paris) 1977;133: 401–15.

[184] Gordon MF, Abrams RI, Rubin DB, et al. Bismuth subsalicylate toxicity as a cause of prolonged encephalopathy with myoclonus. Mov Disord 1995;10:220–2.

[185] Spencer PS. Aluminum and its compounds. In: Spencer PS, Schaumberg HH, Ludolph AC, editors. Experimental and clinical neurotoxicology. 2nd edition. New York: Oxford University Press; 2000. p. 142–51.

[186] Spofforth J. Case of aluminum poisoning. Lancet 1921;1:1301.

[187] McLaughlin AIG, Kazantos G, King E, et al. Pulmonary fibrosis and encephalopathy associated with inhalation of aluminum dust. Br J Ind Med 1962;19:253.

[188] Alfrey AC. Dialysis encephalopathy. In: Yasui M, Strong MJ, Ota K, et al, editors. Mineral and metal neurotoxicity. Boca Raton: CRC Press; 1997. p. 127.

[189] Mahurkar SD, Smith EC, Mamdani BH, et al. Dialysis dementia—the Chicago experience. J Dial 1978;2:447–58.

[190] Lederman RJ, Henry CE. Progressive dialysis encephalopathy. Ann Neurol 1978;4: 199–204.

[191] Burks JS, Alfrey AC, Huddlestone J, et al. A fatal encephalopathy in chronic hemodialysis patients. Lancet 1976;1:764.

[192] Sprague SM, Corwin HL, Tanner CM, et al. Relationship of aluminum to neurocognitive dysfunction in chronic dialysis patients. Arch Intern Med 1988;148:2169–72.

[193] Clarkson TW. The toxicology of mercury. Crit Rev Clin Lab Sci 1997;34:369–403.

[194] Kirchhof JK, Kumral K, Ertekin C. [Acute myoclonia following inhalation of mercury vapors.] Nervenarzt 1963;34:126–9.

[195] Neal PA, Jones RR. Chronic mercurialism in the hatter's fur-cutting industry. JAMA 1938; 110:337–43.

[196] Roullet E, Nizou R, Jedynak P, et al. [Intention and action myoclonus disclosing occupational mercury poisoning.] Rev Neurol (Paris) 1984;140:55–8.

[197] Snyder RD. The involuntary movements of chronic mercury poisoning. Arch Neurol 1972; 152:1443.

[198] Ono K, Komai K, Yamada M. Myoclonic involuntary movement associated with chronic manganese poisoning. J Neurol Sci 2002;199:93–6.

[199] Schneider SM, Rosskopf EN, Leesch JG, et al. United States Department of Agriculture– Agricultural Research Service research on alternatives to methyl bromide: pre-plant and post-harvest. Pest Manag Sci 2003;59:814–26.

[200] Langard S, Rognum T, Flotterod O, et al. Fatal accident resulting from methyl bromide poisoning after fumigation of a neighbouring house; leakage through sewage pipes. J Appl Toxicol 1996;16:445–8.

[201] Goulon M, Nouailhat F, Escourolle R, et al. [Methyl bromide poisoning. 3 cases, 1 fatal. Neruopathological study of one case of coma with myoclonus followed for 5 years.] Rev Neurol (Paris) 1975;131:445–68.

[202] De Haro L, Gastaut JL, Jouglard J, Renacco E. Central and peripheral neurotoxic effects of chronic methyl bromide intoxication. J Toxicol Clin Toxicol 1997;35:29–34.

[203] Hustinx WN, van de Laar RT, van Huffelen AC, et al. Systemic effects of inhalational methyl bromide poisoning: a study of nine cases occupationally exposed due to inadvertent spread during fumigation. Br J Ind Med 1993;50:155–9.

[204] Audry D, Soichot P, Giard MH, et al. [Rare cause of myoclonus with giant SEP's: methyl bromide poisoning. Apropos of a case with unilateral predominance.] Rev Electro-encephalogr Neurophysiol Clin 1985;15:45–52.

[205] Uncini A, Basciani M, Di Muzio A, et al. Methyl bromide myoclonus: an electrophysiological study. Acta Neurol Scand 1990;81:159–64.

[206] Yang RS, Witt KL, Alden CJ, et al. Toxicology of methyl bromide. Rev Environ Contam Toxicol 1995;142:65–85.

[207] Repko JD, Lasley SM. Behavioral, neurological, and toxic effects of methyl chloride: a review of the literature. CRC Crit Rev Toxicol 1979;6:283–302.

[208] Repko JD. Neurotoxicity of methyl chloride. Neurobehav Toxicol Teratol 1981;3:425–9.

[209] Scharnweber HC, Spears GN, Cowles SR. Chronic methyl chloride intoxication in six industrial workers. J Occup Med 1974;16:112–3.

[210] Hartman TL, Wacker W, Roll RM. Methyl chloride intoxication. N Engl J Med 1955;253:552.

[211] McNally WD. Eight cases of methyl chloride intoxication with three deaths. J Ind Hyg Toxicol 1946;28:94.

[212] Welch L, Kirshner H, Heath A, et al. Chronic neuropsychological and neurological impairment following acute exposure to a solvent mixture of toluene and methyl ethyl ketone (MEK). J Toxicol Clin Toxicol 1991;29:435–45.

[213] Orti-Pareja M, Jimenez-Jimenez FJ, Miquel J, et al. Reversible myoclonus, tremor, and ataxia in a patient exposed to methyl ethyl ketone. Neurology 1996;46:272.

[214] Dyro FM. Methyl ethyl ketone polyneuropathy in shoe factory workers. Clin Toxicol 1978;13:371–6.

[215] Sugiyama-Oishi A, Arakawa K, Araki E, et al. [A case of chronic toluene intoxication presenting stimulus-sensitive segmental spinal myoclonus.] No To Shinkei 2000;52:399–403.

[216] Hansen KS, Sharp FR. Gasoline sniffing, lead poisoning, and myoclonus. JAMA 1978;240:1375–6.

[217] Dorndorf W, Kresse M, Christain W, et al. [Dichloroethane poisoning with myoclonic syndrome, seizures and irreversible cerebral defects (author's translation).] Arch Psychiatr Nervenkr 1975;220:373–9.

[218] Doring G, Baumeister FA, Peters J, et al. Butane abuse associated encephalopathy. Klin Padiatr 2002;214:295–8.

[219] Peatfield RC, Boothman BR. Transient myoclonus after exposure to oven cleaner. Mov Disord 1991;6:90–1.

[220] Bratzlavsky M, van der Eeken H. Medullary actions of tetanus toxin: an electrophysiological study in man. Arch Neurol 1976;33:783–5.

[221] Fernandez JM, Ferrandiz M, Larrea L, et al. Cephalic tetanus studied with single fibre EMG. J Neurol Neurosurg Psychiatry 1983;46:862–6.

[222] Warren JD, Kimber TE, Thompson PD. Brainstem myoclonus in generalised tetanus. Mov Disord 2003;18:1204–6.

[223] Pascual-Leone A, Dhuna A. Cocaine-associated multifocal tics. Neurology 1990;40: 999–1000.

[224] Chouinard S, Ford B. Adult onset tic disorders. J Neurol Neurosurg Psychiatry 2000;68: 738–43.

[225] Pulst SM, Walshe TM, Romero JA. Carbon monoxide poisoning with features of Gilles de la Tourette's syndrome. Arch Neurol 1983;40:443–4.

[226] Ko SB, Ahn TB, Kim JM, et al. A case of adult onset tic disorder following carbon monoxide intoxication. Can J Neurol Sci 2004;31:268–70.

[227] Chang LW. Mercury. In: Spencer PS, Schaumburg HH, editors. Experimental and clinical neurotoxicology. Baltimore: Williams & Wilkins; 1980. p. 508–26.

[228] Coulehan JL, Hirsch W, Brillman J, et al. Gasoline sniffing and lead toxicity in Navajo adolescents. Pediatrics 1983;71:113.

[229] Zatuchni J, Hong K. Methyl bromide poisoning seen initially as psychosis. Arch Neurol 1981;38:529.

[230] Taylor JR, Selhorst JB, Houff SA, et al. Chlordecone intoxication in man. I. Clinical observations. Neurology 1978;28:626–30.

[231] Cannon SB, Veazey JM Jr, Jackson RS, et al. Epidemic kepone poisoning in chemical workers. Am J Epidemiol 1978;107:529–37.

[232] Taylor JR. Neurological manifestations in humans exposed to chlordecone: follow-up results. Neurotoxicology 1985;6:231–6.

[233] Taylor JR. Neurological manifestations in humans exposed to chlordecone and follow-up results. Neurotoxicology 1982;3:9–16.

[234] Iwata S, Nomoto M, Fukuda T. Effects of beta-adrenergic blockers on drug-induced tremors. Pharmacol Biochem Behav 1993;44:611.

[235] Hietanen E, Vainio H. Effect of administration route on DDT on acute toxicity and on drug biotransformation in various rodents. Arch Environ Contam Toxicol 1976;4:201.

ELSEVIER
SAUNDERS

NEUROLOGIC
CLINICS

Neurol Clin 23 (2005) 461–484

Amyotrophic Lateral Sclerosis: Possible Role of Environmental Influences

Matthew P. Wicklund, MD

Department of Neurology, Wilford Hall Medical Center, 59MDOS/MMCN,
2200 Bergquist Drive, Suite 1, Lackland Air Force Base, TX 78236, USA

Disease overview

Described by Charcot in 1874, amyotrophic lateral sclerosis (ALS) is a disorder of progressive upper and lower motor neuron degeneration [1]. Lower motor neuron loss manifests as weakness, muscular atrophy, and fasciculations, whereas brisk muscle stretch reflexes, clonus, motor dyscontrol, and Babinski's sign reflect upper motor neuron disease. Sensory and autonomic systems are spared. Although previously believed not to affect cognition, evidence now suggests frontal executive deficits in half of patients who have ALS and frank frontotemporal lobar dementia in a smaller segment [2]. Disease onset occurs approximately equally in the bulbar, cervical, and lumbar regions, with death ensuing within 1 to 6 years [3]. Death occurs most often as a result of respiratory failure. The prognosis for survival in bulbar onset ALS is much shorter on average than in ALS with initial lower extremity onset. Isolated lower motor neuron involvement is called progressive muscular atrophy, whereas solitary upper motor neuron disease carries the moniker of primary lateral sclerosis. Progressive muscular atrophy and primary lateral sclerosis advance more slowly than, but often ultimately transform into, ALS.

The incidence and prevalence of ALS increase with age through the seventh to eighth decades, with men suffering the disorder approximately twice as frequently as females. Epidemiologic studies suggest an increasing incidence of ALS over time. This observed increase likely relates to aging of the world's population, greater precision in diagnosis of ALS, and better case ascertainment [4]. Worldwide, incidence rates of 0.6 to 2.6 per 100,000

The views expressed herein are those of the author and do not reflect the official policy of the United States Air Force or the Department of Defense.

E-mail address: matthew.wicklund@lackland.af.mil

doi:10.1016/j.ncl.2004.12.016   *neurologic.theclinics.com*

and prevalence rates of 1.5 to 8.5 per 100,000 occur nearly uniformly across the globe [5], with a lifetime likelihood of mortality from ALS of approximately 1:1000. Isolated pockets in the Western Pacific, including Guam, the Kii Peninsula of Japan, and western New Guinea, have had markedly elevated incidence rates in the past, sparking research of these populations. More patients who have ALS seem to be born in the spring months [6].

The diagnosis of ALS requires confirmation of upper and lower motor neuron dysfunction. Other neurologic systems should not be affected, and ALS mimickers must be excluded [7,8]. El Escorial World Federation of Neurology criteria for the diagnosis of ALS require evidence of upper and lower motor neuron disease in three of four regions (bulbar, cervical, thoracic, and lumbar). In addition to abnormalities on neurologic examination, MRI, magnetic resonance spectroscopy, magnetic resonance diffusion tensor imaging, and cortical magnetic stimulation may document disease in upper motor neurons [9–11]. Electromyography confirms clinically silent lower motor neuron dysfunction in addition to quantifying the number of remaining motor neurons [12]. Although readily diagnosed clinically, the differential diagnosis of ALS remains broad. Diagnostic considerations requiring exclusion include hyperthyroidism, hyperparathyroidism, brainstem disease, intrinsic and extrinsic disease of the cervical spinal cord, Kennedy's disease, Hirayama's disease, postpolio syndrome, hexosaminidase deficiency, polyradiculopathies and myeloradiculopathies, multifocal motor neuropathy, neuromuscular junction disorders, and inflammatory myopathies [13]. Serology, electromyography, neuroimaging, and mutation analysis exclude these alternative diagnoses.

Currently, treatment options for ALS are limited and mostly ineffective. Riluzole, a glutamate antagonist, is the only agent on the market documented to affect disease progression in ALS. In a published trial, the time to death or respiratory failure (a surrogate marker for death) in the treatment group was 18 months versus 15 months in the placebo group, a benefit of 3 additional months of life [14]. Most of the patients in this trial had moderately advanced disease, and it is believed that treatment early in the course provides up to a year's benefit in terms of life extension. Many patients also are treated with other agents, such as antioxidants, coenzyme Q10, creatine, and minocycline, with hopes that these agents may benefit survival. Lamotrigene, gabapentin, dextromethorphan, selegiline, brain-derived neurotrophic factor, insulin-like growth factor, glial-derived growth factor, clyclophosphamide, levamisole, and amantadine all have proved ineffective in controlled clinical trials.

Although most cases of ALS occur sporadically, approximately 10% are familial [15]. In 1993, mutations were first reported in the gene for copper/zinc superoxide dismutase (*SOD1*), which catalyzes dismutation of the superoxide radical to hydrogen peroxide and oxygen [16]. More than 100 different *SOD1* mutations have since been discovered [17–19]. Most *SOD1* mutations follow autosomal dominant inheritance. Some families that have recessive ALS, however, carry homozygous D90A mutations in the *SOD1* gene [20]. Initially, *SOD1* mutations were believed to exert deleterious effects via diminished enzymatic activity with resultant excitotoxicity. This now is known to be not true. *SOD1* enzyme activity does not correlate with disease expression [21], and *SOD1* knockout mouse models do not develop ALS [22]. Dominant *SOD1* mutations are believed to act via a toxic gain of function as a result of accumulation of abnormal *SOD1* protein products [18]. Genetic testing in sporadic ALS cases estimates 5% to 10% of these cases also carry a genetic underpinning [23,24]. Twelve different chromosomal loci now are known to underlie different genetic forms of ALS, with gene products delineated in at least five [19,25].

Case-control studies

Because of low incidence and prevalence rates, large, randomized, prospective cohort studies are difficult to perform in ALS. Even multiple center studies cannot recruit enough patients over reasonable periods of time. Until studies begin to appear out of the newly formed North American Amyotrophic Lateral Sclerosis Research Group, most research will be conducted on cohorts of smaller sizes, approximately 50 to 200 patients. Much research into the cause of ALS, therefore, has been conducted using case-control studies during the past several decades.

Case-control studies allow evaluation of putative risk factors for disease by retrospectively comparing their presence or absence between patients and matched controls. Patient and control selection and data collection methodology unfortunately may lead to multiple sources of bias. Some forms of bias favor the hypothesis and others decrease its likelihood. Case-control studies also identify only associations and not causal relationships. Selection bias may lead to patient populations derived from samples not reflective of the disease population (eg, patients who have ALS and are referred to a university hospital's neuromuscular center tend to be younger and more atypical in presentation). Nonrespondent bias unwittingly may exclude key portions of the patient or control populations. Inversely, overmatching of patient and control populations might diminish the chance of finding a difference between two populations (eg, patients and controls from the same workplace or households may have similar exposures). Recall bias is difficult to exclude. Patients more commonly recall exposures, whereas controls, with less at stake, more often do not. Interviewers may not be blinded to the patient's condition (ALS patients often appear obviously infirm and debilitated) and might inadvertently probe harder for details from patients than controls (interviewer bias). An inadequate sample size reduces a study's statistical power and constrains the possibility of delineating small, yet key, differences between groups. If the cause of ALS is multifactorial, small differences in only a portion of a population may be diluted and not detected. Finally, multiple statistical determinations increase the likelihood of finding one or more associations based solely on chance. Even with all these limitations, case-control studies still supply the bulwark of the data comprising the knowledge of putative ALS risk factors.

Heavy metals and trace elements

Because of clinical similarities between some heavy metal poisoning cases and ALS and because of the correlation between certain trace elements and clusters of motor neuron disease, early importance was placed on investigation of these factors.

Lead

From Wilson's article in 1907 [26] through today [27], toxicity resulting from lead poisoning has been known to cause a motor polyneuropathy sometimes mimicking ALS [28,29]. Many case-control studies evaluated lead's role in ALS. Several of these studies purport a greater association with lead exposure for patients than for controls [30–36], whereas other studies fail to find such association [37–39]. Investigators also found increased concentrations of lead in cerebrospinal fluid [40,41], plasma [42], blood [36], skeletal muscle [43,44], nerve [44], spinal cord [44,45], and bone [36]. Lead accumulation in these tissues in ALS is of uncertain etiologic significance. Mandybur and Cooper [46] elegantly demonstrated that accumulation of spinal cord lead content is independent of lead intake in rats that have experimental allergic encephalitis. Spinal cords in diseased rats that had experimental allergic encephalitis (whether or not fed a diet high in lead) accumulated twice the lead concentration as control rats. The investigators conclude that lead accumulation in spinal cords might be a manifestation of disease and not of lead intake or exposure. Recently, other investigators find no difference in lead levels in blood [47,48] or toenails (a good source for evaluation of exposures during the previous 6 to 18 months) [49]. Chelation therapy leads to clinical improvement in patients who have lead-associated motor polyneuropathies [28]. However, this treatment modality provides no benefit in sporadic ALS [50–52]. Lead toxicity certainly may cause a syndrome that has features of ALS; but without other symptoms of lead toxicity or a history of lead exposure, testing or treating for lead toxicity is not warranted. There does not seem to be a strong association between lead and the development of ALS.

Mercury

Similar to lead toxicity, acute and chronic mercury poisoning cause an ALS-like syndrome. This has been known for the past half-century [53–56], and reports of this association continue [57]. Two case-control studies discovered that more patients who have ALS report exposure to mercury than controls [31,32], and another case-control study finds greater job exposure to arsenic, manganese, mercury, or other heavy metals [33]. Heavy metal exposure is not more common in patients who have ALS in three case-control studies [37,38,58]. Many humans seem to accumulate mercury in spinal motor neurons by late adulthood, but no difference is found between spinal cords in patients who have ALS and controls [59]. Mercury concentrations in blood, plasma, and red blood cells are not different from those in controls [48]. Unless chronic or acute exposure to mercury is suspected on clinical grounds, screening for mercury seems without merit.

Aluminum

In the middle of the twentieth century, reports of incidence rates 50- to 100-fold higher than elsewhere in the world were noted for ALS in the Western Pacific region. Additionally, a high prevalence of a Parkinsonism-dementia complex (PDC) was intermingled in these populations. The resultant disease came to be known as Guamanian or Western Pacific ALS-PDC. Epidemiologic studies uncovered low amounts of calcium and magnesium and high amounts of aluminum and manganese in the soil and drinking water from these regions [60,61]. Aluminum was detected in neurofibrillary tangles in brains of patients who had ALS-PDC [62]. Cynomolgus monkeys fed low calcium/magnesium and high aluminum diets exhibited intraneuronal aluminum accumulation and neuronal loss consistent with ALS [63]. Intracisternal injection of aluminum in animal models led to a clinical ALS phenotype with motor neuron loss [64–66]. Mice chronically fed low calcium/magnesium and high aluminum diets showed degeneration and reduction in neuronal numbers in spinal cord and cerebral cortex [67] and typical skin changes associated with ALS [68]. Low dietary calcium and magnesium increase intestinal absorption of aluminum. Excessive environmental exposure to aluminum is not confirmed in a recent case-control study [49]. Aluminum may play a role in development of motor neuron disease as a sole agent in some patients or as a contributing factor in patients. There is plausible biologic data using animal models suggesting deleterious effects of aluminum on motor neurons, perhaps enhanced by dietary factors.

Selenium

Kilness and Hochberg observed a cluster of ALS cases in a high selenium environment in 1976 [69]. Kurlander and Patten then documented a higher spinal cord selenium concentration in a single patient compared with three controls [45]. Subsequently, selenium levels were found elevated in blood, spinal cord, liver, and bone of patients who had ALS [70,71]. An Italian case-control study described a high incidence of ALS in a population exposed to drinking water high in selenium content [72]. Recent studies have not replicated findings of elevated blood selenium levels or accumulation of selenium in the toenails in patients who have ALS [47–49]. As with most other heavy metals, selenium may play a role in the pathogenesis of motor neuron disease; however, strong epidemiologic evidence is lacking.

Manganese

Occupational exposure to manganese causing a parkinsonian syndrome was reported first in the 1800s. It has since been well studied [73]. Based on the concept that manganese causes one neurodegenerative disorder, investigations discovered elevated manganese levels in spinal cords of ALS patients who had [45,71]. Manganese concentrations in blood cells from patients who have ALS are significantly lower than in disease controls and healthy people [70]. Case-control studies do not suggest increased occupational exposure to manganese in patients who have ALS [58]. Recent studies fail to document accumulation of manganese in blood or toenails [48,49]. Manganese superoxide dismutase (*SOD2*) is the mitochondrial isoenzyme inactivating superoxide radicals and a cousin to cytosolic *SOD1*. This sole difference between mitochondrial and cytosolic superoxide dismutase spurs curiosity as to the potential pathogenic involvement of manganese in ALS. Thus far, however, no disease-causing mutations have been found in the *SOD2* gene [74].

Other metals and trace elements

Pamphlett et al published an evaluation of cadmium, lead, mercury, copper, zinc, selenium, and manganese blood levels from 20 patients who had ALS and an equal number of partner controls [48]. Cadmium concentrations were elevated to statistically significant levels in patients who had ALS versus controls but with considerable overlap in these values. Copper and zinc are integral components of *SOD1*. Finding mutations in the *SOD1* gene sparked interest into levels of these elements in ALS [75]. Bromine, zinc, rubidium, and iron concentrations in erythrocytes were not different in disease and control groups [70]. Magnesium, chromium, iron, cobalt, zinc, rubidium, cesium, antimony, silver, and copper levels in ALS spinal cord samples did not differ from control spinal cord levels [71]. Finally, using toenail clippings as biomarkers of chronic exposure, concentrations of copper, chromium, cobalt, and iron in 22 patients revealed no differences when compared with 40 controls [49].

Toxins, chemicals, and solvents

In the past, the incidence of ALS in the Western Pacific region was far higher than elsewhere worldwide and remains somewhat elevated today.

Therefore, reports of clusters of ALS cases in a particular household, geographic location, workplace, or occupation lead to speculation concerning common environmental factors afflicting particular populations or geographic locales. A husband and wife may develop ALS. As reports of conjugal ALS remain rare, this occurrence probably reflects the combined odds of both older persons in a marriage developing the same uncommon disease [76,77]. Published reports of clusters in the United States have not always revealed, after further statistical evaluation, any increased endemic incidence rates [78–80]. A more recent, prospective study in the United Kingdom does find a low background rate of ALS studded with pockets of higher incidence [81]. The investigators postulate the geographic distribution of ALS to be nonrandom. Mendell and colleagues published cases of three teachers developing ALS. All taught in the same classroom at an Ohio high school. None had other common exposures in terms of the locations of their homes, hobbies, dietary habits, medications, or family history of neurologic disease. They were not interrelated. An investigation of the school yielded no toxic source. Statistical analysis determined the probability of these three teachers in that school developing ALS to be low ($P < 0.0001$) and the probability of any three teachers dying from ALS at any of Ohio's 878 schools to be low ($P < 0.05$) [82]. One large suspected occupational cluster associated with employment at an Air Force base in Texas was evaluated using a mortality ascertainment study. Using death certificates, investigators found mortality from motor neuron disease, and in particular ALS, not increased in this population compared with statewide ALS death rates. The investigators plan to reinvestigate this population in 10 years because of the potential long latency from toxic exposure to death from ALS [83]. With the advent of the genetic era, some apparent geographic clusters of sporadic ALS have been discovered to be the result of a common genetic defect, likely from a common ancestor [84].

Farming

The pathogenic mechanisms by which employment in the agricultural sector may lead to ALS relate to chemical exposures (fertilizers, insecticides, and herbicides), exposures to animals and their associated diseases, or the physical nature of the work. In 1977, Rosati et al observed an association between employment in farming and an increased risk for ALS in Sardinia, in southern Italy [85]. These findings were expanded for the Sardinia region [86,87] and replicated in the province of Ferrara, in northern Italy [38]. In the northern Italian study, a significant association was found in farmers and persons living in rural areas, but not in those working with agricultural chemicals. Another Italian case-control study, with more than 500 ALS patients, noted both a proportionately higher number of farmers and a greater exposure to chemical products in patients versus controls [88]. A large case-control study in western Washington State in the United States comparing 174 patients and 348 age- and sex-matched controls and provides further evidence of an association between agricultural employment and ALS. This blinded, population-based study derived its control population mostly from random-digit dialing, a method minimizing common geographic or occupational exposures. Although the odds ratio is not robust (OR 2.0; 95% confidence interval [CI] 1.1–3.5), the narrow confidence window adds to this finding's strength [39]. The findings pertain only to men, not to women, but show a dose-response relationship. Men who had the highest exposure rates to agricultural chemicals suffered the highest ORs. Other studies fail to demonstrate this statistical association between agricultural work and ALS [32,34]. The data disclose a mild association between agricultural work and risk for developing ALS. These data do not delineate clearly if this risk relates to chemical exposures, physical exertion, infections, or some other factor.

Solvents

In Deapen and Henderson's study, occupational exposures to toxins are similar in patients and controls, except for those working in plastics manufacturing [37]. Their OR is 3.7 but with broad CIs. A subsequent study by Gunnarsson et al implicates solvents but does not reach statistical significance [89]. The Scottish Motor Neuron Disease Register case-control study, published in 1993, does find a statistically significantly increased risk (OR 3.3; 95% CI, 1.3–10) of exposure to chemicals or solvents, again with wide CIs [35]. Two other studies fail to replicate these weak findings [38,39]. The role of solvent exposure in development of ALS seems small or nonexistent.

Cigarette smoking

A myriad of toxins are associated with cigarette smoking. These toxins might play a role in causing or triggering ALS, possibly by inducing oxidative stress. Contrariwise, smoking previously was believed potentially to have a protective effect on the development of Parkinson's disease and Alzheimer's disease [90]. Early studies found no association between ALS and smoking [32,38,91]. In the late 1990s, three case-control studies obtained positive, although weak, associations between previous or current cigarette smoking and ALS [47,92,93]. Nelson et al find associations between ever smoking cigarettes (OR 2.0, narrow 95% CI of 1.3–3.2) or current smoking (threefold risk). They also delineated significant trends suggesting increased risk for ALS with duration of smoking and number of cigarette pack-years. The only prospective study was in New England. This study assesses the relation between cigarette smoking and ALS mortality among participants in the Cancer Prevention Study II and has conflicting results. In 291 woman and 330 men who died from ALS between 1989 and

1998, the relative risk (RR) for death from ALS in current smokers compared with those who never smoked is 1.67 (95% CI, 1.24–2.24) in females and 0.69 (95% CI, 0.49–0.99) in males. These diametrically opposed results suggest cigarette smoking may increase the likelihood of ALS in women but not men (and may even be protective) [94]. Thus, the jury is still out regarding tobacco abuse and ALS risk. The best data suggest a mild risk associated with smoking, but the only prospective study hints toward a protective benefit in men.

Gulf War service

After a decade of conjecture over claims of increased illness in military veterans who served in the 1990–1991 Persian Gulf War, two studies observed an increased incidence of ALS in military personnel who were deployed to the Persian Gulf region. Horner et al derived an increased RR for all deployed personnel (RR 1.92; 95% CI, 1.29–2.84), deployed active-duty military personnel (RR 2.15; 95% CI, 1.38–3.36), deployed Air Force members (RR 2.68; 95% CI, 1.24–5.78), and deployed Army troops (RR 2.04; 95% CI, 1.10–3.77) [95]. Subgroup analyses found elevated risks did not reach statistical significance for populations of deployed Marine, Army National Guard, or Navy personnel. Haley studied ALS in young Gulf War veterans (age less than 45 years). He reports ALS incidence rates in young veterans exceed that expected from age-specific United States population death rates [96].

Early studies of Persian Gulf War veterans failed to find increased rates of illness. One found no excess of unexplained hospitalizations [97]. Deployed veterans had a slightly, yet significantly, higher death rate after deployment, but most of this increased mortality was related to accidents and not disease [98]. A later review of hospitalization records looked specifically at systemic lupus erythematosus, fibromyalgia, and ALS [99]. That study concludes that Gulf War veterans were hospitalized slightly more often for fibromyalgia, but not for lupus. The data for ALS were inconclusive because of small numbers and wide CIs. In 2001, a case-control study drawing from Department of Veterans Affairs and the Social Security Administration databases found a nonsignificant deficit of deaths resulting from ALS (RR 0.59; 95% CI, 0.21–1.66) [100]. The epidemiologic strength of these studies suffers from their small numbers of ALS cases and several potential methodologic issues—some of which are unavoidable [101].

Thorough electrophysiologic evaluations of Gulf War veterans who had neuromuscular symptoms fail to discern objective measurable abnormalities in veterans in the United States [102] or the United Kingdom [103]. Cases of ALS were not found in these series [104]. Several environmental factors are purported possibly to initiate or cause ALS in military personnel deployed to the Persian Gulf: pesticides, chemical weapons, immunizations, medications, radiation exposure, physical exertion, trauma, genetic predisposition, or some unique interplay of these factors. Thus far, none has strong evidence supporting causation. A recent examination of archived records of hospitalizations in United States military facilities in the Kuwait theater of operations and European evacuation facilities shows no increase in the OR for oil well fire smoke exposure or possible nerve agent exposure [105].

Elsewhere in this issue of *Neurologic Clinics*, Gronseth explores the possible role of toxins in the Gulf War syndrome in more detail. In late 2004, the Research Advisory Committee on Gulf War Veterans' Illnesses, a congressionally chartered panel of scientific experts and veterans, released its first major report on Gulf War illnesses. The report concludes that a substantial proportion of Gulf War veterans suffer from unexplained illnesses; these illnesses are not explained by stress or psychiatric illness in most cases; ill veterans exhibit an excess of ALS; research supports a probable link to neurotoxic exposures; treatments are needed urgently; and further research is imperative for military missions and homeland security [106].

Infections

One prominent early theory concerning the cause of ALS was that an underlying viral agent causes the disease directly, indirectly, or in a latent state. An early case-control study found a history of polio in 5 of 80 patients who had ALS and none in 78 controls [32]. However, recent, large case-control studies fail to find any association between previous polio infection and ALS risk [107,108], and a review of the epidemiologic literature comes to the same determination [109]. Detection of enterovirus nucleic acid sequences via polymerase chain reaction in cerebrospinal fluid [110] and neuronal cell bodies of spinal cords [111] from ALS patients has reignited interest in this mechanism of disease. Other researchers have been unable to reproduce these findings [112,113]. Retroviral infection may cause motor neuron disease with either lower or upper and lower motor neuron involvement. This occurs in HTLV-1 infection [114] and in HIV disease [115,116]. Treatment of the underlying HIV infection transiently or completely can reverse the associated motor neuron disease [115–117]. A poliomyelitis-like syndrome with an asymmetric lower motor neuronopathy may accompany West Nile virus infection, with or without meningoencephalitis [118]. Hepatitis C infection also may produce a pure motor axonal polyneuropathy without cryoglobulinemia that is at least somewhat responsive to therapy of the underlying viral infection [119]. Lower motor neuron involvement occasionally accompanies the prion disorders, Creutzfeldt-Jakob disease, and Gerstmann-Sträussler-Scheinker disease [120]. With reports that Lyme disease rarely presents as a motor neuronopathy [121] and that spirochetes have been cultured from cases of ALS [122], bacterial infections are postulated as potential causes or triggers of ALS [123]. Approaching the issue of a bacterial etiology from a treatment perspective, a trial of ceftriaxone therapy in ALS lacked efficacy [124]. The antibiotic, minocycline, shows benefit in slowing ALS in mouse models, but this positive effect is not believed a result of the drug's antibacterial effects, rather its neuroprotective actions [125–127]. There now is a placebo-controlled trial of minocycline as therapy for human ALS [128]. More investigation is required before a bacterial theory gains credulity. At this time, any relation between infections and the cause of ALS must be viewed as speculative and unsubstantiated.

Neoplasms

Patients who have ALS also can develop cancer. An association between lymphoma and a lower motor neuron disorder is reported. Some cases present signs of classic ALS with evidence of upper and lower motor neuron disease [129]. Patients who have other cancers also manifest ALS-like symptoms [130]. Infrequently, patients who initially present with primary lateral sclerosis and breast cancer eventually develop upper and lower motor neuronal dysfunction [131]. Motor neuron disease also may be a manifestation of a paraneoplastic syndrome. Anti-Hu antibodies [132] and anti-Yo antibodies [133] are reported associated with cases of motor neuron disease. These cases remain rare in the literature. Vigliani et al published a case-control study of patients who had ALS and cancer using patients who had ALS but not cancer as controls [134]. In their study, patients who had ALS and who either did or did not have cancer did not significantly differ clinically. Patients who had ALS and cancer died from motor neuron disease, irrespective of cancer progression. Treatment with antitumor therapy did not influence the course of their ALS. Although exceptional cases of a lower motor neuron disorder may be the result of underlying cancers, most cases of ALS and cancer coexist by chance.

Electrical shock and electromagnetic fields

Instances of myeloradiculopathy as a delayed neurologic consequence of electrical injuries spurred conjecture as to the association between electrical trauma and ALS [135]. Two case-control studies from the 1980s describe a greater association with electrical injury in patients who have ALS compared with controls [37,136]. A more recent nationwide Danish mortality study conducted a comparison of all men employed in utility companies from 1900 through 1993 and compared them to national death rates from different causes. This utility worker study finds a twofold increase in mortality from ALS and a tenfold increase in deaths from electrical accidents. The investigators postulate that increased exposure to electrical shocks and electromagnetic fields (EMFs) may be associated causally with the excess mortality from ALS [137]. The Scottish Motor Neuron Disease Register study finds no such association between ALS and electrical injury in Scotland [35].

Toward the end of the previous millennium and during the past few years, a flourish of interest in EMF exposure and neurodegenerative disorders has emerged. Researchers hypothesized that electrical injuries may parallel EMF exposure, thus serving as a surrogate marker. Davanipour et al conducted a case-control study investigating lifetime occupational exposure to EMFs in 28 patients who had ALS [138]. The ORs for total occupational exposure and average occupational exposure to EMFs in patients who had at least 20 years of work experience were 7.5 (95% CI, 1.4–38.1) and 5.5 (95% CI, 1.3–22.5), respectively. The broad CIs weaken the strength of this association in this small population. When the comparison was extended to all patients who had ALS regardless of total work experience, the ORs did not meet statistical significance. Savitz and colleagues performed a mortality study of United States utility workers and a case-control study of the neurodegenerative disorders, Parkinson's disease, Alzheimer's disease, and ALS in these same workers [139,140]. Both studies find weak associations between ALS and extent of EMF exposure. A Scandinavian case-referent study finds ALS associated with a history of electrical occupation (OR 2.30; 95% CI, 1.29–4.09) but not with EMF exposure as estimated by a job-exposure matrix [141]. Contradictory results are reported in two publications using predominantly the same Swedish study populations. Håkansson et al report a RR of 2.2 (95% CI,1.0–4.7) for EMF exposure and ALS, whereas Feychting et al fail to discover any such association [142,143]. Plausible biologic mechanisms linking EMFs to the onset of ALS remain poorly understood. If EMFs do elevate the risk for ALS, at this time that increased risk seems relatively small.

Physical factors

Physical exertion, participation in athletics, bodily trauma, bone fractures, and surgeries all are posited as antecedent events more common in patients who have ALS than in controls. Famous athletes have developed ALS, and their popularity may highlight this association in peoples' minds, despite no true association or causation. This prominence of athletes in a culture's collective mind has led to use of the term, Lou Gehrig's disease, for ALS in the United States. Possible mechanisms underlying this relationship include increased exposure to ambient toxins, greater contact of neural tissues with immune surveillance systems, augmented absorption or bodily distribution of toxins, and neuronal fatigue and stress. Many studies support this general hypothesis [31,33,35,37,38,47,88,91,144], whereas others are not able to substantiate the association [34,108, 145,146]. Physical exertion and trauma remain one mechanism that possibly underlies the increased risk for ALS in Gulf War veterans. An intriguing recent development is the clustering of ALS in Italian soccer players. Between 1960 and 1997, approximately 24,000 men played professional soccer, of whom eight already have died from ALS [147]. The true number of players suffering or dying from ALS actually is believed greater than 30 [148]. The expected number of cases in the Italian general population in the age group of the soccer players is less than one case. Disease onset in these athletes is young, usually in their 40s. The mechanism of disease onset in these soccer players is not yet known. They suffer more head trauma and bone fractures and are more physically active than the general population. The literature provides some evidence for the involvement of head injury in patients who have ALS [91,149]. It is not clear if these athletes use performance-enhancing drugs at a greater rate than the general population, but this is a safe assumption. Therefore, a toxic cause also should be considered. Another hypothesis posits the existence of a genetic factor initially providing athletic excellence only to culminate in premature neuronal degeneration. No such gene is yet known. Currently, the association between physical exertion and trauma and the development of ALS remains captivating but without powerful epidemiologic support or a proven pathogenic mechanism.

Diet

Ingestion of certain foods, toxins associated with foods, or toxins within foods might predispose to development of ALS. Felmus et al, in Texas, investigated this concept in their early case-control series. They found consumption of large quantities of milk was associated with patients who had ALS [31,32]. Milk, as a prominent source of calcium, might affect absorption or body stores of heavy metals and could alter parathyroid function. Parathyroid disease causes weakness, exercise intolerance, and muscle atrophy [150] but is now known not to be associated with ALS [151]. Two recent case-control studies fail to find an association with milk ingestion or with any particular food [33,145]. A recent, large case-control study from Washington State in the United States finds high amounts of dietary fat intake correlates somewhat with ALS (OR 2.7; 95% CI, 0.9–8.0), whereas high dietary fiber intake seems protective (OR 0.3; 95% CI, 0.1–0.7) [152]. High glutamate intake also is linked to an increased risk for ALS (OR 3.2; 95% CI,1.2–8.0). Consumption of dietary or supplemental antioxidant vitamins does not decrease this hazard. These glutamate findings align with the glutamate excitotoxicity theory of ALS, whereas the data on fats and fiber fit well with a model related to toxin ingestion.

Motor neuron diseases are well known adverse consequences of dietary consumption of toxins. Lathyrism is a neurologic disorder that has predominant upper motor neuron dysfunction associated with the use of the chickling pea (Lathyrus sativa) in foodstuffs. A drought-resistant crop, the chickling pea contains abundant quantities of β-N-oxalyl-L-α, β-diaminopropionic acid, a glutamate analog, which is believed to inflict its neuronal damaging effect via excitation of the α-amino-3-hydroxy-5-methylisoxazole-4-propionate–activated receptors [153]. Another neurologic disorder, Konzo, is a tropical myelopathy presenting with abrupt onset of spastic paraplegia [154]. Consumption of flour from insufficiently processed cassava leads to excessive dietary cyanide exposure and resultant disease. Additionally, an atypical parkinsonism in the French West Indies is associated with consumption of herbal teas and fruits from the Annonaceae family, which contain neurotoxic benzyltetrahydroisoquinoline alkaloids [155]. Four of 30 patients who had this atypical parkinsonism had associated motor neuron disease. The neuronal toxicity of benzyltetrahydroisoquinolines is believed mediated through either glutamate toxicity or free radical formation.

Western Pacific amyotrophic lateral sclerosis

Three foci in the Western Pacific—Guam, the Kii Peninsula of Japan, and western New Guinea—were determined to have markedly elevated rates of ALS in the middle of the twentieth century [156]. In the 1940s and 1950s, the annual incidence rates for the Chamorro natives on the island of Guam were 50 per 100,000, with incidence rates in certain municipalities or districts as high as 250 per 100,000 [157]. These Guamanian ALS incidence rates were as much as 100-fold higher than age-adjusted worldwide incidence rates. Prevalence rates reached nearly 1 in 600 Guamanian Chamorros for all ages and almost 1 in 100 for persons in their 40s and 50s. Native Chamorros, who called their ALS syndrome by the name of lytico, also were aware of a concomitant disease running in their populations, a PDC with the Chamorran name of bodig. These two diseases may occur concurrently in the same patient or same family, leading to the term ALS-PDC. Although incidence rates for ALS in the Western Pacific have decreased substantially over time, distinct foci continue to exceed worldwide values [158]. Post-mortem pathologic specimens of patients who have ALS or PDC reveal pyknosis and loss of anterior horn cells in the spinal cord and neurofibrillary degeneration in the cortex [159].

Investigators propose three main theories to explain the high incidence of Western Pacific ALS: a genetic underpinning in this isolated island population due to familial aggregation of cases of ALS and PDC [160]; dietary consumption of a plant neurotoxin from the cycad plant in the form of cycad flour [161,162]; and exposure to drinking water and agricultural soil low in calcium and high in aluminum content [63]. Although Western Pacific ALS occurs 7 to 28 times more frequently in siblings than in the Chamorro population as a whole, ALS also transpires more often in spousal pairs [163,164]. This risk for ALS in susceptible sibships still is significantly lower than is expected by a monogenic mendelian model. Polygenic inheritance, without an environmental trigger, also is unlikely. Thus, the increased incidence of ALS in family members related either by blood or marriage fits better with a shared environmental exposure than with a purely genetic cause. Even with a substantial influx of other races onto the island of Guam, resulting in intermixing of gene pools during the past 50 years, much more generational time would have had to pass to explain the marked decline in incidence [165]. Evaluation of the case registry on Guam by Zhang et al determines that the cycad neurotoxin hypothesis better conforms to the data than the low calcium, high aluminum hypothesis [163].

Whiting initially suggested that ALS on Guam might be related to ingestion of the seed of the false sago palm (*Cycas circinalis*) [166]. Much attention was given to cycasin, a potent hepatotoxic and carcinogenic component of the cycad seed. Spencer et al subsequently proposed that β-N-methylamino-L-alanine (BMAA) actually may be the offending agent in cycad seeds [161]. This group orally administered BMAA to cynomolgus monkeys, inducing neurologic dysfunction with upper and lower motor neuron involvement. These monkeys also developed chromatolytic and degenerative changes of motor neurons in the cerebral cortex and spinal cord [162]. The main exposure of the native Chamorro people to these toxins was through eating flour made from the cycad seeds. The Chamorro people subjected the cycad seeds for flour to multiple washings for detoxification, as they knew these seeds to be acutely toxic. Processed cycad flour contains little BMAA [167]. Therefore, humans would need to eat massive quantities of flour-based foods on a daily basis. With this information, cycad flour fell out of favor as a potential source for a neurotoxin in Guamanian ALS.

The exact substance in cycad seeds exerting the neurotoxic effect is debated [168]. Recently, however, the mechanism by which the Chamorro people were exposed to these neurotoxins may have been identified. ALS-PDC seems to be the product of biomagnification of neurotoxins up through the food chain [169]. Guamanian flying foxes (*Pteropus mariannus mariannus*) consume large quantities of the BMAA-laden sarcotesta of cycad seeds. Museum specimens of Guamanian flying foxes contain high levels of BMAA, levels 1000 times more concentrated than in cycad seed flour [170]. The Chamorro people traditionally feasted on flying foxes, and consumption of a single flying fox may have resulted in a dose of BMAA equivalent to 174 to 1014 kg of processed cycad flour. Traditional feasting on flying foxes therefore may be the entry route for massive quantities of a neurotoxin, with subsequent development of ALS-PDC. Cox et al detail this biomagnification further by documenting the following progressive concentrating effect on BMAA upward through the food chain: (1)

free-living cyanobacteria produce 0.3 μg/g BMAA; (2) cyanobacteria living as symbionts in cycad roots produce 2 to 37 μg/g BMAA; (3) cycad seeds contain mean levels of 1161 μg/g BMAA in their fleshy outer most seed layer; and (4) flying fox tissues accumulate mean levels of 3556 μg/g BMAA [171]. Frontal cortex from six Chamorro patients who died from ALS-PDC contained mean BMAA levels of 6 μg/g. Mean BMAA levels in frontal cortex at autopsy from two Canadian patients who had Alzheimer's disease were 6.6 μg/g, whereas BMAA was undetectable in frontal cortex in postmortem evaluation of 13 patients who did not have neurodegenerative diseases. Finally, BMAA exists in free and bound forms in bacterial, plant, animal, and human tissues. Protein-bound BMAA levels may be one to two orders of magnitude higher than free BMAA levels in cyanobacteria and cycad seeds. Protein-bound BMAA levels in brain tissues from Guamanian ALS-PDC patients range from 60- 130- fold higher than free levels [172]. BMAA bound to protein may function as an endogenous neurotoxic reservoir and may be neuroprotective. Large doses of a neurotoxin might be acutely absorbed and sequestered in protein-bound form, consequently only to be discharged slowly into the surrounding brain milieu.

Biomagnification of neurotoxins seems a strong candidate to explain ALS-PDC of Guam. Further investigations into biomagnification of other neurotoxins in ALS and other neurodegenerative disorders may yield unexpectedly exciting answers.

Summary

This treatise briefly discusses the genetic features of ALS and reviews environmental exposures in sporadic ALS. At least 10 genetic foci are responsible for cases of familial motor neuron disease and more are yet to be discovered. Research into sporadic ALS suggests that abundant factors apparently participate in the disease process. A singular cause and unifying pathogenesis for sporadic ALS remain elusive. As with weakness in muscle disease and nerve dysfunction in polyneuropathies, a multitude of genetic, toxic, autoimmune, infectious, and systemic processes seem to be at play. The ALS syndrome likely will not be dissimilar.

References

[1] Rowland LP, Shneider NA. Amyotrophic lateral sclerosis. N Engl J Med 2001;344: 1688–700.

[2] Lomen-Hoerth C, Murphy J, Langmore S, et al. Are amyotrophic lateral sclerosis patients cognitively normal? Neurology 2003;60:1094–7.

[3] Leigh PN, Ray-Chaudhury K. Motor neuron disease. J Neurol Neurosurg Psychiatry 1994; 57:886–96.

[4] Govoni V, Granieri E, Capone J, et al. Incidence of amyotrophic lateral sclerosis in the local health district of Ferrara, Italy, 1964–1998. Neuroepidemiology 2003;22:229–34.

[5] Chancellor AM, Warlow CP. Adult onset motor neuron disease: worldwide mortality, incidence and distribution since 1950. J Neurol Neurosurg Psychiatry 1992;55:1106–15.

[6] Ajdacic-Gross V, Wang J, Gutzwiller F. Season of birth in amyotrophic lateral sclerosis. Eur J Epidemiol 1998;14:359–61.

[7] Brooks BR. El Escorial World Federation of Neurology criteria for the diagnosis of amyotrophic lateral sclerosis. J Neurol Sci 1994;124(Suppl):96–107.

[8] Brooks BR, Miller RG, Swash M, et al. World Federation of Neurology Research Group on Motor Neuron Diseases. El Escorial revisited: revised criteria for the diagnosis of amyotrophic lateral sclerosis. Amyotroph Lateral Scler Other Motor Neuron Disord 2000;1:293–9.

[9] Chan S, Shungu DC, Douglas-Akinwande A, et al. Motor neuron diseases: comparison of single-voxel proton MR spectroscopy of the motor cortex with MR imaging of the brain. Radiology 1999;212:763–9.

[10] Triggs WJ, Menkes D, Onorato J, et al. Transcranial magnetic stimulation identifies upper motor neuron involvement in motor neuron disease. Neurology 1999;53:605–11.

[11] Sach M, Winkler G, Glauche V, et al. Diffusion tensor MRI of early upper motor neuron involvement in amyotrophic lateral sclerosis. Brain 2004;127:340–50.

[12] Olney RK, Yuen EC, Engstrom JW. Statistical motor unit number estimation: reproducibility and sources of error in patients with amyotrophic lateral sclerosis. Muscle Nerve 2000;23:193–7.

[13] Ross MA. Acquired motor neuron disorders. Neurol Clin 1997;3:481–500.

[14] Bensimon G, Lacomblez L, Meinenger V. A controlled trial of riluzole in amyotrophic lateral sclerosis. N Engl J Med 1994;330:585–91.

[15] Siddique T, Pericak-Vance MA, Brooks BR, et al. Linkage analysis in familial amyotrophic lateral sclerosis. Neurology 1989;39:919–25.

[16] Rosen DR, Siddique T, Patterson D, et al. Mutations in copper/zinc superoxide dismutase gene are associated with familial amyotrophic lateral sclerosis. Nature 1993;362:59–62.

[17] Siddique T, Lalani I. Genetic aspects of amyotrophic lateral sclerosis. In: Pourmand R, Yadollah H, editors. Neuromuscular disorders. Philadelphia: Williams and Wilkins; 2001. p. 21–32.

[18] Majoor-Krakauer D, Willems PJ, Hofman A. Genetic epidemiology of amyotrophic lateral sclerosis. Clin Genet 2003;63:83–101.

[19] Washington University, St. Louis, Neuromuscular Disease Center website. Hereditary motor syndromes page. Available at: www.neuro.wustl.edu/neuromuscular/synmot.html# Hereditaryals. Accessed October 15, 2004.

[20] Al-Chalabi A, Anderson PM, Chioza B, et al. Recessive amyotrophic lateral sclerosis families with the D90A SOD1 mutation share a common founder: evidence for a linked protective factor. Hum Mol Genet 1998;7:2045–50.

[21] Ratovitski T, Corson LB, Strain J, et al. Variation in the biochemical/biophysical properties of mutant superoxide dismutase 1 enzymes and the rate of disease progression in familial amyotrophic lateral sclerosis kindreds. Hum Mol Genet 1999;8:1451–60.

[22] Reaume AG, Elliott JL, Hoffman EK, et al. Motor neurons in Cu/Zn superoxide dismutase-deficient mice develop normally but exhibit enhanced cell death after axonal injury. Nat Genet 1996;13:43–7.

[23] Jones CT, Swingler RJ, Simpson SA, et al. Superoxide dismutase mutations in an unselected cohort of Scottish amyotrophic lateral sclerosis patients. J Med Genet 1995; 32:290–2.

[24] Jackson M, Al-Chalabi A, Enayat ZE, et al. Copper/zinc superoxide dismutase 1 and sporadic amyotrophic lateral sclerosis: analysis of 155 cases and identification of a novel insertion mutation. Ann Neurol 1997;42:803–7.

[25] Puls I, Jonnakuty C, LaMonte BH, et al. Mutant Dynactin in motor neuron disease. Nat Genet 2003;33:455–6.

[26] Wilson SAK. The amyotrophy of chronic lead poisoning—amyotrophic lateral sclerosis of toxic origin. Rev Neurol Psychiat 1907;5:441–55.

[27] Mishra D, Agrawal A, Gupta VK. Distal spinal muscular atrophy of upper limb (Hirayama disease) associated with high serum lead levels. Indian Pediatr 2003;40:780–3.

[28] Livesley B, Sissons CE. Chronic lead intoxication mimicking motor neurone disease. BMJ 1968;4:387–8.

[29] Boothby JA, DeJesus PV, Rowland LP. Reversible forms of motor neuron disease: lead "neuritis." Arch Neurol 1974;31:18–23.

[30] Campbell AMG, Williams ER, Barltrop D. Motor neurone disease and exposure to lead. J Neurol Neurosurg Psychiatry 1970;33:877–85.

[31] Felmus MT, Patten BM, Swanke L. Antecedent events in amyotrophic lateral sclerosis. Neurology 1976;26:167–72.

[32] Pierce-Ruhland R, Patten BM. Repeat study of antecedent events in motor neuron disease. Ann Clin Res 1981;13:102–7.

[33] Roelofs-Iverson RA, Mulder DW, Elveback LR, et al. ALS and heavy metals: a pilot case-control study. Neurology 1984;34:393–5.

[34] Armon C, Kurland LT, Daube JR, et al. Epidemiologic correlates of sporadic amyotrophic lateral sclerosis. Neurology 1991;41:1077–84.

[35] Chancellor AM, Slattery JM, Fraser H, et al. Risk factors for motor neuron disease: a case-control study based on patients from the Scottish Motor Neuron Disease Register. J Neurol Neurosurg Psychiatry 1993;56:1200–6.

[36] Kamel F, Umbach DM, Munsat TL, et al. Lead exposure and amyotrophic lateral sclerosis. Epidemiology 2002;13:311–9.

[37] Deapen DM, Henderson BE. A case-control study of amyotrophic lateral sclerosis. Am J Epidemiol 1986;123:790–9.

[38] Granieri E, Carreras M, Tola R, et al. Motor neuron disease in the province of Ferrrara, Italy, in 1964–1982. Neurology 1988;38:1604–8.

[39] McGuire V, Longstreth WT, Nelson LM, et al. Occupational exposures and amyotrophic lateral sclerosis: a population-based case-control study. Am J Epidemiol 1997;145:1076–88.

[40] Conradi S, Ronnevi L-O, Vesterberg O. Abnormal tissue distribution of lead in amyotrophic lateral sclerosis. J Neurol Sci 1976;29:259–65.

[41] Conradi S, Ronnevi L-O, Vesterberg O. Abnormal distribution of lead in amyotrophic lateral sclerosis: reestimation of lead in the cerebrospinal fluid. J Neurol Sci 1980;48:413–8.

[42] Conradi S, Ronnevi L-O, Vesterberg O. Increased plasma levels of lead in patients with amyotrophic lateral sclerosis compared with control subjects as determined by flameless atomic absorption spectrophotometry. J Neurol Neurosurg Psychiatry 1978;41:389–93.

[43] Petkau A, Sawatzky A, Hillier CR, et al. Lead content of neuromuscular tissue in amyotrophic lateral sclerosis: case report and other considerations. Br J Ind Med 1974;31:275–87.

[44] Conradi S, Ronnevi L-O, Vesterberg O. Lead concentration in skeletal muscle in amyotrophic lateral sclerosis patients and control subjects. J Neurol Neurosurg Psychiatry 1978;41:1001–4.

[45] Kurlander HM, Patten BM. Metals in spinal cord tissue of patients dying of motor neuron disease. Ann Neurol 1979;6:21–4.

[46] Mandybur TI, Cooper GP. Increased spinal cord lead content in amyotrophic lateral sclerosis–possibly a secondary phenomenon. Med Hypotheses 1979;5:1313–5.

[47] Vinceti M, Guidetti D, Bergomi M, et al. Lead, cadmium, and selenium in the blood of patients with sporadic amyotrophic lateral sclerosis. Ital J Neurol Sci 1997;18:87–92.

[48] Pamphlett R, McQuilty R, Zarkos K. Blood levels of toxic and essential metals in motor neuron disease. Neurotoxicology 2001;22:401–10.

[49] Bergomi M, Vinceti M, Nacci G, et al. Environmental exposure to trace elements and risk of amyotrophic lateral sclerosis: a population-based case-control study. Environ Res 2002;89:116–23.

[50] Currier RD, Haerer AF. Amyotrophic lateral sclerosis and metal toxins. Arch Environ Health 1968;17:712–9.

[51] House AO, Abbott RJ, Davidson DLW, et al. Response to penicillamine of lead concentrations in CSF and blood of patients with motor neurone disease. BMJ 1978;2:1684.

[52] Conradi S, Ronnevi LO, Nise G, et al. Long-time penicillamine treatment in amyotrophic lateral sclerosis with parallel determination of lead in blood, plasma and urine. Acta Neurol Scand 1982;65:203–11.

[53] Brown IA. Chronic mercurialism. A cause of the clinical syndrome of amyotrophic lateral sclerosis. Arch Neurol Psychol 1954;72:674–81.

[54] Kantarjian AD. A syndrome clinically resembling amyotrophic lateral sclerosis following chronic mercurialism. Neurology 1961;11:639–44.

[55] Barber TE. Inorganic mercury intoxication reminiscent of amyotrophic lateral sclerosis. J Occup Med 1978;20:667–9.

[56] Adams CA, Ziegler DK, Lin JT. Mercury intoxication simulating amyotrophic lateral sclerosis. JAMA 1983;250:642–3.

[57] Schwarz S, Husstedt IW, Bertram HP, et al. Amyotrophic lateral sclerosis after accidental injection of mercury. J Neurol Neurosurg Psychiatry 1996;60:698.

[58] Gresham LS, Molgaard CA, Golbeck AL, et al. Amyotrophic lateral sclerosis and occupational heavy metal exposure: a case control study. Neuroepidemiology 1986;5:29–38.

[59] Pamphlett R, Waley P. Mercury in human spinal motor neurons. Acta Neuropathol 1998; 96:515–9.

[60] Yase Y. The pathogenesis of amyotrophic lateral sclerosis. Lancet 1972;2(7772):292–6.

[61] Garruto RM, Yanagihara R, Gajdusek DC, et al. Concentration of heavy metals and essential minerals in garden soil and drinking water in the Western Pacific. In: Chen KM, Yase Y, editors. Amyotrophic lateral sclerosis in Asia and Oceania. Shyan-Fu Chou: National Taiwan University, Taipei; 1984. p. 265–329.

[62] Perl DP, Gajdusek DC, Garruto RM, et al. Intraneuronal aluminum accumulation in amyotrophic lateral sclerosis and parkinsonism-dementia of Guam. Science 1982;217: 1053–5.

[63] Garruto RM, Shankar SK, Yanagihara R, et al. Low-calcium, high-aluminum diet-induced motor neuron pathology in cynomolgus monkeys. Acta Neuropathol 1989;78:210–9.

[64] Strong MJ, Garruto RM. Chronic aluminum-induced motor neuron degeneration: clinical, neuropathological and molecular biological aspects. Can J Neurol 1991;18(Suppl 3): 428–31.

[65] Wakayama I, Nerurkar VR, Strong MJ, et al. Comparative study of chronic aluminum-induced neurofilamentous aggregates with intracytoplasmic inclusions of amyotrophic lateral sclerosis. Acta Neuropathol 1996;92:545–54.

[66] Tanridag T, Coskun T, Hürdag C, et al. Motor neuron degeneration due to aluminum deposition in the spinal cord: a light microscopical study. Acta Histochem 1999;101: 193–201.

[67] Kihira T, Yoshida S, Yase Y, et al. Chronic low-Ca/Mg high-Al diet induces neuronal loss. Neuropathology 2002;22:152–60.

[68] Kihira T, Yoshida S, Kondo T, et al. ALS-like skin changes in mice on a chronic low-Ca/Mg high-Al diet. J Neurol Sci 2004;219:7–14.

[69] Kilness AW, Hochberg FH. Amyotrophic lateral sclerosis in a high selenium environment. JAMA 1976;237:2843–4.

[70] Nagata H, Miyata S, Nakamura S, et al. Heavy metal concentrations in blood cells in patients with amyotrophic lateral sclerosis. J Neurol Sci 1985;67:173–8.

[71] Mitchell JD, East BW, Harris IA, et al. Manganese, selenium and other trace elements in spinal cord, liver and bone in motor neurone disease. Eur Neurol 1991;31:7–11.

[72] Vinceti M, Guidetti D, Pinotti M, et al. Amyotrophic lateral sclerosis after long-term exposure to drinking water with high selenium content. Epidemiology 1996;7:529–32.

[73] Cotzias GC, Horiuchi K, Fuenzalida S, et al. Chronic manganese poisoning: clearance of tissue manganese concentrations with persistence of the neurological picture. Neurology 1968;18:376–82.

[74] Parboosingh JS, Rouleau GA, Meninger V, et al. Absence of mutations in the Mn superoxide dismutase or catalase genes in familial amyotrophic lateral sclerosis. Neuromuscul Disord 1995;5:7–10.

[75] Perry G, Sayre LM, Atwood CS, et al. The role of iron and copper in the aetiology of neurodegenerative disorders: therapeutic implications. CNS Drugs 2002;16:339–52.

[76] Chad D, Mitsumoto H, Adelman LS, et al. Conjugal motor neurone disease. Neurology 1982;32:306–7.

[77] Camu W, Cadilhac J, Billiard M. Conjugal amyotrophic lateral sclerosis: a report on two couples from southern France. Neurology 1994;44:547–8.

[78] Sienko DG, Davis JP, Taylor JA, et al. Amyotrophic lateral sclerosis: a case control study following detection of a cluster in a small Wisconsin community. Arch Neurol 1990;47: 38–41.

[79] Armon C, Daube JR, O'Brien PC, et al. When is an apparent excess of neurologic cases epidemiologically significant? Neurology 1991;41:1713–8.

[80] Proctor SP, Feldman RG, Wolf PA, et al. A perceived cluster of amyotrophic lateral sclerosis in a Massachusetts community. Neuroepidemiology 1992;1:277–81.

[81] Mitchell JD, Gatrell AC, Al-Hamad A, et al. Geographical epidemiology of residence of patients with motor neuron disease in Lancashire and South Cumbria. J Neurol Neurosurg Psychiatry 1998;65:842–7.

[82] Hyser CL, Kissel JT, Mendell JR. Three cases of amyotrophic lateral sclerosis in a common occupational environment. J Neurol 1987;234:443–4.

[83] Mundt DJ, Dell LD, Luippold RS, et al. Cause-specific mortality among Kelly Air Force Base civilian employees, 1981–2001. J Occup Environ Med 2002;44:989–96.

[84] Ceroni M, Malasina A, Poloni TE, et al. Clustering of ALS patients in central Italy due to the occurrence of the L84F SOD1 gene mutation. Neurology 1999;53:1064–71.

[85] Rosati G, Pinna L, Granieri E, et al. Studies on epidemiological, clinical and etiological aspects of ALS disease in Sardinia, Southern Italy. Acta Neurol Scand 1977;55: 231–44.

[86] Giagheddu M, Puggioni G, Masala C, et al. Epidemiologic study of amyotrophic lateral sclerosis in Sardinia, Italy. Acta Neurol Scand 1983;68:394–404.

[87] Granieri E, Rosati G, Paolino E, et al. The risk of amyotrophic lateral sclerosis among laborers in Sardinia, Italy: a case-control study [abstract]. J Neurol 1985;232(Suppl):241.

[88] Chiò A, Meineri P, Tribolo A, et al. Risk factors in motor neuron disease: a case-control study. Neuroepidemiology 1991;10:174–84.

[89] Gunnarsson LG, Bodin L, Soderfeldt B, et al. A case control study of motor neurone disease: its relation to solvents. Br J Ind Med 1992;49:791–8.

[90] Morens DM, Gradinetti A, Reed D, et al. Cigarette smoking and protection from Parkinson's disease: false association or etiologic clue. Neurology 1995;45:1041–51.

[91] Kondo K, Tsubaki T. Case-control studies of motor neuron disease: association with mechanical injuries. Arch Neurol 1981;38:220–6.

[92] Kamel F, Umbach DM, Munsat TL, et al. Association of cigarette smoking with amyotrophic lateral sclerosis. Neuroepidemiology 1999;18:194–202.

[93] Nelson LM, McGuire V, Longstreth WT, et al. Population-based case-control study of amyotrophic lateral sclerosis in Western Washington State. I. Cigarette smoking and alcohol consumption. Am J Epidemiol 2000;151:156–63.

[94] Weisskopf MG, McCullough ML, Calle EE, et al. Prospective study of cigarette smoking and amyotrophic lateral sclerosis. Am J Epidemiol 2004;160:26–33.

[95] Horner RD, Kamins KG, Feussner JR, et al. Occurrence of amyotrophic lateral sclerosis among Gulf War veterans. Neurology 2003;61:742–9.

[96] Haley RW. Excess incidence of ALS in young Gulf War veterans. Neurology 2003;61: 750–6.

[97] Gray GC, Coate BD, Anderson CM, et al. The postwar hospitalization experience of US veterans of the Persian Gulf War. N Engl J Med 1996;335:1505–13.

[98] Kang HK, Bullman TA. Mortality among US veterans of the Persian Gulf War. N Engl J Med 1996;335:1498–504.

[99] Smith TC, Gray GC, Knoke JD. Is systemic lupus erythematosus, amyotrophic lateral sclerosis, or fibromyalgia associated with Persian Gulf War service? An examination of Department of Defense hospitalization data. Am J Epidemiol 2000; 151:1053–9.

[100] Kang HK, Bullman TA. Mortality among US veterans of the Persian Gulf War: 7-year follow up. Am J Epidemiol 2001;154:399–405.

[101] Rose MR. Gulf War service is an uncertain trigger for ALS [editorial]. Neurology 2003;61: 730–1.

[102] Amato AA, McVey A, Cha C, et al. Evaluation of neuromuscular symptoms in veterans of the Persian Gulf War. Neurology 1997;48:4–12.

[103] Sharief MK, Priddin J, Delamont RS, et al. Neurophysiologic analysis of neuromuscular symptoms in UK Gulf War veterans. Neurology 2002;59:1518–25.

[104] Barohn RJ, Rowland LP. Neurology and Gulf War veterans [editorial]. Neurology 2002; 59:1484–5.

[105] Smith TC, Corbeil TE, Ryan MAK, et al. In-theater hospitalizations of US and allied personnel during the 1991 Gulf War. Am J Epidemiol 2004;159:1064–76.

[106] Research Advisory Committee on Gulf War Veterans' Illnesses Media Release. Washington, DC—(November 15, 2004). Available at: http://www1.va.gov/rac-gwvi/docs/Pressrelease_Releaseof2004Report_Nov152004.pdf.

[107] Morikawa F, Okumura H, Tashiro K, et al. Motor neuron disease and past poliomyelitis. Geographic study in Hokaido, the northern-most island of Japan. J Neurol 1993;240: 13–6.

[108] Cruz DC, Nelson LM, McGuire, et al. Physical trauma and family history of neurodegerative diseases in amyotrophic lateral sclerosis: a population-based case-control study. Neuroepidemiology 1999;18:101–10.

[109] Okumura H, Kurland LT, Waring SC. Amyotrophic lateral sclerosis and polio: is there an association? Ann N Y Acad Sci 1995;753:245–56.

[110] Leparc-Goffart I, Julien J, Fuchs F, et al. Evidence for the presence of poliovirus genomic sequences in the CSF of patients with post-polio syndrome. J Clin Microbiol 1996;34: 2023–36.

[111] Berger MM, Kopp N, Vital C, et al. Detection and cellular localization of enterovirus RNA sequences in spinal cord of patients with ALS. Neurology 2000;54:20–5.

[112] Swanson NR, Fox SA, Mastaglia FL. Search for persistent infection with poliovirus or other enteroviruses in amyotrophic lateral sclerosis-motor neuron disease. Neuromuscul Disord 1995;5:457–65.

[113] Muir P, Nicholson F, Spencer GT, et al. Enterovirus infection of the central nervous system of humans: lack of an association with chronic neurological disease. J Gen Virol 1996;77: 1469–76.

[114] Roman GC. Neuroepidemiology of amyotrophic lateral sclerosis: clues to aetiology and pathogenesis. J Neurol Neurosurg Psychiatry 1996;61:131–7.

[115] Moulignier A, Moulonguet A, Pialoux G, et al. Reversible ALS-like disorder in HIV infection. Neurology 2001;57:995–1001.

[116] MacGowan DJ, Scelsa SN, Waldron M. An ALS-like syndrome with new HIV infection and complete response to antiretroviral therapy. Neurology 2001;57:1094–7.

[117] Calza L, Manfredi R, Freo E, et al. Transient reversal of HIV-associated motor neuron disease following the introduction of highly active antiretroviral therapy. J Chemother 2004;16:98–101.

[118] Leis AA, Stokic DS, Webb RM, et al. Clinical spectrum of muscle weakness in human West Nile virus infection. Muscle Nerve 2003;28:302–8.

[119] Costa J, Resende C, de Carvalho M. Motor-axonal polyneuropathy with hepatitis C virus. Eur J Neurol 2003;10:183–5.

[120] Worrall BB, Rowland LP, Chin SS-M, et al. Amyotrophy in prion diseases. Arch Neurol 2000;57:33–8.

[121] Hemmer B, Glocker FX, Kaiser R, et al. Generalised motor neuron disease as an unusual manifestation of Borrelia burgdorferi infection. J Neurol Neurosurg Psychiatry 1997;63: 257–8.

[122] Mattman LH. Cell deficient forms: stealth pathogens. 3rd edition. Boca Raton (FL): CRC Press; 2001.

[123] Koch AL. Cell wall-deficient (CWD) bacterial pathogens: could amyotrophic lateral sclerosis (ALS) be due to one? Crit Rev Microbiol 2003;29:215–21.

[124] Robberecht W. Lack of improvement with ceftriaxone in motor neuron disease. Lancet 1992;340:1096–7.

[125] Zhu S, Stavroskaya IG, Drozda M, et al. Minocycline inhibits cytochrome c release and delays progression of amyotrophic lateral sclerosis in mice. Nature 2002;417:74–8.

[126] Van Den Bosch I, Tilkin P, Lemmens G, et al. Minocycline delays disease onset and mortality in a transgenic model of ALS. Neuroreport 2002;13:1067–70.

[127] Kris J, Nguyen MD, Julien JP. Minocycline slows disease progression in a mouse model of amyotrophic lateral sclerosis. Neurobiol Dis 2002;10:268–78.

[128] Gordon PH, Moore DH, Gelinas DF, et al. Placebo-controlled phase I/II studies of minocycline in amyotrophic lateral sclerosis. Neurology 2004;62:1845–7.

[129] Younger DS, Rowland LP, Hays AP, et al. Lymphoma, motor neuron disease, and amyotrophic lateral sclerosis. Ann Neurol 1991;29:78–86.

[130] Gordon PH, Rowland LP, Younger DS, et al. Lymphoproliferative disorders and motor neuron disease: an update. Neurology 1997;48:1671–8.

[131] Forsythe PA, Dalmau J, Graus F, et al. Motor neuron syndromes in cancer patients. Ann Neurol 1997;41:722–30.

[132] Verma A, Berger JR, Snodgrass S, et al. Motor neuron disease: a paraneoplastic process associated with anti-hu antibody and small-cell lung carcinoma. Ann Neurol 1996;40:112–6.

[133] Khwaja S, Sripathi N, Ahmad BK, et al. Paraneoplastic motor neuron disease with type 1 Purkinje cell antibodies. Muscle Nerve 1998;21:943–5.

[134] Vigliani MC, Polo P, Chio A, et al. Patients with amyotrophic lateral sclerosis and cancer do not differ clinically from patients with sporadic amyotrophic lateral sclerosis. J Neurol 2000;247:778–82.

[135] Farrell DF, Starr A. Delayed neurological sequelae of electrical injuries. Neurology 1968; 18:601–6.

[136] Gawel M, Zaiwalla A, Rose FC. Antecedent events in motor neuron disease. J Neurol Neurosurg Psychiatry 1983;46:1041–3.

[137] Johansen C, Olsen JH. Mortality from amyotrophic lateral sclerosis, other chronic disorders, and electric shocks among utility workers. Am J Epidemiol 1998;148:362–8.

[138] Davanipour Z, Sobel E, Bowman JD, et al. Amyotrophic lateral sclerosis and occupational exposure to electromagnetic fields. Bioelectromagnetics 1997;18:28–35.

[139] Savitz DA, Checkoway H, Loomis DP. Magnetic field exposure and neurodegenerative disease mortality among electric utility workers. Epidemiology 1998;9:398–404.

[140] Savitz DA, Loomis DP, Tse C-KT. Electrical occupations and neurodegenerative disease: analysis of US mortality data. Arch Environ Health 1998;53:71–4.

[141] Noonan CW, Reif JS, Yost M, et al. Occupational exposure to magnetic fields in case-referent studies of neurodegenerative diseases. Scand J Work Environ Health 2002;28:42–8.

[142] Håkansson N, Gustavsson P, Johansen C, et al. Neurodegenerative diseases in welders and other workers exposed to high levels of magnetic fields. Epidemiology 2003;14:420–6.

[143] Feychting M, Jonsson F, Pedersen NL, et al. Occupational magnetic field exposure and neurodegenerative disease. Epidemiology 2003;14:413–9.

[144] Scarmeas N, Shih T, Stern Y, et al. Premorbid weight, body mass, and varsity athletics in ALS. Neurology 2002;59:773–5.

[145] Savettieri G, Salemi G, Arcara A, et al. A case-control study of amyotrophic lateral sclerosis. Neuroepidemiology 1991;10:242–5.

[146] Longstreth WT, McGuire V, Koepsell TD, et al. Risk of amyotrophic lateral sclerosis and history of physical activity: a population-based case-control study. Arch Neurol 1998;55: 201–6.

[147] Beretta S, Carri MT, Beghi E, et al. The sinister side of Italian soccer. Lancet Neurol 2003; 2:656–7.

[148] Piazza O, Sirén A-L, Ehrenreich H. Soccer, neurotrauma and amyotrophic lateral sclerosis: is there a connection? Curr Med Res Opin 2004;20:505–8.

[149] Strickland D, Smith SA, Dolliff G, et al. Physical activity, trauma, and ALS: a case-control study. Acta Neurol Scand 1996;94:45–50.

[150] Patten BM, Bilezikian JP, Mallette LE, et al. Neuromuscular disease in primary hyperparathyroidism. Ann Intern Med 1974;80:182–93.

[151] Jackson CE, Amato AA, Bryan WW, et al. Primary hyperparathyroidism and ALS: is there a relation? Neurology 1998;50:1795–9.

[152] Nelson LM, Matkin C, Longstreth WT, et al. Population-based case-control study of amyotrophic lateral sclerosis in Western Washington State. II. Diet. Am J Epidemiol 2000; 151:164–73.

[153] Getahun H, Lambein F, Vanhoorne M, et al. Food-aid cereals to reduce neurolathyrism related to grass-pea preparations during famine. Lancet 2003;362:1808–10.

[154] Tylleskär T, Banea M, Bikangi N, et al. Cassava cyanogens and konzo, an upper motoneuron disease found in Africa. Lancet 1992;339(8787):208–11. Erratum in: Lancet 1992;339(8790):440.

[155] Caparros-Lefevre D, Elbaz A. Possible relation of atypical parkinsonism in the French West Indies with consumption of tropical plants: a case-control study. Lancet 1999;354: 281–6.

[156] Mitchell JD. Amyotrophic lateral sclerosis: toxins and environment. Amyotroph Lateral Scler Other Motor Neuron Disord 2000;1:235–50.

[157] Kurland LT, Mulder DW. Epidemiologic investigations of amyotrophic lateral sclerosis. 1. Preliminary report on geographic distribution, with special reference to the Mariana Islands, including clinical and pathological observations. Neurology 1954; 4:355–448.

[158] Yoshida S, Uebayashi Y, Kihira T, et al. Epidemiology of motor neuron disease in the Kii Peninsula of Japan, 1989–1993: active or disappearing focus? J Neurol Sci 1998;155: 146–55.

[159] Anderson FH, Richardson EP, Okazaki H, et al. Neurofibrillary degeneration on Guam: frequency in Chamorros and non Chamorros with no known neurological disease. Brain 1979;102:65–77.

[160] Armon C. Environmental risk factors for amyotrophic lateral sclerosis. Neuroepidemiology 2001;20:2–6.

[161] Spencer PS, Nunn PB, Hugon J, et al. Motor neuron disease on Guam: possible role of a food neurotoxin. Lancet 1986;1:965.

[162] Spencer PS, Nunn PB, Hugon J, et al. Guam amyotrophic lateral sclerosis-parkinsonism-dementia linked to a plant excitant neurotoxin. Science 1987;237:517–22.

[163] Zhang ZX, Anderson DW, Mantel N, et al. Motor neuron disease on Guam: geographic and familial occurrence, 1956–85. Acta Neurol Scand 1996;94:51–9.

[164] Plato CC, Galasko D, Garruto RM, et al. ALS and PDC of Guam: forty-year follow up. Neurology 2002;58:765–73.

[165] Plato CC, Garruto RM, Galasko D, et al. Amyotrophic lateral sclerosis and parkinsonism-dementia complex of Guam: changing incidence rates during the past 60 years. Am J Epidemiol 2003;157:149–57.

[166] Whiting MG. Toxicity of cycads. Econ Bot 1963;17:271–302.

[167] Duncan MW, Steele JC, Kopin IJ, et al. 2-amino-3-(methylamino)-propanoic acid (BMAA) in cycad flour: an unlikely cause of amyotrophic lateral sclerosis and parkinsonia-dementia complex of Guam. Neurology 1990;40:767–72.

[168] Khabazian I, Bains JS, Williams DE, et al. Isolation of various forms of sterol β-D-glucoside from the seed of *Cycas circinalis*: neurotoxicity and implications for ALS-parkinsonism dementia complex. J Neurochem 2002;82:516–28.

[169] Cox PA, Sacks OW. Cycad neurotoxins, consumption of flying foxes, and ALS-PDC disease in Guam. Neurology 2002;58:956–9.

[170] Banack SA, Cox PA. Biomagnification of cycad neurotoxins in flying foxes: implications for ALS-PDC in Guam. Neurology 2003;61:387–9.

[171] Cox PA, Banack SA, Murch SJ. Biomagnification of cyanobacterial neurotoxins and neurodegenerative disease among the Chamorro people of Guam. Proc Natl Acad Sci USA 2003;100:13380–3.

[172] Murch SJ, Cox PA, Banack SA. A mechanism for slow release of biomagnified cyano-bacterial neurotoxins and neurodegenerative disease in Guam. Proc Natl Acad Sci USA 2004;101:12228–31.

ELSEVIER
SAUNDERS

NEUROLOGIC
CLINICS

Neurol Clin 23 (2005) 485–521

Neurodegenerative Memory Disorders: A Potential Role of Environmental Toxins

Allison Caban-Holt, PhD[a], Michelle Mattingly, PhD[b],
Gregory Cooper, MD, PhD[a,b,c],
Frederick A. Schmitt, PhD[a,b,d],*

[a]*Sanders-Brown Center on Aging, University of Kentucky Medical Center, Lexington,
KY 40536, USA*
[b]*Department of Neurology, University of Kentucky Medical Center, Lexington,
KY 40536, USA*
[c]*Lexington Clinic Department of Neurology, Lexington, Kentucky 40536*
[d]*Departments of Psychiatry, Psychology, and Behavioral Science, University of Kentucky
Medical Center, Lexington, KY 40536, USA*

Age-associated neurodegenerative disorders are widely recognized by clinicians, researchers, and epidemiologists as sharing common features, including the accumulation of altered proteins within the brain and an average age of onset after the sixth decade. These disorders appear to encompass both inherited and sporadic forms. A recently published review [1] highlights the clinical features, genetics, risk factors, and potential treatment approaches of these disorders across the spectrum of Alzheimer's disease (AD), Parkinson's disease (PD), and amyotrophic lateral sclerosis (ALS). As Mayeux [1] notes in his summary, epidemiologic studies of neurodegenerative disorders are shifting their focus away from descriptive studies (disease incidence and prevalence) to the analyses of genetic and environmental factors that may expand our understanding of causality. As causes and risks factors for neurodegenerative disorders are identified, more effective treatment approaches may develop as well. Environmental factors such as neurotoxins have been evaluated as risks for the dementias and

This work was supported by the National Institute on Aging grants 5P50AG005144 and 1R01AG19241.

* Corresponding author. Alzheimer's Disease Research Center and Department of Neurology, University of Kentucky Medical Center, L445 KY Clinic, 800 Rose Street, Lexington, KY 40536-0284.

E-mail address: fascom@email.uky.edu (F.A. Schmitt).

motor neuron disease, but most studies to date have remained more descriptive in nature.

The present review provides a summary of the research literature that evaluates putative environmental exposure to toxins and its potential association with these neurodegenerative disorders. It should be remembered, however, that much of what we know about toxins and neurodegeneration is derived from laboratory models and epidemiologic research. Therefore, causality is often difficult to infer when these data are generalized to populations or applied to individual patients.

Demographics of dementia

Alzheimer's disease is by far the most common form of adult onset dementia, affecting over 4 million individuals in the United States. With the aging of our society, it has been estimated that approximately 14 million individuals in the US alone will have AD by the year 2050 [2] unless preventive measures are found. The economic burden of AD is estimated to be over 100 billion dollars per year [3]. AD is not the only adult onset dementia but its prevalence reflects approximately 60% to 75% of all cases, given that AD often coexists with other dementia disorders. Prevalence estimates for dementia with Lewy bodies (DLB) and vascular dementia (VaD) suggest that these are the second most common dementias (20% and 16%, respectively) followed by AD with PD and AD with stroke (8% each). Other dementing conditions such as Pick's disease, corticobasal degeneration, and primary progressive aphasia, for example, account for an additional 5% of cases, with PD plus dementia reflecting another 3% of prevalent cases [4].

Epidemiologic studies have consistently shown that the prevalence and incidence of AD increase dramatically after age 65. Population-based epidemiologic studies published before 1998 have been reviewed in two meta-analyses [5,6] and will not be discussed in detail here. Furthermore, important epidemiologic concepts and study design issues related to determining factors for elevated AD risk, along with potential protective factors, are elegantly summarized in reviews by Kukull and Ganguli [7] and Garabrant [8]. However, several important points raised by Kukull and Ganguli [7] and Garabrant [8] are relevant to this review of neurotoxins as risk factors for dementing disorders. First, without a biological measure for diagnosing AD or other dementias, the methods that are used to determine the presence of dementia generally involve the use of operational clinical criteria that encompass tests of mental functioning and clinical examinations of patient symptoms and functional skills. As a result, the identification of a case is less than perfectly accurate even though AD diagnosis is no longer a diagnosis of exclusion [9,10]. Second, additional sources of error and bias arise in studies depending on the sampling strategies (in addition to case ascertainment methods), how well the selected sample reflects the total population of interest, and how the population sample was obtained. Third, disease severity may result in underestimates in a given population. For example, early or mild AD may not be detected, or if it is specifically studied, it may result in estimates that differ from epidemiologic studies in which moderate or severe cases are identified. Finally, the design of the epidemiologic study that intends to evaluate risk factors for dementia can result in important sources of potential bias. Prospective longitudinal studies suffer from biases, including the loss of subjects to follow-up because of dropout, death (especially before the dementia evolves or is detected), and how exposure is defined. These factors could therefore underestimate the incidence (development of the dementia) in a given study, as could the variability in actual and measured exposure to a potential risk factor. Case-control studies have similar sources of bias, including the definition of a case, how exposure is determined, and because these studies compare groups of individuals with a given disease versus similar persons without the disease, the study may suffer from selection bias (the groups differ from the general population), misestimation of age, duration, and degree of exposure, or recall bias (which could reduce or inflate the exposure to an assumed risk factor).

Added sources of bias in studies that prospectively attempt to define risk factors linked to dementia and other neurodegenerative disorders are highlighted by reports that AD often is unrecognized, particularly in the mild stages, by physicians and family members of the patient [11,12]. As a result of methodological components, studies of environmental toxins and dementia risk can be expensive, time consuming, and difficult to replicate, and the interpretation of results may reflect unrecognized sources of bias [13]. In the case of dementia, an age-associated condition, a potentially complex spectrum of risks, subject factors, and genetic predispositions clearly require careful attention to study design if associations between environmental toxins and neurodegeneration are to be uncovered [14].

Dementia diagnosis and screening

The evaluation of the demented patient has received a great deal of attention in the past two decades and will not be summarized in this review. Readers are referred to excellent reviews of AD diagnosis and management by Morris' [15] handbook reference, Grossberg and Desai [16], and Cummings [17]. These reviews contain standard approaches for the evaluation of suspected neurodegenerative disorders, clinical criteria, and treatment. Dementia is defined as "an acquired and sustained deterioration of memory and other intellectual functions in an alert patient. Dementia results from brain dysfunction and is a symptom of many diseases" [15]. Relevant to the evaluation of the literature on environmental toxins and dementia, the American Academy of Neurology practice parameter [9] summarizes the usefulness of current diagnostic criteria for degenerative disorders. The reliability of AD diagnostic criteria ranges from 0.51 to 0.73, and inter-rater reliability is as high as 95% between the initial diagnosis and the diagnosis after 1 year, with a sensitivity of approximately 80% and a specificity of approximately 70%. For non-AD dementias, diagnostic criteria fare less well with generally low sensitivity but high specificity [9]. Clearly, studies attempting to ascertain risk factors for neurodegenerative or dementing disorders could be greatly influenced by the relatively low prevalence of various neurodegenerative disorders, how screening procedures are implemented [18], and the selection, application, screening procedures, and limitations of diagnostic criteria in a given study.

Environmental exposure and Alzheimer's disease

As noted previously, AD is the most common disease process of pathologic aging. AD is a multifactorial disease, and numerous hypotheses have been proposed to explain its causes, including genetic defects, oxidative stress, β-amyloid toxicity, and environmental factors [19–22]. Over the past several years, an abundance of research has focused on the exploration of environmental factors such as solvents, metals, pesticides, and magnetic field exposure in the neurodegenerative process. Therefore, this review provides an overview of the literature as it pertains to environmental toxins and neurodegeneration, with reference to solvents, metals, pesticides, magnetic field exposure, and smoking.

Solvents and Alzheimer's disease

It is recognized that exposure to solvents can be neurotoxic [23]. However, an association between solvent exposure and neurodegeneration, particularly AD, has yet to be established. Three epidemiologic studies [24–26] did not find a relationship between lifetime occupational exposure to solvents and AD. Graves et al [24] used a case-control design to compare 89 subjects with probable AD with 89 controls and obtained their lifetime job histories with an industrial hygienist rating exposure for each job. An increased risk for developing AD was noted with the increasing number of years of solvent exposure; however, an inverse relationship between exposure intensity and AD was reported. Palmer et al [25] compared individuals diagnosed with dementia based on computed tomography records with controls with brain cancer or another non-disabling disorder on lifetime occupational exposure to organic solvents. Their findings did not yield a positive association between occupational exposure to solvents and dementia. Shalat et al [26], using a case-control design, evaluated the effect of occupational history and subsequent diagnosis of AD on a total of 98 case and 162 control subjects. The 98 cases were all men from the Geriatric Research, Education, and Clinical Center at the Edith N. Rogers Memorial Veterans Hospital in Bedford, MA. These men had been diagnosed with Alzheimer's type dementia between July 1975 and July 1985, based on criteria of the Diagnostic and Statistical Manual III-R (DSM-III-R) [27] and the National Institute of Neurologic, Communicative Disorders, and Stroke-Alzheimer's Disease and Related Disorders Association (NINCDS-ADRDA) [28]. Control subjects were selected from Massachusetts voter registration lists and matched by gender, year of birth, and town of residence. No increased risk for the development of AD was evident with a history of occupational exposure to organic solvents or lead.

In contrast to the above findings, Freed and Kandel [29] and Kukull et al [30] provide data suggesting a possible relationship between occupational exposure and dementia diagnosis. The authors [29] provide evidence from a single-case study, a case series study, and a preliminary case-control study of the relationship between chronic exposure in the workplace and later development of dementia. Specifically, in the single-case study, serum levels of perchlorethylene (745 parts per billion [ppb]) elevated to approximately 15 times that seen in a normal population were found in a man who worked as a dry cleaner for over 30 years and was subsequently diagnosed with probable AD. Their case series used 80 AD patients screened post hoc for occupational exposure based on their performance on a delayed match-to-sample recognition memory test. Analyses of the memory performances in these individuals showed a pattern of greater decline in delayed (72 hr) recognition in those AD cases with a history of occupational exposure (based on family member interviews). A medical records review found that four of five individuals had been exposed to metal vapors (primarily copper), and the fifth case had been exposed to solvent. All of the subjects had histories of memory impairment, coronary artery disease, left temporal slow wave activity on electroencephalography, cortical atrophy on CT scans, and impaired short-term memory and word-finding problems on neuropsychologic testing. Neurologic findings also showed extrapyramidal signs, including impaired gait, coordination, and posture. Therefore, the authors pointed out the need to further study metals as potential contributors to the AD process. The final data set reported by Freed and Kandel [29] considered data of long-term occupational exposure to a variety of compounds (eg, metals and solvents) from 150 patients diagnosed with AD. Occupational exposure was defined as a minimum of 2000 hours in the workplace, based on questionnaires completed by the patients' family members. The authors found that 55 of the 150 patients with AD (37%) met the operational definition for long-term occupational exposure, whereas only 7 of the 57 (12%) healthy controls met the same operational definition.

Kukull et al [30] conducted a community-based case-control study with 139 individuals diagnosed with AD based on the NINCDS-ADRDA criteria and 243 controls randomly drawn from the Group Health Cooperative population (case-control design). Results of the study were interpreted as demonstrating a moderate-to-strong association between solvent exposure and AD, with a greater effect in men and more years of exposure. Specifically, a history of exposure to one or more solvent groups (benzene and toluene, phenols and alcohols, and ketones plus other solvents) resulted in an adjusted

AD odds ratio (OR) of 2.3 (95% confidence interval [CI], 1.1–4.7); however, among men the odds ratio increased to 6.0 (95% CI, 2.1–17.2).

Heavy metals

Many metals such as iron, copper, and manganese are essential for normal brain function. However, many of these same elements have also been implicated in neurotoxicity and subsequent neurodegeneration, specifically AD. Iron, in particular appears to be important, given theories concerning AD pathophysiology that link oxidative stress to neurodegeneration [20,21].

Aluminum

Klatzo et al [31] were the first to present a hypothesis linking aluminum to the cause of AD. They found that injecting aluminum salts into the brains of rabbits resulted in neurofibrillary changes. Subsequent work by Crapper et al [32] replicated this finding in cats and demonstrated that aluminum concentration was increased in AD patients. Furthermore, Beal et al [33] found a reduction of up to 40% in choline acetyltransferease activity in the entorhinal cortex and hippocampus, as well as a reduction in serotonin and noradrenaline as a result of aluminum-induced neurofibrillary degeneration in their rabbit model of AD.

Crapper et al [32,34] provided the first reports of neurotoxic concentrations of aluminum in the brains of AD patients. Based on these early findings, it was been suggested that aluminum exposure represented a risk factor for the development of AD. Additional data showed that aluminum could be detected in the characteristic neuropathologic hallmarks of AD (senile plaques and neurofibrillary tangles [35–37]) lending further support to a link between AD and aluminum. Evidence was also reported [38] suggesting that aluminum potentiates oxidative and inflammatory events in the brain, leading to tissue damage. Although no direct relationship has been established between aluminum and AD, numerous studies suggest that aluminum may exacerbate events associated with AD. In contrast, many authors have presented results that do not support the aluminum hypothesis [39,40], having found no increase in AD risk with aluminum exposure. The most solid epidemiologic evidence comes from the case-control study by Graves et al [24] in Seattle, Washington. In 178 matched cases of AD and controls, ORs adjusted for age and education ranged from 0.89 (low) to 2.04 (high) for aluminum exposure duration (neither value was statistically significant). Furthermore, the intensity of exposure showed an inverse and nonsignificant relationship with an OR of 4.52 for low exposure and 0.76 for high levels of aluminum exposure.

Neuropathologic investigations such as the one by Candy et al [41] demonstrated the presence of minuscule insoluble aluminum silicate granules in the brain of patients with AD. These granules were described as being surrounded by amyloid protein plaques, suggesting to the authors that these granules represented an early or initiating factor in plaque formation. In addition, Ward and Mason [42] found higher concentrations of aluminum in certain brain regions of autopsy samples from patients with AD. In contrast, the extensive work (and review) on aluminum in the brains of AD patients by Markesbery and Ehmann [20] as well as other investigators has tried to answer the question of aluminum as a primary factor in AD, in contrast to aluminum as a secondary mechanism. As covered in their reviews [20,21], aluminum is not directly toxic to hippocampal neurons in vitro, but aluminum tends to accumulate in degenerating neurons (and therefore represents a marker of neurodegeneration).

Other clinical data come from the role of aluminum in the development of Alzheimer-like symptoms in patients with renal failure, although these findings have also been inconsistent [43–45]. Generally, aluminum toxicity has been documented in patients with impaired renal functions secondary to aluminum accumulation through hemodialysis fluids and aluminum-containing pharmaceutical agents administered for the treatment of hypophosphatemia [46]. The primary symptoms of this well-known complication of dialysis, dialysis encephalopathy, consist of disordered speech, dementia, convulsions, myoclonus, and accompanying anemia and osteomalacia. Although some of these symptoms are evident in patients with AD, dialysis encephalopathy does not result in pathologic neurofibrillary tangles [46], which are a hallmark of AD.

Many epidemiologic studies have examined the possible link between exposure to aluminum in drinking water and the incidence of AD [47–49]. In drinking water, aluminum sulfate is used in water treatment to remove suspended particles and to reduce the dose of chlorine. The ingestion of aluminum in drinking water has been suggested to have a positive relationship to the occurrence of AD [50–55]. Martyn et al [56] found the risk of AD to be 1.5 times higher in districts where the mean aluminum levels in tap water exceeded 0.11 mg/l than in districts where the concentration was less than 0.01 mg/l. In contrast, Wettstein et al [57] found no relationship to an increased risk of AD in their study of 800 male octogenarians consuming drinking water with aluminum concentration up to 98 mg/L. Interestingly, the regular ingestion of aluminum through daily antacid consumption suplies thousands of times the amount of aluminum ingested through drinking water. Yet the findings of epidemiologic studies of AD and antacid exposure have been largely negative. For example, a Canadian population-based case-control study [58] found no association between the use of aluminum-containing antacids and AD in 285 cases clinically diagnosed with probable AD compared with 535 controls. Flaten et al [59] obtained similar findings, with no association between antacid use and AD mortality.

The neurotoxic effects of aluminum through occupational exposure have also been studied in different groups of workers [60,61]. Although numerous studies [62–68] have attempted to demonstrate a possible link between the inhalation of aluminum dust and neurologic disorders, no study has yet to develop a causal link between aluminum inhalation and AD. Polizzi et al [50] compared retired foundry workers with nonexposed workers, and found that retired foundry workers had cognitive test scores suggestive of mild cognitive impairment [69,70]. They subsequently speculated that aluminum affects primarily the entorhinal cortex through the absorption of the metal through the olfactory bulb, resulting in symptoms compatible with mild cognitive impairment, a potential prodrome for AD [50]. Graves et al [24] and Salib and Hiller [71] published two epidemiologic studies that attempted to evaluate the relationship between AD and occupational exposure to aluminum. These studies taken together suggest that lifetime occupational exposure to aluminum does not appear to be a strong risk factor for AD, with ORs of approximately 1.0.

In summary, earlier evidence implicated aluminum in the development of AD; however, the aluminum hypothesis appears to have fallen out of favor as a major component of AD pathophysiology. Early studies [72] demonstrated evidence of elevated levels of aluminum in the brains of AD patients, and one small single-blind clinical trial [73] with an aluminum chelating agent (desferrioxamine) showed a reduced rate of decline in the activities of daily living in treated AD cases. Subsequent studies [74] continued to demonstrate small but significant elevations of aluminum in the AD hippocampus, inferior parietal lobule, and superior and middle temporal gyri compared with corresponding control tissues. In contrast, other studies [75,76] have failed to find differences between aluminum levels in AD brain compared with age-matched controls. Therefore, aluminum has an unclear causative role in AD neurodegeneration but may contribute to neurodegeneration through mechanisms such as its promotion of oxidative stress and, therefore, may play a secondary role in this disease [21].

Copper, iron, lead, manganese, and zinc

The oxidative stress hypothesis is believed to be a major mechanism accounting for cumulative neurodegeneration in AD [77–79]. Metals such as iron and copper act as catalysts in oxygen free-radical generation and may therefore increase the risk for AD [77,80]. Deibel et al [77] compared 10 AD brain specimens and 11 age-matched control subjects and found a significant decrease in copper along with significant increases in zinc and iron in the hippocampus and amygdala, areas with evidence of considerable histopathologic alterations in AD. Lovell et al [81] reported similar results in their study of metal concentration in the rims and cores of senile plaques and neuropil of the amygdala of nine AD and five control subjects. They found statistically significant increases in iron and zinc in the rims and cores of senile plaques in the AD amygdala compared with AD neuropil and elevated copper in the rim of senile plaques. Zinc was noticeably elevated in the neuropil of AD subjects when compared with the controls. In contrast, mouse models of AD pathology have suggested that increasing amounts of copper appear to reduce β-amyloid concentrations, resulting in fewer pathogenic β-amyloid plaques [82,83], whereas the cholesterol-fed rabbit model of AD shows that copper-fed (0.12 parts per million [ppm]) animals developed structures in the brain resembling β-amyloid plaques and showed reduced classical conditioning performance [84].

Molina et al [85] ascertained serum and cerebrospinal fluid (CSF) levels of numerous metals in 26 patients with AD and 28 matched controls. Serum levels of zinc and CSF and serum levels of iron, copper, and manganese did not differ significantly between the two groups, whereas CSF zinc levels were decreased in AD patients compared with controls. It was hypothesized that the main finding of decreased CSF zinc levels suggested that low CSF zinc levels were related to the presence of oxidative stress processes or possibly the interaction of β-amyloid or amyloid precursor protein with zinc, resulting in a depletion of zinc levels [86]. Therefore, Cuajungco and Lees [86] argue that zinc is associated with AD pathology through its ability to precipitate β-amyloid and influence various exogenous and endogenous risk factors for AD pathology. In contrast, Price et al [87] found that zinc supplementation at normal concentrations appeared to slow down the progression of AD. However, a number of studies [77,88,89] have resulted in contradictory findings, with evidence of increased zinc in the brain or CSF of individuals with Alzheimer's disease. The importance of zinc as a risk factor for neurodegeneration rests on data suggesting that zinc may play a role in brain-based oxidative stress as well as its observed effects of direct neuronal toxicity [21].

Mercury has been suggested as a factor in the formation of neurofibrillary tangles [90]. Thompson et al [91] and Pendergrass et al [92] demonstrated elevations of mercury in the nucleus basalis of Meynert in greater than 80% of AD brains studied. Webb [93] suggests that mercury inactivates enzymes by slowing down the repair and metabolism of vital functions, which in turn may result in neurofibrillary tangles and memory loss of AD. In sum, there may be an association between mercury and AD, but the strongest data to date suggest that it is not related to the pathogenesis of AD based on a careful study of dental amalgams. Saxe et al [94] derived direct estimates of mercury vapor exposure from dental amalgams in 33 autopsied normal elderly and 68 autopsied AD cases. Using intraoral video recordings of dental restorations, they measured (1) amalgam location, (2) surface area, (3) time in the mouth, (4) type of filling, (5) the degree of opposing dentition (as an index of abrasion leading to release of mercury), and (6) other environmental sources of mercury exposure (eg, occupation and diet). They then evaluated brain tissues (eight regions in each hemisphere) using instrumental and radiochemical neutron analysis to determine the mercury load in the tissue. Even though the control cases were, on average, 4 years older than the AD cases, no differences in dental exposure, and more importantly, mercury levels were found between the two groups. In fact, when the data were analyzed for olfactory tissue, controls (30.9 ng/g) had higher mean values of mercury than did AD cases (14.0 ng/g). As a result, the data were interpreted as providing no support for the hypothesis that dental amalgams, and therefore mercury, were involved in AD pathogenesis.

Inorganic (eg, lead paint) and organic (ie, tetraethyl lead) lead have been investigated as possible risk factors for AD. Two cases [95] of workers with long-term occupational exposure to lead demonstrated neuropathologic features of AD at autopsy, with one individual reporting a history of dementia for many years before his death. In contrast, no consistent evidence is available to support a relationship between increased levels of manganese and the development of AD [95].

Pesticides

Rural areas appear to account for a higher incidence of AD cases than urban settings [96,97]. Growth and productivity in these rural communities have resulted in the increased use of pesticides [98]. Many families of pesticides are known to contain neurotoxic properties [98] that cause serious central nervous system damage (eg, carbamates, organophosphates, organochlorines, and bipyridyles [99]). Organophosphates are known inhibitors of acetylcholine, bipyridyles are able to generate free radicals that cross the blood-brain barrier, and organochlorines are capable of impairing mitochondrial function and producing free radicals [100–105]. As such, it has been hypothesized that pesticides may contribute to the cholinergic system dysfunction and production of free radicals present in AD [98].

Epidemiologic data suggest an OR of 2.17 for AD as derived from the Canadian Study of Health and Aging [58] with respect to occupational exposure to pesticides. More recently, Gauthier et al [98] conducted an epidemiologic study by randomly selecting subjects from the Saguenay-Lac Saint-Jean, Quebec, region to evaluate their long-term exposure to pesticides and a possible association between pesticide exposure and AD. In their study, AD was not significantly related to long-term exposure to herbicides and insecticides. In contrast, a cohort study of French elderly found an association between past occupational exposure to pesticides and low cognitive performance, with an increased risk of developing AD or PD [106]. This elevated risk was exclusively found in men who worked predominantly in vineyards. Based on these studies, more work clearly is needed to ascertain the impact of exposure, dose, and duration of specific pesticides.

Magnetic fields

Although no documented causal relationship between occupational electromagnetic field (EMF) exposure and AD has been found, a link between occupations involving exposure to electric and magnetic fields and the subsequent development of AD has been hypothesized. Some research findings [107] suggest that EMF exposure may contribute to an increased production of β-amyloid in the brain, which might eventually result in AD. In southern California and Finland, Sobel et al [107] used a case-control method to analyze a sample of 387 AD patients and 475 hospital patients, vascular dementia cases, and community controls. After evaluating exposure through surrogate interviews, they found an association between AD and employment in occupations (seamstress, tailor, and dressmaker) associated with elevated EMF exposure, with an OR of 3.0 when the Finnish and Southern California cases were combined, and with a higher OR (3.8) for women, however, the OR varied greatly. Based on the first Finnish group (AD and vascular cases) medium to high EMF exposure was associated with an OR of 2.9 with a 95% CI, of 0.7 to 12.2, with women having greater risk with exposure (women OR 7.3, men OR 0.7). In the second series (AD and hospital controls), the EMF exposure OR for all cases was 3.1 (95% CI, 0.7–8.9), with women at a higher risk (OR 3.3) than men (OR 2.5). In the Southern California series of subjects, the OR was 3.0 (95% CI, 0.8–11.1), with women again showing an elevated risk (OR 4.2) than men (OR 2.7). Part of the difficulty with these analyses rests on the fact that there were only 36 AD cases with medium to high EMF exposure and 16 controls in the combined sample.

However, a larger study by Savitz et al [108] found only modest associations between EMF occupational exposure and AD, with an adjusted OR of 1.2 (95% CI, 1.0–1.4) in a sample of electrical workers who died during the period between 1985 and 1991. This study ascertained 256 cases of AD and randomly matched 768 controls of a larger sample of men who had occupations associated with electrical field exposure. Furthermore, the odds of AD did not change because of age, year of death, or social class. In a related study, Savitz et al [109] examined mortality in men employed at five large electric utility companies in the United States who had worked for more than 5 months at these facilities during the years 1950 to 1986. Death certificates were obtained on over 20,000 men and estimated their exposure to magnetic fields in microtesla years. Causes of death were further reviewed by evaluating any mention of neurodegenerative disorders on the death certificate (mentioned cause, 56 cases of AD) as well as any neurodegenerative disorder listed as the cause of death (underlying cause, 24 AD cases). Analyses were adjusted for several factors including solvent and polychlorinated biphenyl exposure. Overall, AD was not strongly associated with EMF exposure based on years of employment (risk ratios of 1.0–1.4 for mentioned cause and 0.9–2.1 for underlying cause). The highest risk ratio (RR) for AD was found for 9 cases (RR, 2.0, 95% CI, 0.6–7.0) who had more than 19.9 years of exposure (microtesla years) during their careers.

A positive relationship between EMF occupational exposure and AD has also been reported by Feychting et al [110] and Hakansson et al [111]. Feychting et al conducted a cohort study by evaluating all "economically active individuals" in the Swedish 1980 census and following them for neurodegenerative disease mortality from 1981 through 1995. EMF exposure was determined by development of a job exposure matrix based on magnetic field measurements. Findings indicated an increased risk of AD (based on mortality records) observed among exposed men both in 1970 and 1980, with a relative risk of 2.3. The associations were most pronounced for early onset AD mortality or with follow-up limited to 10 years after the last known exposure. Hakansson et al [111] completed a cohort study with a large population of resistance welders who were exposed to high levels of extremely low-frequency magnetic fields. These welders completed spot, flash, butt, projection, and seam welding with high electrical currents. They found an increased risk of AD (and ALS but not PD) in workers exposed to extremely low-frequency magnetic fields. One potential factor that confounds the findings of this study is that welders were also exposed to heavy metal vapors and solvents.

Smoking

Studies evaluating smoking as a risk for AD have demonstrated a "protective effect," an unrelated effect, or a modestly increased risk for AD. Lee [112] conducted a meta-analysis of 13 case-control studies from 1984 through 1993 and found a significant 40% reduction in the risk of AD among smokers. Ott et al [113] used a cohort study design involving 6870 persons over the age of 55 with approximately 2 years of follow-up to compare former smokers with "never" smokers and observed an increased relative risk of 1.4 for AD. Their results also showed that current smokers had an increased relative risk for AD of 2.2 relative to never smokers. Ott et al therefore demonstrated a doubling of risk for AD among smokers, with men at a greater risk than women. These investigators [113] subsequently assessed the simultaneous effects of smoking and apolipoprotein E genotype. For those individuals with an E4 allele, in either current smokers or former smokers, smoking had no effect. However, among persons without an E4 allele, the risk of AD caused by smoking appeared to be elevated. Merchant et al [114] and Launer et al [115] found results similar to the study by Ott et al [113], with no association found between former smokers and never smokers and AD and a modestly increased risk seen with current smokers to never smokers. Merchant et al [114] also demonstrated an increased risk with non-E4-containing genotypes and a null association between smoking and AD among those carrying the E4 allele.

A more recent report from the Honolulu-Asia Aging Study by Tyas et al [116] studied the association between dementia and mid-life smoking of 3232 men. Pack years were derived for each participant and then grouped into light (less than 26.8 pack years), medium (26.8 to 40.5 pack years), heavy (40.6 to 55.5 pack years), and very heavy (55.6 to 156 pack years) smokers. Dementia diagnosis was based on DSM-III-R [27] and NINCDS-ADRDA [28] criteria and the accuracy of the clinical diagnosis was validated in some cases (218) with autopsy examination in which approximately 67% of the clinical AD cases met neuropathologic criteria for AD. After adjustments for age, education, and apolipoprotein E genotype, AD risk increased at the medium (OR 2.18) and heavy (OR 2.40) levels of smoking. These derived risks agree well with the data from the Rotterdam study [113] demonstrating a doubling of AD risk with smoking. However, very heavy smoking did not increase the risk of AD (OR 1.08), and the authors suggested that this lack of elevated dementia risk might have been because of a "hardy survivor effect." More importantly, however, the data from Tyas et al [116] also included estimates of smoking and the presence of neuritic plaques, a hallmark of AD neuropathology, in the brain. Medium and heavy smokers had more neocortical neuritic plaques at autopsy than those men who had never smoked. In contrast, data from the Multi-Institutional Research in AD Genetic Epidemiology Study by Bachman et al [117] did not find an elevated risk for AD in white and African American smokers in a sample of 2779 individuals. In this study, current and past smokers were compared with nonsmokers for risk of AD. In whites the risk for AD in smokers after adjusting for age and education was 0.88 (OR), whereas it was 1.0 for African Americans.

Clearly, the data on smoking as a risk for AD are conflicting and reflect study design and population differences. Additionally, as neurodegeneration in AD is believed to involve oxidative stress, no information is available from these studies about diet and antioxidant supplements that may moderate the risk of AD with smoking, especially given the findings that antioxidant levels are affected by smoking [118–120] and may also moderate oxidative damage in smokers [121,122]. As a result, smoking as an environmental toxin and AD risk will require more careful study to more clearly define their association.

Parkinson's disease and environmental toxins

In PD, the main pathologic change is the loss of pigmented neurons in the substantia nigra [123]. These neurons project their axons to the striatum and use dopamine as their neurotransmitter. A reduction of the striatal dopamine represents the primary neurochemical alteration in PD. Another primary feature is the presence of cytoplasmic inclusions called Lewy bodies within the nigral dopaminergic neurons as well as in other areas of the brain such as the locus ceruleus, the dorsal motor nucleus of the vagus, the sympathetic ganglia, and the cerebral cortex. The loss of nigrostriatal dopaminergic projection neurons is largely responsible for the extrapyramidal movement disorder and may also be responsible for cognitive changes such as impaired dual task performances [124]. Because the function of Lewy bodies in the processes resulting in PD is unknown and Lewy bodies are often seen in postmortem AD cases, it is believed may suggest an overlap in these clinical entities [123,125].

The typical symptoms of PD are resting tremor, slowness in movements, rigidity, postural instability, loss of facial expression, gait disturbance, micrographia, constipation, and excessive sweating. Over time, the disease can cause depression, personality changes, dementia, sleep disturbance, speech impairment, and sexual dysfunction [1]. PD is typically idiopathic [123], however, age appears to be the most apparent risk factor for developing PD. PD is rare before the age of 50 and increases with age thereafter.

The rate of dementia incidence in idiopathic PD ranges between 10% and 15%. Mayeaux et al [126] reviewed the clinical records of a cohort of patients with PD in a major medical center and estimated the overall incidence rate of dementia in this cohort to be 69 per 1000 person years of observation. Furthermore, these authors found that by age 85 more than 65% of the surviving cohort was demented. The age-specific rates of dementia in the cohort group were significantly greater than for a similarly aged sample of healthy elderly individuals. As with AD, multiple studies have evaluated potential risk factors including environmental toxin exposure as a contributing factor for PD.

Parkinson's disease dementia

In terms of dementia in PD, autopsy data show that cortical Lewy bodies are present but that they differ in their distribution from those seen in AD [124,127,128]. The major clinical difference reported by Mayeaux et al [129] between PD patients with and without dementia was a later age at the onset of motor manifestations. In multiple logistic regression analyses, significant predictors of dementia in PD were lack of education, severity of motor deficit, and PD onset at an age greater than 60 [130,131]. These findings are similar to those of Levy et al [132] who showed that an increased risk of incident dementia in PD is associated with the age and severity of extrapyramidal signs, but this association is primarily related to their combined effect rather than separate effects. Interestingly, Marder et al [133] found that a family history of dementia was present in 30% of their demented PD patients but only 5.6% of their nondemented group. Thus PD patients with a family history of dementia may be predisposed to developing dementia during the course of PD. Overall, the age at onset of PD, motor symptoms, lower education level, and family history of dementia may increase the chances of PD patients becoming demented. McKeith and Burn [124] suggest that the precise diagnosis of a dementia syndrome in PD is problematic, particularly in the early stages. They state, "Minor performance deficits in set-shifting, retrieval of learned material, and reduced verbal fluency are very frequent and usually do not warrant a diagnosis of dementia...because they fail to impact substantially on the person's day-to-day functioning...Cognitive screening tools that have been developed for the detection of AD...are poorly sensitive to the subtle subcortical deficits."

Parkinson's disease versus dementia with Lewy bodies

A variant of PD and AD, termed dementia with Lewy bodies (DLB), is defined by the presence of Lewy bodies throughout the neocortex and brainstem. In this disorder, cortical Lewy bodies are frequently accompanied by neuritic plaques and neurofibrillary tangles as seen in AD [134]. McKeith and Burn [124] point out that a few cortical Lewy bodies can be found in most PD cases, even those without dementia, suggesting that the distribution and density of cortical Lewy bodies are important in determining their effects on clinical symptoms, rather than simply their presence. The researchers define DLB as a dementing disorder with prominent neuropsychiatric features, which are associated with the degeneration of cortical neurons, particularly in frontal, anterior cingulate, insular, and temporal regions. DLB presents mainly in late life, with a mean age of onset between 75 and 80 years [127].

Searches of the current literature yielded little data exploring connections between DLB and neurotoxins. Perhaps the pathological and clinical similarities inherent in PD and DLB may be obscuring the conclusions of toxicologic studies of these diseases, thus making it particularly difficult to differentiate the unique effects of environmental toxins on each of these diseases. Consequently, our knowledge of DLB and its potential connection to toxins is awaiting additional epidemiologic and toxicologic investigations. Thus, the present review focuses on the significantly larger literature on PD with dementia and environmental toxins, rather than on DLB and toxins.

Environmental toxins and Parkinson's disease

In terms of environmental toxins, those related to agricultural work have been closely studied in relation to neurodegenerative diseases. Of particular interest to researchers have been herbicides, pesticides, fungicides, and to a lesser extent rural living in general and well water consumption. Unfortunately, the literature in these areas is fraught with contradictory findings, probably because of the methodological differences that exist between studies.

Parkinson's disease and herbicides

Herbicidal compounds have generally been explored as a potential risk factor for PD. Gorell et al [135], in a case-control study, found a significant association between PD and occupational exposure to herbicides (OR 4.10, 95% CI). One herbicide in particular that has been closely examined is paraquat. Used extensively during the mid 20th Century, this herbicide has been found to be associated with PD incidence [136]. A study by Li and Sun [137] theorized that paraquat leads to oxidative stress, which results in the death of dopaminergic neurons. Paraquat has been shown to induce parkinsonian symptoms such as increased rigidity, bradykinesia, and tremor [138]. Further implicating the potential danger of this specific herbicide are the findings of a study by Liou et al [139] that show PD risk was highest in those who had used paraquat (OR 4.74) compared with other herbicides

(OR 2.17) and control subjects who had no exposure to pesticides (OR 1.00). However, Kuopio et al [140] did not find an association between exposure to herbicides and PD.

Parkinson's disease and fungicides

The neurotoxic effect of Maneb, a manganese-containing dithiocarbamate fungicide, is the inhibition of the activity of the mitochondrial respiratory chain. It has been shown in animal studies to enhance the toxicity of the herbicide paraquat toward the nigrostriatal neurons [141]. Thus, the combination of fungicides and herbicides may pose an even higher risk for PD than exposure to either one individually.

Parkinson's disease and pesticides

Baldereschi et al [142] showed that occupational pesticide exposure is significantly associated with PD (OR 3.33). Furthermore, their results suggest that by virtue of obtaining a pesticide use license, regardless of the actual amount of time spent in contact with pesticides, pesticide is related to an increased risk of PD. Additional evidence comes from a cohort study of French elderly that describes a significant association, in men only, between PD and occupational exposure to pesticides (adjusted RR 5.63 [106]).

The neurotoxic effect of rotenone, a plant-derived pesticide, is to increase the formation of cytoplasmic inclusions in the substantia nigra neurons and α-synuclein aggregation. Data from rat studies [143] demonstrate that rotenone promotes degeneration of the dopaminergic neurons and induces parkinsonian symptoms.

Organochlorine pesticides, such as Dieldrin, are believed to increase α-synuclein formation, reactive oxygen species formation, and lipid peroxidation [144]. Other investigators have found contrary results. Corrigan et al [145] analyzed frozen samples of human substantia nigra using gas chromatography with electron capture detection. These investigators found that organochlorines did not produce a direct toxic action on the dopaminergic system but may contribute to PD through cytochrome P-450 polymorphism. They compared the concentrations of organochlorine compounds in the tissues of the substantia nigra of patients diagnosed with PD, AD, cortical Lewy body dementia, and nondemented nonparkinsonian controls. It was found that the levels of organochlorine compounds were significantly higher in the brains of PD patients but not in those of the other groups. These results suggest that organochlorine insecticides do not produce a direct toxic effect on the dopaminergic tracts of the substantia nigra and may contribute to the development of PD in those rendered susceptible by virtue of a cytochrome P-450 polymorphism, excessive exposure, or other factors. Taylor et al [146] found no association between exposure to pesticides or herbicides and PD.

Parkinson's disease and farm work and rural living

Employment in agriculture and living in a rural environment have both been examined in regard to environmental toxins and neurodegeneration. Similar to the risks for lung diseases that appear to be associated with agriculture [147], it has been speculated that working on a farm may be related to neurodegeneration because of the potential for increased exposure to pesticides, herbicides, and fungicides, which are used in the large scale growth and harvesting of vegetation. Research from the Honolulu Heart Program/Honolulu-Asia Aging Study [148] found that working on a farm increased the relative risk of PD from 1.0 to 1.9 (in individuals who worked 20 years on plantations in Honolulu). Conversely, Kuopio et al [140] did not find an association between farm and rural work as an occupation and PD. Rural residence has also been examined as a potential risk factor for toxin exposure because people live closer to areas where pesticides, herbicides, and fungicides may be spread, and the higher likelihood of using well water for drinking. A study by Gorell et al [135] concluded that farming is a risk factor for PD (OR 2.79, 95% CI); however rural or farm residence was not found to increase the risk of the disease. Other research has found no difference in the history of rural residence, farm residence, previous farming activity, or employment in agricultural work between PD patients and control subjects in Germany [149]; yet, it has been shown that the risk for PD appears to be elevated for those living in a rural area (OR 3.62 [149]). The results of research on well water are in direct opposition. DePalma et al [149] found that well water increases the risk of PD to 2.09 (OR). However, this finding of increased risk of PD was associated with well water in African Americans only, whereas other investigators [135,149] have not found such an association between well water and increased PD risk. As a result, the data in this area remain unclear and contradictory. Additional investigation is needed in this area to elucidate the connections between these factors.

Parkinson's disease and methyl-4-phenyl-1,2,3,6-tetrahydropyridine

In 1983, Langston et al [150] reported on a series of narcotic addicts in northern California who developed parkinsonism after exposure to 1-methyl-4-phenyl-1,2,3,6-tetrahydropyridine (MPTP). MPTP was formed as a byproduct during the synthesis of a meperidine derivative. With the exception of its relatively rapid onset, the syndrome experienced by these individuals has been indistinguishable from idiopathic PD. In subsequent studies, MPTP was found to exert its toxic effect in the central nervous system after being oxidized by monoamine oxidase-B to 1-methyl-4-phenyl-pyridinium (MPP+) [151]. MPP+ is concentrated in mitochondria and blocks oxidative phosphorylation and ATP production [152], leading to cell death. Hence, these chance occurrences have significantly informed our knowledge of the mechanisms related to the development of PD.

Parkinson's disease and metals

Heavy metals have been implicated in the development of PD because high concentrations of iron, zinc, and aluminum have been found in the substantia nigra tissue of PD patients compared with controls [153]. Gorell et al [154] found an increased risk of PD with exposure to combinations of metals (eg, lead-copper, lead-iron, and iron-copper) compared with any metal alone. This study determined that short-term exposure to metals (20 years or less) was not statistically related to the development of PD.

Parkinson's disease and manganese

Manganese is well-known for its neurotoxic effects in humans, such as extrapyramidal symptoms and neuropsychiatric difficulties [155]. Symptoms of manganese exposure syndrome reportedly include extrapyramidal and neuropsychiatric symptoms. As summarized by Zatta et al [155], the clinical features of manganese neurotoxicity involve (1) an early phase consisting of fatigue, headache, muscle cramps, loss of appetite, apathy, insomnia, diminished libido, and psychotic reactions (aggression and emotional lability); (2) extrapyramidal signs, including monotone speech, expressionless face, impaired writing dexterity, and antero- and retropulsion; and (3) an established phase in which individuals present with dystonia and a "cock-walk" gait.

Manganese is present in the pesticide Maneb and in the engine anti-knock compound MMT (methylcyclopentadienyl manganese tricarbonyl), which is used in gasoline. Gorell et al [154] found that 20 years' of exposure to manganese increases PD risk by 10.61 (OR). This finding was replicated more recently by Gorell et al [156], who reported that persons with more than 20 years' of exposure had a significantly increased risk of developing PD (OR 10.63, 95% CI, 1.07–105.99).

Parkinson's disease and copper sulfate

Twenty years' exposure to copper increases the risk of PD by 2.49 (95% CI, 1.06–5.89) as reported by Gorell et al in two separate studies [154,156]. This finding was confirmed by DePalma et al [150] in which copper exposure increased the odds of PD by 2.69.

Parkinson's disease and mercury, iron, and zinc

Gorell et al [154] found no association between PD and exposure to mercury or iron. There is also little available evidence implying a direct link between an abundance of zinc and PD [155]. In fact, Jiménez-Jiménez et al [157] found low zinc levels in the cerebrospinal fluid of PD patients but not in controls.

Parkinson's disease and aluminum

One of the proposed mechanisms in PD by which metals may produce an effect is through oxidative stress, a mechanism that, as discussed above, is also implicated in AD. Investigators have studied the effects of the presence of aluminum and zinc on the oxidative stress induced by the neurotoxin 6-hydroxydopamine (6-OHDA) in the mitochondria from the brains of rats [158]. It has been found that the consumption of O_2 during 6-OHDA auto-oxidation was significantly decreased in the presence of aluminum and zinc. Uversky et al [153] propose that oxidative stress may result from increased levels of redox-active metal ions within the substantia nigra as metal accumulation occurs. The authors conducted a systematic analysis of the effect of various metal ions on the structural and aggregation properties of human recombinant α-synuclein in vitro. α-Synuclein is a presynaptic protein that has been shown to be a component of the Lewy body and may trigger Lewy body formation in PD and DLB [159]. They concluded that aluminum was the most effective of the metals examined in accelerating the rate of α-synuclein fibril formation. Taken together, these results suggest that aluminum, through its promotion of α-synuclein and fibril formation may play a substantial role in the development of PD and DLB.

One pathway by which PD patients may encounter aluminum may be through aluminum-containing antacids. Altschuler [160] re-examined the work of Strang [161], who studied 200 PD patients and 200 controls and found that there was a significantly higher incidence of ulcers in the PD patients compared with the controls. Altschuler [160] states that the use of aluminum-containing antacids may intensify the absorption of aluminum, but few other data are available to support this hypothesis.

Parkinson's disease and carbon monoxide poisoning

Shuichi et al [162], using an animal model, found that increases in extracellular dopamine accompanied with the enhancement of its oxidative metabolism in rat striatum exposed to CO had a deleterious effect on the striatal dopamine system. This finding would suggest that CO could be related to the development or progression of PD, although Kuopio et al [140] did not find an association between CO poisoning and PD.

Parkinson's disease and solvents

DePalma et al [149] found that exposure to solvents alone was not associated with PD. Research by Pezzoli et al [163] concluded that exposure to hydrocarbon solvents is a risk factor for the earlier onset of symptoms of PD and more severe disease throughout its course. However, Jacques et al [164] dispute the findings of Pezzoli et al's study, stating that the study design and conclusions were misconstrued.

Parkinson's disease and magnetic fields

Savitz et al [108] looked at the occurrence of neurodegenerative disease in male electrical workers in the United States. The researchers examined the death certificates of men over the age of 20, who were employed primarily in an electrical occupation and who died between 1985 and 1991. No evidence was found that suggests any demographic variable considered (eg, age, race, year of death, social class) had any affect on the development of PD. However, looking at specific occupations yielded an interesting finding. Men who were employed as power plant operators were at a higher risk of developing PD (adjusted OR 2.1, 95% CI, 0.9–4.7). In another study by Savitz et al [109] that looked at disease mortality by duration of employment in electrical occupations, the findings for PD risk were inconsistent, with no clear association between the length of employment and PD being demonstrated. The only significant finding was shown in eight men who were exposed for a period of 10–20 years or longer to 0.490–0.888 microtesla years of electromagnetic field (EMF), whose underlying cause of death was PD. The adjusted rate ratio for this group was found to be 2.4 (95% CI, 1.0–5.8). However, no strong findings were shown for men who had undergone similar EMF exposure whose cause of death from PD was mentioned on their death certificate or for men whose EMF exposure was at a higher level or for a greater length of time. Thus, there is little evidence that EMF has a substantial affect on PD risk.

Parkinson's disease and smoking

Research on cigarette smoking and PD is one area that has been widely researched and yields consistent findings across studies. Overall, cigarette smoking appears to be a protective factor against developing PD. Gorell et al [156] showed that smoking more than 30 packs per year was associated with a decreased chance of developing PD (OR 0.42, 95% CI, 0.25–0.71). In monozygotic and dizygotic twin pairs in which at least one twin had PD, the risk of developing PD was inversely related to the amount of cigarette smoking [165]. In an animal model of PD initiated by MPTP intoxication, exposure to cigarette smoke led to a decrease in the loss of dopaminergic neurons in substantia nigra. Taken together, such results suggest that frequent nicotine exposure may have a neuroprotective effect on the dopaminergic nigrostriatal system [166]. Although the mechanism by which nicotine produces its effect is not known, several have been hypothesized. One mechanism that has been proposed is through the ability of nicotine to block the effects of two endogenous or exogenous dopaminergic proneurotoxicants, 1,2,3,4-tetrahydroisoquinoline and 1,2,3,4-tetrahydro-β-carboline [1,167]. Alternatively, nicotine may also act by stimulating a neurotrophic factor, fibroblast growth factor-2, which is believed to protect the dopamine-containing cells in the substantia nigra [1,168]. DiMonte et al [123] reviews the mechanisms behind the association between smoking and neuroprotection with regard to PD. Two possible mechanisms they propose are that nicotine may be neuroprotective in itself or nicotine may inhibit monoamine oxidase activity and dopamine turnover, thereby preventing nigrostriatal damage.

Frontotemporal dementia and Pick's disease

Frontotemporal dementia (FTD) involves the progressive dysfunction of the anterior temporal and frontal lobes. The usual presenting features in FTD relate to cognitive function, but personality and behavioral symptoms are prominent. Behavioral features include the loss of personal and social awareness, disinhibition, dampening of affect, and loss of insight. The neuropsychologic profile of FTD is characterized by impairment in executive and attentional abilities disproportionate to the degree of memory impairment. This clinical pattern is opposite to that found in AD, in which memory functions are more impaired than executive abilities [169].

Three patterns of behavior and cognitive dysfunction were outlined in sets of formal criteria for the diagnosis of FTD. The first pattern, labeled FTD, is characterized by the classic behavioral symptoms associated with FTD and Pick's disease. The other two syndromes, called semantic dementia and progressive nonfluent aphasia, are characterized primarily by disorders of language and semantic knowledge [169].

Progressive nonfluent aphasia is a second clinical syndrome identified in FTD. Progressive nonfluent aphasia involves primarily unilateral left frontal, left frontoparietal, or left frontotemporal degeneration and is characterized by dysfunction in expressive language [169]. Semantic dementia is a third clinical syndrome identified in FTD. In semantic dementia there is a progressive loss of semantic knowledge. Because content becomes progressively devoid, this syndrome is characterized by frequent vague references to people, objects, and places. Semantic dementia is characterized as a fluent aphasia. The loss of word meaning is apparent in anomia and impaired comprehension [169]. Given the rarity of these disorders, no epidemiologic data are yet available from the standpoint of environmental exposure and FTD, with the exception of zinc.

Pick's disease and zinc

Wallwork [170] proposes that zinc concentration and metabolism may lead to neurodegeneration. Evidence from Constantinidis and Tissot [171] found that hippocampi from patients with Pick's disease contained 25% more zinc than normal controls. The researchers suggest that the excess hippocampal zinc may interfere in glutamate metabolism, causing some of the symptoms of the disease. However, Ehmann et al [172] found that hippocampal zinc concentrations in patients with Pick's disease were similar to controls. The authors suggest that this conflict may be caused by the difficulty of diagnosing this disease.

Amyotrophic lateral sclerosis

ALS is a well-known motor neuron disease caused by the gradual degeneration of nerve cells in the brain and spinal cord [173]. Investigations of environmental risks for ALS have been ongoing and have recently received greater public attention because of speculation about exposure during the Desert Storm campaign.

Amyotrophic lateral sclerosis and metals

Using a case-control study design, Gresham et al [174] examined the association between occupational heavy metal exposure and the risk of developing ALS in 66 ALS patients and 66 age- and gender-matched controls. The participants responded to questionnaires that probed for occupational heavy metal exposure (ie, aluminum, lead, lead alkyl, magnesium, mercury, mercury alkyl, nickel, and selenium), medical events (eg, polio, thyroid, and other conditions), and travel history (including travel to the southern and western Pacific). Women were excluded from the analyses because of the low numbers of women who had been potentially exposed to heavy metals during their occupational service. The analyses determined that, in men only, there was no association between heavy metal exposure and ALS. Furthermore, no increased risk was found with increased exposure to lead or mercury. The authors deduced that given the disparity between men and women in terms of occupational exposure to metals, it is not likely that occupational exposure to metals would be a primary causative factor in the development of ALS.

Amyotrophic lateral sclerosis and magnetic fields

Work by Savitz et al [108] has provided some evidence for the hypothesis that EMF exposure increases the risk of ALS. The investigators studied a population of men whose occupations exposed them to EMF. It was determined that working in electrical occupations increased the risk of ALS. Specifically, telephone installers and repairers (adjusted OR 2.2), electrical equipment repairers (adjusted OR 3.9), supervisors, power installers, and repairers (adjusted OR 2.9), and power plant operators (adjusted OR 4.8) were all found to be at a greater risk of developing ALS. A related study by Savitz et al [109] compared mortality rates of men exposed to EMF through their occupations with the risk of ALS. Again, several significant findings were shown. In cases in which ALS was listed as the cause of death, the risk of ALS increased with the number of years of exposure to EMF (0 to $\leq$5 years RR 1.0, 5–20 years RR 1.8, and $\geq$20 years RR 2.4). Furthermore, in the group with the greatest number of years of working in electrical occupations ($\geq$20 years), those with the highest levels of exposure were shown to have the highest risk of developing ALS (0.000–0.386 microtesla years, RR 1.0; 0.386–1.060 microtesla years, RR 1.9; 1.060–2.033 microtesla years, RR 2.3; and 2.033–14.547 microtesla-years, RR 2.4). Similar patterns of risk were shown for men in whom the underlying cause of death was ALS. In terms of the number of years of exposure, those with longer employment in exposed occupations were more likely to develop ALS (0 to ≤5 years RR 1.0, 5–20 years RR 2.0, and ≥20 years RR 3.1). In this group as well, among the men who underwent the longest length of exposure, those with the highest levels of exposure were at greater risk of ALS (0.000–0.386 microtesla years, RR 1.0; 0.386–1.060 microtesla years, RR 2.3; and 1.060–2.033 microtesla years, RR 3.0). The data from these two studies suggest that men who are exposed to EMF at higher levels and for longer periods of time are at the greatest risk of developing ALS. If this is the case, additional research into the mechanisms by which these neurodegenerative changes are affected by EMF is needed.

Amyotrophic lateral sclerosis and the Persian Gulf War

After the Persian Gulf War ended in 1991, veterans began reporting a number of inexplicable symptoms including memory loss, headaches, joint pains, chronic fatigue, nervous system disorders, limb weakness, paresthesias, and sexual dysfunction [173,175,176]. Reports of troops coming into contact with potentially neurotoxic chemicals during their deployment (eg, insect repellants, flea collars, medications containing pyridostigmine bromide, and other substances) [177,178] have spurred several investigations. Investigations by the military and by research scientists have looked into these phenomena to determine whether these symptoms are indicative of a diagnosable syndrome or have a determinant cause. Gray et al [179] studied the health of the US Naval Mobile Construction Battalion (NMCB) after the Persian Gulf War using questionnaire methods. Compared with those who did not go to the Persian Gulf, NMCB personnel who spent time in the Gulf reported a higher prevalence of four physician-diagnosed multisymptom conditions: chronic fatigue syndrome, posttraumatic stress disorder, multiple chemical sensitivity, and irritable bowel syndrome.

A nationwide epidemiologic study conducted by Horner et al [176] identified all of the new occurrences of ALS among Gulf War veterans in the mobilized Reserves and National Guard since their initial deployment in 1990. Deployed military personnel were defined as those who served in the Gulf region during Operation Desert Shield and Desert Storm or in the period after Desert Storm. The study included 2,482,333 veterans, of whom 696,118 were deployed to the Gulf region. It was shown that the risk ratio for the development of ALS for deployed military was almost twice that of the nondeployed (1.92), with an age-adjusted relative risk of 2.41. In another study [180] of 690,000 Gulf War veterans who were followed for 8 years, findings show that by 1998, the observed incidence of ALS was 3.19 times higher than what was expected given the age distribution of the Gulf War veteran population and the age-specific death rates of the US population.

There have been several critiques of the aforementioned studies. Rose [181] explains that the degree of excess risk is not significant given the small number of ALS cases in the young, healthy military personnel being studied. In a correspondence note, Armon [182] critiqued the research of Horner et al [176], stating that the "lower-than-usual number of cases identified in the non-deployed veterans would make even a 'usual' number of cases in the deployed veterans appear excessive." The critique goes on to explain that the study design did not take the confounding effect of smoking frequency into consideration in their analyses.

Furthermore, other researchers suggest their own data do not corroborate the findings of elevated risk resulting from Gulf War deployment. Smith et al [173] studied deployed (n = 551,841) and nondeployed (n = 1,478,704) Gulf War veterans. The authors found a risk ratio of 1.66 (CI, 0.62–4.44) for deployed veterans developing ALS. They imply that their statistical power to detect risk factor associations with ALS hospitalizations was low, as demonstrated by the broad CI around the risk ratio. Overall, the authors reported that the ALS outcomes were "sparse," despite having a large subject pool.

Another case-control study of general neuromuscular symptoms of European Gulf War veterans did not demonstrate significant findings. Sharief et al [178] looked at reports of symptoms of neuromuscular dysfunction in Gulf War veterans with more than four symptoms (Gulf-ill, n = 49) consisting of 26 healthy (Gulf-well) veterans, 13 symptomatic Bosnian veterans (Bosnian-ill), and 22 symptomatic troops who had not been deployed to the Gulf (Era-ill) in a random sample selected from a larger cohort. Numerous procedures were administered to the study population including a clinical assessment, nerve conduction studies, quantitative sensory and autonomic function tests, and needle and single-fiber electromyogram. Although some troops reported symptoms that might be related to conditions such as carpal tunnel syndrome or ulnar neuropathy, common neurologic syndromes not specifically related to active service in the Gulf region, overall results showed no objective evidence of peripheral neurologic disorders in Gulf War veterans who described neuromuscular symptoms. Taken as a whole, the current literature in this area appears to give conflicting accounts as to whether deployment in the Gulf region is associated with neuromuscular dysfunction, including ALS. However, the preponderance of the research thus far does not support Gulf War deployment as a contributing factor in the development of ALS.

Parkinsonism-dementia complex and amyotrophic lateral sclerosis on the island of Guam

Over the past 60 years or more, a puzzling neurologic phenomena has been observed in the Western Pacific Ocean region. Specifically, the Chamorro people of Guam and other Marianas Islands have experienced a highly elevated rate of neurodegenerative diseases, with a complex that neuro-pathologically demonstrates a combination of ALS, parkinsonism, and dementia complex (termed ALS/PDC) being the most prevalent of the diseases recorded [183]. Significant investigation has been conducted in an attempt to understand the reasons for the large number of neurologic disease occurrences in this region.

Neuropathology of the amyotrophic lateral sclerosis/parkinsonism, dementia complex

Descriptions of the ALS/PDC of Guam have evolved. An early investigation by Kurland et al [184] describes two distinct diseases, ALS and PDC, occurring in epidemic proportions in the Guamanian population. On microscopic examination, the brains of persons diagnosed with PDC showed intraganglionic fibrillary changes and scattered intracytoplasmic granulovas-cular bodies but no plaques, Pick, or Lewy bodies. The authors also describe diffuse loss of ganglion cells and reactive gliosis, particularly in the substantia nigra and globus pallidus. The presence of the neurofibrillary tangles distin-guishes PDC from idiopathic PD, Creutzfeldt-Jakob disease, Shy-Drager syndrome, and supranuclear palsy [186]. However, in a number of their autop-sied PDC cases, there were clinical features of ALS in addition to the PDC. Specifically, in terms of pathology findings for these subjects, the authors stated, "in addition to Parkinsonism-dementia complex, there was also degen-eration of motor neurons and demyelination of the pyramidal tracts throughout the brain and spinal cord." Kurland et al [184] conducted histo-logic examinations of Chamorro cases of ALS and reported classical changes expected in ALS as well as Alzheimer's fibrillary changes and Simchowicz's granulovascular bodies but in a distribution less than that observed in PDC. Overall, there were a number of Chamorro cases, which, on pathological ex-amination, did not clearly fit into a diagnostic category for ALS or PDC but were a combination of ALS, PDC, and AD. The diagnosis for these persons has been termed ALS/PDC to incorporate the totality of their brain pathology.

Recent research by Morris et al [186] has brought the exploration of the Guamanian neurodegenerative phenomena full circle by suggesting, as in earlier research, that the Guamanian ALS and PDC may be separate diseases, in which the ALS of Guam is classical ALS rather than a form unique to the Chamorro people. In their study, the authors reviewed 45 cases of motor neuron disease seen on Guam between 1983 and 1998 and categorized them according to their clinical and pathological similarity to classical motor neuron disease in other areas of the world. Clinically, they found that the majority of the Guamanian patients studied met the criteria for ALS, with progressive bulbar and limb upper and lower motor neuron involvement without sensory signs or evidence of compressive pathology. Their data also supported findings that tau neurofibrillary degeneration in the ALS patients on Guam occurred at a higher level than in asymptomatic whites of similar age; yet, in the Chamorro cases, the neurofibrillary degeneration was not associated with significant nerve cell loss, clinical dementia, or extrapyramidal syndromes, a finding that contrasts with the features of typical PDC. The authors conclude that tau disorders may produce both diseases with the neurofibrillary tangle symptomology, varying from classical ALS in this population, resulting from some unknown factor specific to Guam or the Chamorro people. Pérez-Tur et al [187] undertook a genetic study of the *TAU* gene in five Chamorro participants (two with PDC, one with ALS, and two normal controls). The results showed no abnormalities in the sequence of the *TAU* gene in any of the study groups. The findings suggest that *TAU* gene abnormalities may not be the primary cause of PDC or ALS in the Chamorro people, but rather that some environmental factor is a more likely cause of the high incidence of neurodegenerative diseases in Guam. Taken together, the evidence in this area is not conclusive about whether ALS and PDC of Guam are separate or combined diseases or what role the *TAU* gene plays in the development of these neurologic disorders.

Amyotrophic lateral sclerosis/parkinsonism, dementia complex of Guam, and metals

There has been significant speculation about the cause of the high rate of ALS/PDC on Guam. Gellein et al [188] analyzed brain tissues of Guamanian patients with ALS (n = 8), PDC (n = 4), and normal controls (n = 5) to determine whether concentrations of various metals are related to the disease incidence. The authors speculated that some metals in the Guamanian environment may be deficient (eg, magnesium and calcium), whereas other metals may be highly "bioavailable" (eg, aluminum). The significant findings of the Gellein et al [188] study were that in the Guamanian study population, ALS patients had significantly higher concentrations of cadmium in their gray and white matter than patients with PDC and controls. The other significant finding was that PDC patients were shown to have more zinc in their gray matter than ALS patients or controls. Interestingly, no differences were found in this study between the three groups for levels of cobalt, copper, iron, manganese, rubidium, or vanadium. The authors suggest that the limited number of subjects, formalin tissue preparation methods, diagnostic difficulties, and low power of the statistical tests used may have contributed to the lack of findings for other significant metal concentration differences between the groups. Thus, metals may play a role in the development of PDC; however, more evidence for this hypothesis needs to be gathered.

Amyotrophic lateral sclerosis/parkinsonism, dementia complex of Guam, and cyad

Another potential environmental culprit for the high occurrence of ALS/PDC on the island of Guam is cyad, the seed of the false sago palm, which is unique to the Western Pacific. The cyad seed has been used by the Chamorro people as a food source as well as a topical medicine for skin lesions [185]. The cyad seed contains several toxins, two of which have been closely studied cycasin, a potent cytotoxin and carcinogen, and β-methylamino-L-alanine (BMAA) [185]. Large doses of isomers of BMAA have been shown to be related to muscle weakness in rhesus monkeys [189]. However, other animal studies have not shown such results. Perry et al [183] administered large doses of BMAA (15.5 g/kg of the L-isomer) to mice over a period of 11 weeks. They found that during the course of the experimental protocol all mice that were given BMAA maintained their weight and did not exhibit any behavioral abnormalities. On microscopic examination of the brain and spinal cord, no pathological changes were seen in any of the mice. Specifically, there was no evidence of neuropathologic changes suggesting ALS or PD. Research by Wilson et al [190] suggests that BMAA may not be the cyad toxin responsible for the ALS/PDC seen on Guam. These investigators fed mice pellets made of washed cyad flour. High-performance liquid chromatography-mass spectrometry failed to show significant amounts of BMAA, cycasin, methylazoxymethanol, or β-N-oxalylamino-L-alanine (the compound responsible for lathyrism [191]), all potentially neurotoxic compounds. However, they did identify another compound in the cyad flour that they propose may be the responsible agent for the cyad-induced neurodegeneration, β-sitosterol-β-D-glucoside. Khabazian et al [192] found that mice fed with cyad seed flour containing isolated sterol glucosides showed behavioral and neuropathologic outcomes. Thus, some investigators disagree that BMAA in cyad is the cause of the neurodegenerative diseases on Guam. Evidence seems to be gathering that implicates sterol glucosides as the responsible toxin found in cyad seeds.

Overall, evidence continues to suggest that the consumption of the cyad in some form is responsible for ALS/PDC. Patients with PDC have been shown to have a preference for local food and lead a more traditional lifestyle, which includes the consumption of cyad flour and fruit-eating bats [185,193]. It is believed that the Chamorro people may be particularly exposed to toxic amounts of the cyad toxins through the consumption of fruit bats (called flying foxes), which are part of the traditional celebratory diet. Flying foxes eat the cyad seed, the toxins of which accumulate in high doses in the fat molecules of the fruit bats [194,195].

Additional evidence for the relationship of ALS/PDC to bat consumption comes from studies that have charted the changes in the flying fox population and the rates of ALS/PDC on Guam. Cox and Sachs [195] compared the recorded rates of ALS to the flying fox population size. They found that when the native flying fox population on Guam declined and the importation of flying foxes from Western Samoa (where there are no indigenous cyad seeds) occurred during the 1970s, the rates of ALS on Guam also began to decline. Furthermore, the rapid modernization and westernization of Guam in the late 1960s had a profound effect on the eating habits of the local population [196]. Present day Chamorro now eat a diet that is much more western in style and are not exposed to cyad through flour or fruit-bats to the same extent as they had been in earlier times. Thus, in the Guamanian population, the rates of exposure to cyad toxins through diet appear to coincide with "socioeconomic, ethnographic, and ecologic changes brought about by the rapid westernization of Guam" [195], lending more support to the cyad seed as a factor contributing to the high incidence of ALS/PDC on the island of Guam. Additional dietary and exposure data may shed further light on this potential environmental risk.

Summary

The hypothesis that neurotoxins may play a role in neurodegenerative disorders remains an elusive one, given that epidemiologic studies often provide conflicting results. Although these conflicting results may result from methodological differences within and between studies, the complexity of chemical disruption of the central nervous system cannot be ignored in attempts to evaluate this hypothesis in different neurodegenerative disorders. Spencer [197] provides a detailed review of the complex processes involved in defining the neurotoxic potential of naturally occurring and synthetic agents. Even concepts such as exposure and dose, as often reported in studies attempting to evaluate the risk imparted by a potential compound, can be deceptive. For example, although dose reflects "that amount of chemical transferred to the exposed subject" [197], factors such as time and concentration in the organism, the ability to access the central nervous system, and how a compound reaches the central nervous system (routes of administration) or secondarily affects other organ systems leading to central nervous system disruption are clearly important to the concept of neurotoxic risk in neurodegenerative disorders.

These factors would appear to explain the observed disagreements between studies using animal or neuronal models of neurotoxicity and population-based studies in humans. The importance of these factors and how a potential neurotoxin is investigated are clearly seen in the data on AD and aluminum. In contrast, the impact of MTPT on the central nervous system is more direct and compelling. Added complexity in the study of neurotoxins in human neurodegeneration is derived from data showing that agents may have additive, potentiating, synergistic, or antagonistic effects [196]. Therefore, data from studies evaluating EMF risks could be readily confounded by the presence or absence of heavy metals (eg, arc welding).

Other factors that may conceal neurotoxic causes for a given disorder focus on additional features such as genetic predispositions, physiologic changes that occur with aging, and even nutritional status that can support or hinder the affect of a given agent on the central nervous system. Finally, many studies that investigate exposure risk do not readily incorporate the five criteria proposed by Schaumburg [198] for establishing causation. For example, if we apply Schaumburg's first criterion, epidemiologic studies often determine the presence of an agent through history, yet they cannot readily confirm exposure based on environmental or clinical chemical analyses to fulfill this criterion for causation [198,199]. Additional limitations in research design along with the populations and methods that are used to study neurotoxins in human neurodegenerative disorders often fail to meet other criteria such as linking the severity and onset with duration and exposure level. Therefore, although studies of agents such as MTPT provide compelling models of neurotoxins and neurodegeneration in humans, disorders such as ALS, PD, and particularly AD will require additional effort if research is to determine the contribution (presence or absence) of neurotoxins to these neurologic disorders.

Acknowledgments

The authors thank Kara Bottiggi for editorial assistance during the development of this manuscript.

References

[1] Mayeaux R. Epidemiology of neurodegeneration. Annu Rev Neurosci 2003;26:81–104.

[2] D'Epiro P. Keeping current in Alzheimer's disease. Patient Care 1999;13:127–39.

[3] Richards SS, Hendrie HC. Diagnosis, management and treatment of Alzheimer's disease: a guide for the internist. Arch Intern Med 1999;159:789–801.

[4] Morris JC. Differential diagnosis of Alzheimer's disease. Clin Geriatr Med 1994;10:257–76.

[5] Jorm AF, Jolley D. The incidence of dementia: a meta-analysis. Neurology 1998;51:728–33.

[6] Gao S, Hendrie HC, Hall KS, et al. The relationship between age, sex, and the incidence of dementia and Alzheimer's disease: a meta-analysis. Arch Gen Psychiatry 1998;55:809–15.

[7] Kukull WA, Ganguli M. Epidemiology of dementia: concepts and overview. Neurol Clin 2000;18(4):923–50.

[8] Garabrant DH. Epidemiologic principles in the evaluation of suspected neurotoxic disorders. Neurol Clin 2000;18(3):631–48.

[9] Knopman DS, DeKosky ST, Cummings JL, et al. Practice parameter: diagnosis of dementia (an evidence-based review): report of the Quality Standards Subcommittee of the American Academy of Neurology. Neurology 2001;56:1143–53.

[10] Petersen RC, Stevens JC, Ganguli M, et al. Practice parameter: early detection of dementia (an evidence-based review): report of the Quality Standards Subcommittee of the American Academy of Neurology. Neurology 2001;56:1133–42.

[11] Callahan CM, Hendrie HC, Tierney WM. Documentation and evaluation of cognitive impairment in elderly primary care patients. Ann Intern Med 1995;122:422–9.

[12] Boise L, Neal MB, Kaye J. Dementia assessment in primary care: results from a study in three managed care systems. J Gerontol A Biol Sci Med Sci 2004;59:621–6.

[13] Kukull WA. The association between smoking and Alzheimer's disease: effects of study design bias. Biol Psychiatry 2001;49:194–9.

[14] Schmitt FA, Ranseen JD. Neuropsychological toxicology and aging. In: Cooper RL, Goldman JM, Harbin TJ, editors. Aging and environmental toxicology: biological and behavioral perspectives. Baltimore (MD): Johns Hopkins Press; 1991. p. 246–71.

[15] Morris JC. Evaluation of the demented patient. In: Morris JC, editor. Handbook of dementing illnesses. New York: Marcel Dekker; 1994. p. 71–88.

[16] Grossberg GT, Desai AK. Management of Alzheimer's disease. J Gerontol A Biol Sci Med Sci 2003;58(4):331–53.

[17] Cummings JL, editor. The neuropsychiatry of Alzheimer's disease and related disorders. Independence (KY): Martin Dunitz; 2003.

[18] Zhou XH, Higgs RE. Assessing the relative accuracies of two screening tests in the presence of verification bias. Stat Med 2000;19(11–12):1697–705.

[19] Markesbery WR. The role of oxidative stress in Alzheimer disease. Arch Neurol 1999;56: 1449–552.

[20] Markesbery WR, Ehmann WD. Brain trace elements in Alzheimer disease. In: Terry RD, Katzman R, Bick L, editors. Alzheimer disease. New York: Raven Press Ltd.; 1994. p. 353–67.

[21] Markesbery WR, Ehmann WD. Oxidative stress in Alzheimer disease. In: Terry RD, Katzman R, Bick KL, et al, editors. Alzheimer disease. 2nd edition. Philadelphia: Lippincott, Williams, & Wilkins; 1999. p. 401–14.

[22] Selkoe DJ. Toward a comprehensive theory for Alzheimer's disease; hypothesis: Alzheimer's disease is caused by the cerebral accumulation and cytotoxicity of amyloid beta-protein. Ann N Y Acad Sci 2000;924:17–25.

[23] Arlien-Soborg P, Hansen L, Ladefoged O, et al. Report on a conference on organic solvents and the nervous system. Neurotoxicol Teratol 1992;14(1):81–2.

[24] Graves AB, Rosner D, Echeverria D, et al. Occupational exposure to solvents and aluminum and estimated risk of Alzheimer's disease. Occup Environ Med 1998;55: 627–33.

[25] Palmer K, Inskip H, Martyn C, et al. Dementia and occupational exposure to organic solvents. Occup Environ Med 1998;55:712–5.

[26] Shalat SL, Seltzer B, Baker EL. Occupational risk factors and Alzheimer's disease: a case-control study. J Occup Med 1988;30(12):934–6.

[27] American Psychiatric Association. Diagnostic and statistical manual of mental disorders. 3rd edition. Washington (DC): American Psychiatric Association; 1980.

[28] McKhann G, Drachman D, Folstein M, et al. Clinical diagnosis of Alzheimer's disease: report of the NINCDS ADRDA work group under the auspices of Department of Health and Human Services Task Force on Alzheimer's disease. Neurology 1984;34(7):939–44.

[29] Freed DM, Kandel E. Long-term occupational exposure and diagnosis of dementia. Neurotoxicology 1988;9(3):391–400.

[30] Kukull WA, Larson EB, Bowen JD, et al. Solvent exposure as a risk factor for Alzheimer's disease: a case-control study. Am J Epidemiol 1995;141(11):1059–79.

[31] Klatzo I, Wisniewski H, Streicher E. Experimental production of neurofibrillary degeneration: light microscopic observations. J Neuropathol Exp Neurol 1965;24:187–99.

[32] Crapper DR, Krishnan SS, Dalton AJ. Brain aluminum distribution in Alzheimer's disease and experimental neurofibrillary degeneration. Trans Am Neurol Assoc 1973;98:17–20.

[33] Beal MF, Mazurek MF, Ellison DW, et al. Neurochemical characteristics of aluminum-induced neurofibrillary degeneration in rabbits. Neuroscience 1989;29(2):339–46.

[34] Crapper DR, Krishnan SS, Quittkat S. Aluminum, neurofibrillary degeneration and Alzheimer's disease. Brain 1976;99(1):67–80.

[35] Itzhaki RF. Possible factors in the etiology of Alzheimer's disease. Mol Neurobiol 1994;9: 1–13.

[36] Yokel RA. The toxicology of aluminum in the brain: a review. Neurotoxicology 2000;21(5): 813–28.

[37] Braak H, Braak E. Neuropathological staging of Alzheimer-related changes. Acta Neuropathol (Berl) 1991;82:239–59.

[38] Campbell A. The potential role of aluminum in Alzheimer's disease. Nephrol Dial Transplant 2002;17(Suppl 2):S17–20.

[39] Zatta P. Controversial aspects of aluminum (III) accumulation and subcompartmentation in Alzheimer's disease. J Trace Elem Med Biol 1993;10:120–8.

[40] Munoz DG. Is exposure to aluminum, a risk factor for the development of Alzheimer's disease?–no. Arch Neurol 1998;55(5):737–9.

[41] Candy JM, Oakley AE, Klinowski J, et al. Aluminosilicates and senile plaque formation in Alzheimer's disease. Lancet 1986;1(8477):354–7.

[42] Ward N, Mason J. Neutron activation analysis techniques for identifying elemental status in Alzheimer's disease. Journal of Radioanalytical and Nuclear Chemistry 1987;113:515–26.

[43] Altmann P, Shanesha U, Hamon C, et al. Disturbance of cerebral function by aluminum in haemodialysis patients without overt aluminum toxicity. Lancet 1989;2(8653):7–12.

[44] Candy JM, McArthur FK, Oakley AE, et al. Aluminum accumulation in relation to senile plaque and neurofibrillary tangle formation in the brains of patients with renal failure. J Neurol Sci 1992;107(2):210–8.

[45] Harrington CR, Wishlik CM, McArthur FK, et al. Alzheimer's-disease-like changes in tau protein processing: association with aluminum accumulation in brains of renal dialysis patients. Lancet 1994;343(8904):993–7.

[46] Soni MG, White SM, Flamm WG, et al. Safety evaluation of dietary aluminum. Regul Toxicol Pharmacol 2001;33:66–79.

[47] World Health Organization/International Programme on Chemical Safety. Aluminum, environmental health criteria, 194. Geneva: WHO; 1997 p. 1–152.

[48] Schupf N. Aluminum in drinking water and Alzheimer's disease: methodological problem. In: Gitelman HJ, editor. Proceedings of the Second International Conference on Aluminum and Health. Tampa (FL): Aluminum Association (WA); 1992. p. 53–59.

[49] Agency for Toxic Substances and Disease Registry. Toxicological profile for aluminum and compounds. ATSDR TP-91/01, 1992;77:83.

[50] Polizzi S, Pria E, Ferrara M, et al. Neurotoxic effects of aluminum among foundry workers and Alzheimer's disease. Neurotoxicology 2002;23:761–74.

[51] Neri LC, Hewitt D. Aluminum, Alzheimer's disease, and drinking water. Lancet 1991;338(8763):1592–3.

[52] Rondeau V, Commenges D, Jacqmin-Gadda H, et al. Relation between aluminum concentrations in drinking water and Alzheimer's disease: an 8-year follow-up study. Am J Epidemiol 2000;152(1):288–90.

[53] Forbes WF, Gentleman JF, Maxwell CJ. Concerning the role of aluminum in causing dementia. Exp Gerontol 1995;30(1):23–32.

[54] McLachlan DR, Bergeron C, Smith JE, et al. Risk for neuropathologically confirmed Alzheimer's disease and residual aluminum in municipal drinking water employing weighted residential histories. Neurology 1996;46(2):401–5.

[55] Gauthier E, Fortier I, Courchesne F, et al. Aluminum forms in drinking water and risk of Alzheimer's disease. Environ Res 2000;84(3):234–46.

[56] Martyn CN, Barker DJ, Osmond C, et al. Geographical relation between Alzheimer's disease and aluminum in drinking water. Lancet 1989;14(1):59–62.

[57] Wettstein A, Aeppli J, Gautschi K, et al. Failure to find a relationship between mnestic skills of octogenarians and aluminum in drinking water. Int Arch Occup Environ Health 1991;63(2):97–103.

[58] The Canadian study of health and aging: risk factors for Alzheimer's disease in Canada. Neurology 1994;44:2073–80.

[59] Flaten TP, Glattre E, Viste A, et al. Mortality from dementia among gastroduodenal ulcer patients. Epidemiol Community Health 1991;45(3):203–6.

[60] Sjogren B. Occupational exposure to dust: inflammation and ischaemic heart disease. Occup Environ Med 1997;54(7):466–9.

[61] McLachlan D. Aluminum and the risk for Alzheimer's disease. Environmetrics 1995;6:233–75.

[62] McLaughlin AI, Kazantzis G, King E, et al. Pulmonary fibrosis and encephalopathy associated with the inhalation of aluminum dust. Br J Ind Med 1962;19:253–63.

[63] Longstreth WT Jr, Rosenstock L, Heyer NJ. Potroom palsy: neurologic disorder in three aluminum smelter workers. Arch Intern Med 1985;145(11):1972–5.

[64] White DM, Longstreth WT Jr, Rosenstock L, et al. Neurologic syndrome in 25 workers from an aluminum smelting plant. Arch Intern Med 1993;153(7):1443–8.

[65] Langauer-Lewowicka H, Braszczynska Z. Evaluation of the combined effect of various harmful physical and chemical factors on the nervous system. Acta Neurochir (Wien) 1983; 17(1):91–6.

[66] Rifat SL, Eastwood MR, McLachlan DR, et al. Effect of exposure of miners to aluminum powder. Lancet 1990;336(8724):1162–5.

[67] Kilburn KH. Neurobehavioral impairment and symptoms associated with aluminum remelting. Arch Environ Health 1998;53(5):329–35.

[68] Sim M, Dick R, Russo J, et al. Are aluminum potroom workers at increased risk of neurological disorders? Occup Environ Med 1997;54(4):229–35.

[69] Zaudig M. A new systematic method of measurement and diagnosis of "mild cognitive impairment" and dementia according to ICD-10 and DSM-III-R criteria. Int Psychogeriatr 1992;4(Suppl 2):S203–19.

[70] Krasuki J, Alexander G, Horvitz B, et al. Volumes of medial temporal lobe structures inpatients with Alzheimer's disease and mild cognitive impairment and in healthy controls. Biol Psychiatry 1998;43(1):194–9.

[71] Salib E, Hiller V. A case-control study of Alzheimer's disease and aluminum occupation. Br J Psychiatry 1996;168(2):244–9.

[72] Crapper DR, Krishnan SS, De Boni U, et al. Aluminum: a possible neurotoxic agent in Alzheimer's disease. Trans Am Neurol Assoc 1975;100:154–6.

[73] Crapper, McLachlan DR, Dalton AJ, Kruck TP, et al. Intramuscular desferrioxamine in patients with Alzheimer's disease. Lancet 1991;337:1304–8.

[74] Xu N, Majidi V, Markesbery WR, et al. Brain aluminum in Alzheimer's disease using an improved GFAAS method. Neurotoxicology 1992;14(4):735–43.

[75] McDermott JR, Smith AI, Iqbal K, et al. Brain aluminum in aging and Alzheimer disease. Neurology 1979;29(6):809–14.

[76] Bjertness E, Candy JM, Torvik A, et al. Content of brain aluminum is not elevated in Alzheimer disease. Alzheimer's Dis Assoc Disord 1996;10(3):171–4.

[77] Deibel MA, Ehmann WD, Marksbery WR. Copper, iron, and zinc imbalances in severely degenerated brain regions in Alzheimer's disease: possible relation to oxidative stress. J Neurol Sci 1996;143:137–42.

[78] Butterfield DA, Hensley K, Harris M, et al. Beta-Amyloid peptide free radical fragments initiate synaptosomal lipoperoxidation in a sequence-specific fashion: implications in Alzheimer's disease. Biochem Biophys Res Commun 1994;200:710–5.

[79] Butterfield DA. Amyloid beta-peptide (1–42)-induced oxidative stress and neurotoxicity: implications for neurodegeneration in Alzheimer's disease brain; a review. Free Radic Res 2002;36:1307–13.

[80] Mortimer JA, Hutton JT. Epidemiology and etiology of Alzheimer's disease. In: Hutton JT, Kenny AD, editors. Senile dementia of the Alzheimer type. New York: A.R. Liss; 1985. p. 177–96.

[81] Lovell MA, Robertson JD, Teesdale WJ, et al. Copper, iron, and zinc in Alzheimer's disease senile plaques. J Neurol Sci 1998;158:47–52.

[82] Senior K. Copper may have a positive effect on Alzheimer's disease. Lancet Neurol 2004; 3(1):1–2.

[83] Phinney AL, Horne P, Yang J, et al. Mouse models of Alzheimer's disease: the long and filamentous road. Neurol Res 2003;25(6):590–600.

[84] Sparks DL, Schreurs BG. Trace amounts of copper in water induce β-amyloid plaques and learning deficits in a rabbit model of Alzheimer's disease. Proc Natl Acad Sci U S A 2003; 100:11065–9.

[85] Molina JA, Jimenez-Jimenez FJ, Aguilar MV, et al. Cerebrospinal fluid levels of transition metals in patients with Alzheimer's disease. J Neural Transm 1998;105:479–88.

[86] Cuajungco MP, Lees GJ. Zinc metabolism in the brain: relevance to human neurodegenerative disorders. Neurobiol Dis 1997;4:137–69.

[87] Price D, Davis P, Morris J, et al. The distribution of tangles, plaques, and related immunohistochemical markers in healthy aging and Alzheimer's disease. Neurobiol Aging 1991;12:295–312.

[88] Rulon LL, Robertson JD, Lovell MA, et al. Serum zinc levels and Alzheimer's disease. Biol Trace Elem Res 2000;75:79–85.

[89] Gonzalez C, Martin T, Cacho J, et al. Serum zinc, copper, insulin, and lipids in Alzheimer's disease epsilon 4 apolipoprotein E allele carriers. Eur J Clin Invest 1999;29:637–42.

[90] Ely JTA. Mercury induced Alzheimer's disease: accelerating incidence? Bull Environ Contam Toxicol 2001;67:800–6.

[91] Thompson C, Markesbery W, Ehmann W, et al. Regional brain trace element studies in Alzheimer's disease. Neurotoxicology 1988;9:1–7.

[92] Pendergrass JC, Haley BE, Vimy MJ, et al. Mercury vapor inhalation inhibits binding of GTP to tubulin in rat brain: similarity to a molecular lesion in Alzheimer diseased brain. Neurotoxicology 1997;18(2):315–24.

[93] Webb J. Enzyme and metabolic inhibitors. New York: Academic Press; 1963.

[94] Saxe S, Wekstein M, Kryscio R, et al. Alzheimer's disease, dental amalgam and mercury. J Am Dent Assoc 1999;130:191–9.

[95] Gautrin D, Gauthier S. Alzheimer's disease: environmental factors and etiologic hypotheses. Can J Neurol Sci 1989;16:375–87.

[96] Shibayama H, Kashara Y, Kobsayashi H. Prevalence of dementia in Japanese elderly population. Acta Psychiatr Scand 1986;74:144–51.

[97] Jean H, Emard JF, Thouez JP, et al. Alzheimer's disease: preliminary study of spatial distribution at birth place. Soc Sci Med 1996;42:871–8.

[98] Gauthier E, Fortier I, Courchesne F, et al. Environmental pesticide exposure as a risk factor for Alzheimer's disease: a case-control study. Environ Res 2001;86:37–45.

[99] Blain PG. Aspects of pesticide toxicology. Adverse Drug React. Acute Poison Rev 1990;9:37–68.

[100] Fukuto TR. Mechanism of action of organophosphorus and carbmate insecticides. Environ Health Perspect 1990;87:245–54.

[101] Bardin PG, Van Eden SF, Moolman A, et al. Organophosphate and carbmate poisoning. Arch Intern Med 1994;154:1433–41.

[102] Elroy-Stein O, Bernstein Y, Groner Y. Over production of human Cu/Zn-superoxide dismutase in transfected cells: extenuation of paraquat-mediated cyctoxicity and enhancement of lipid peroxidation. EMBO J 1986;5:615–22.

[103] Corasaniti M, Defilippo R, Rodino P. Evidence that paraquat is able to cross the blood brain-barrier to a different extent in rats of various age. Funct Neurol 1991;6:385–91.

[104] Kimbrough RD, Gaines TB, Linder RE. The ultrastructure of livers of rats fed DDT and Dieldrin. Arch Environ Health 1971;22:460–7.

[105] Fleming L, Mann JB, Bean J, et al. Parkinson's disease and brain levels of organochlorine pesticides. Ann Neurol 1994;36:100–3.

[106] Baldi I, Lebailly P, Mohammed-Brahim B, et al. Neurodegenerative diseases and exposure to pesticides in the elderly. Am J Epidemiol 2003;157:409–14.

[107] Sobel E, Davanipour Z, Sulkava R, et al. Occupation with exposure to electromagnetic fields: a possible risk factor for Alzheimer's disease. Am J Epidemiol 1995;142(5):515–24.

[108] Savitz DA, Loomis DP, Tse CJ. Electrical occupations and neurodegenerative disease: analysis of US mortality data. Arch Environ Health 1998;53:71–4.

[109] Savitz DA, Checkoway H, Loomis DP. Magnetic field exposure and neurodegenerative disease mortality among electric utility workers. Epidemiology 1998;9(4):398–404.

[110] Feychting M, Jonsson F, Pedersen NL, et al. Occupational magnetic field exposure and neurodegenerative disease. Epidemiology 2003;14(4):413–9.

[111] Hakansson N, Gustavsson P, Johansen C, et al. Neurodegenerative diseases in welders and other workers exposed to high levels of magnetic fields. Epidemiology 2003;14(4):420–6.

[112] Lee PN. Smoking and Alzheimer's disease: a review of the epidemiological evidence. Neuroepidemiology 1994;13(4):131–44.

[113] Ott A, Slooter AJ, Hofman A, et al. Smoking and risk of dementia and Alzheimer's disease in a population-based cohort study: the Rotterdam study. Lancet 1998;351(9119):1840–3.

[114] Merchant C, Tang MX, Albert S, et al. The influence of smoking on the risk of Alzheimer's disease. Neurology 1999;52(7):1408–12.

[115] Launer L, Andersen K, Dewey M, et al. for the European Studies of Dementia Incidence Research Group and Work Groups. Rates and risk factors for dementia and Alzheimer's disease: results from EURODEM pooled analyses. Neurology 1999;52(1):78–84.

[116] Tyas SL, White LR, Petrovitch H, et al. Mid-life smoking and late-life dementia: the Honolulu-Asia aging study. Neurobiol Aging 2003;24:589–96.

[117] Bachman DL, Green RC, Benke KS, et al. Comparisons of Alzheimer's disease risk factors in white and African American families. Neurology 2003;60:1372–4.

[118] Fuller CJ, May MA, Martin KJ. The effect of vitamin E and vitamin C supplementation on LDL oxidizability and neutrophil respiratory burst in young smokers. J Am Coll Nutr 2000;19(3):361–9.

[119] Traber MG, Winklhofer-Roob BM, Roob JM, et al. Vitamin E kinetics in smokers and nonsmokers. Free Radic Biol Med 2001;31(11):1368–74.

[120] Stamatelopoulos KS, Lekakis JP, Papamichael CM, et al. Oral administration of ascorbic acid attenuates endothelial dysfunction after short-term cigarette smoking. Int J Vitam Nutr Res 2003;73(6):417–22.

[121] Panda K, Chattopadhyay R, Chattopadhyay DJ, et al. Vitamin C prevents cigarette smoke-induced oxidative damage in vivo. Free Radic Biol Med 2000;29(2):115–24.

[122] Kim HS, Lee BM. Protective effects of antioxidant supplementation on plasma lipid peroxidation in smokers. J Toxicol Environ Health A 2001;63(8):583–98.

[123] DiMonte D, Lavasani M, Manning-Bog A. Environmental factors in Parkinson's disease. Neurotoxicology 2002;23:487–502.

[124] McKeith I, Burn D. Spectrum of Parkinson's disease, Parkinson's dementia, and Lewy body dementia. Neurol Clin 2000;18(4):865–83.

[125] Jellinger KA. α–Synuclein pathology in Parkinson's and Alzheimer's disease brain: incidence and topographic distribution; a pilot study. Acta Neuropathol (Berl) 2003;106: 191–201.

[126] Mayeaux R, Chen J, Mirabello E, et al. An estimate of the incidence of dementia in idiopathic Parkinson's disease. Neurology 1990;40(10):1513–7.

[127] Campbell S, Stephens S, Ballard C. Dementia with Lewy bodies: clinical features and treatment. Drugs Aging 2001;18(6):397–407.

[128] Wagner M, Bachman D. Neuropsychological features of diffuse Lewy Body disease. Arch Clin Neuropsychol 1996;11(3):175–84.

[129] Mayeaux R, Denaro J, Hemenegildo N, et al. A population-based investigation of Parkinson's disease with and without dementia: relationship to age and gender. Arch Neurol 1992;49(5):492–7.

[130] Glatt S, Hubble J, Lyons K, et al. Risk factors for dementia in Parkinson's disease: effect of education. Neuroepidemiology 1996;15(1):20–5.

[131] Hubble J, Kurth J, Glatt S, et al. Gene-toxin interaction as a putative risk factor for Parkinson's disease with dementia. Neuroepidemiology 1998;17(2):96–104.

[132] Levy G, Schupf N, Tang M, et al. Combined effects of age and severity on the risk of dementia in Parkinson's disease. Ann Neurol 2002;51(6):722–9.

[133] Marder K, Flood P, Cote L, et al. A pilot study of risk factors for dementia in Parkinson's disease. Mov Disord 1990;5(2):156–61.

[134] Kotzbauer P, Trojanowski J, Lee V. Lewy body pathology in Alzheimer's disease. J Mol Neurosci 2001;17:225–32.

[135] Gorell J, Johnson C, Rybicki B, et al. The risk of Parkinson's disease with exposure to pesticides, farming, well water, and rural living. Neurology 1998;50(5):1346–50.

[136] Lewin R. Parkinson's disease: an environmental cause? Science 1985;230:257–8.

[137] Li X, Sun A. Paraquat induced activation of transcription factor AP-1 and apoptosis in PC12 cells. J Neural Transm 1999;106:1–21.

[138] Barbeau A, Dalliare L, Buu N, et al. Comparative behavioral, biochemical, and pigmentary effects of MPTP, MPP +, and paraquat in Rara Pipiens. Life Sci 1985;37:1529–38.

[139] Liou H, Tasi M, Chen C, et al. Environmental risk factors and Parkinson's disease: a case control study in Taiwan. Neurology 1997;48(6):1583–8.

[140] Kuopio A, Marttila R, Helenius H, et al. Environmental risk factors in Parkinson's disease. Mov Disord 1999;14(6):928–39.

[141] Collins M, Neafsey E. Potential neurotoxic "agents provocateurs" in Parkinson's disease. Neurotoxicol Teratol 2002;24(5):571–7.

[142] Baldereschi M, DiCarlo A, Vanni P, et al. Lifestyle-related risk factors for Parkinson's disease: a population-based study. Acta Neurol Scand 2003;108:239–44.

[143] Alam M, Schmidt W. Rotenone destroys dopaminergic neurons and induces parkinsonian symptoms in rats. Behav Brain Res 2002;136(1):317–24.

[144] Liu B, Gao HM, Hong JS. Parkinson's disease and exposure to infectious agents and pesticides and the occurrence of brain injuries role of neuroinflammation. Environ Health Perspect 2003;11(8):1065–73.

[145] Corrigan F, Weinburg C, Shore R, et al. Organochlorine insecticides in substantia nigra in Parkinson's disease. J Toxicol Environ Health 2000;59(4):229–34.

[146] Taylor C, Saint-Hilaire M, Cupples L, et al. Environmental, medical, and family history risk factors for Parkinson's disease: a New England-based case control study. Am J Med Genet 1999;88:742–9.

[147] Kirkhorn SR, Garry VF. Agricultural lung diseases. Environmental Health Perspect 2000; 108:705–12.

[148] Petrovitch H, Ross GW, Abbott RD, et al. Plantation work and risk of Parkinson disease in a population-based longitudinal study. Arch Neurol 2002;59:1787–92.

[149] DePalma G, Mozzoni P, Mutti A, et al. Case-control study interactions between genetic and environmental factors in Parkinson's disease. Lancet 1998;352:1986–7.

[150] Langston JW, Ballard PA, Tetrud JW, et al. Chronic parkinsonism in humans due to a product of meperidine-analog synthesis. Science 1983;219:979–80.

[151] Salach JI, Singer TP, Castagnoli N, et al. Oxidation of the neurotoxic amine MPTP by monoamine oxidases A and B and suicide inactivation of the enzymes MPTP. Biochem Biophys Res Commun 1984;125:831–5.

[152] Nicklas WJ, Byas I, Heikkila RE. Inhibition of NADH-linked oxidation in brain mitochondria by 1-methyl-4-phenyl-1, 2, 3, 6 tetrahydropyridine. Life Sci 1985;36:2503–8.

[153] Uversky VN, Li J, Finke AL. Metal-triggered structural transformations, aggregation, and fibrillation of human α–synuclein. J Biol Chem 2001;276(47):44284–96.

[154] Gorell J, Johnson C, Rybicki B, et al. Occupational exposures to metals as risk factors for Parkinson's disease. Neurology 1997;48(3):650–8.

[155] Zatta P, Lucchini R, van Rensburg S, et al. The role of metals in neurodegenerative processes: aluminum, manganese, and zinc. Brain Res Bull 2003;62:15–28.

[156] Gorell J, Peterson E, Rybicki B, et al. Multiple risk factors for Parkinson's disease. J Neurol Sci 2004;217(2):169–74.

[157] Jiménez-Jiménez F, Molina J, Aguilar M, et al. Cerebrospinal fluid levels of transition metals in patients with Parkinson's disease. J Neural Transm 1998;105:497–505.

[158] Mendez-Alvarez E, Soto-Otero R, Hermida-Ameijeiras A, et al. Effects of aluminum and zinc on the oxidative stress caused by 6-hydroxydopamine autoxidation: relevance for the pathogenesis of Parkinson's disease. Biochim Biophys Acta 2001;1586:155–68.

[159] Spillantini MG, Schmidt ML, Jakes R, et al. α–Synuclein in Lewy bodies. Nature 1997;388: 839–40.

[160] Altschuler E. Aluminum-containing antacids as a cause of idiopathic Parkinson's disease. Med Hypotheses 1999;53(1):22–3.

[161] Strang RR. The association of gastro-duodenal ulceration and Parkinson's disease. Med J Aust 1965;52:842–3.

[162] Shuichi H, Mukai T, Kurosaki K, et al. Modification of the striatal dopaminergic neuron system by carbon monoxide exposure in free-moving rats, as determined by in vivo brain microdialysis. Arch Toxicol 2002;76:596–605.

[163] Pezzoli G, Canesi M, Antonini A, et al. Hydrocarbon exposure and Parkinson's disease. Neurology 2000;55(5):667–73.

[164] Jaques A, Gamble J, Tsai S. Hydrocarbon exposure and Parkinson's disease [letter]. Neurology 2001;57(2):371.

[165] Tanner C, Goldman S, Aston D, et al. Smoking and Parknson's disease in twins. Neurology 2002;58:581–8.

[166] Parain K, Hapdey C, Rousselet E, et al. Cigarette smoke and nicotine protect dopaminergic neurons against the 1-methyl-4-phenyl-1,2,3,6-tetrahydropyridine parkinsonian toxin. Brain Res 2003;984:224–32.

[167] Soto-Otero R, Mendez-Alvarez E, Sanchez-Sellero I, et al. Reduction of rat brain levels of the endogenous dopaminergic proneurotoxinx 1,2,3,4-tetrehydroisoquinoline and 1,2,3,4-tetrahydro-bet-carboline by cigarette smoke. Neurosci Lett 2001;298(3):187–90.

[168] Maggio R, Riva M, Vaglini F, et al. Nicotine prevents experimental parkinsonism in rodents and induces striatal increase of neurotrophic factors. J Neurochem 1998;71(6): 2439–46.

[169] Rosen H, Lengenfelder J, Miller B. Frontotemportal dementia. Neurol Clin 2000;18(4): 979–92.

[170] Wallwork J. Zinc and the central nervous system. Prog Food Nutr Sci 1987;11(2):203–47.

[171] Constantinidis J, Tissot R. Role of glutamate and zinc in the hippocampal lesions of Pick's disease. In: Dichiara G, Gessa G, editors. Glutamate as a neurotransmitter. New York: Raven Press; 1981. p. 413–22.

[172] Ehmann W, Alauddin M, Hossain T, et al. Brain trace elements in Pick's disease. Ann Neurol 1984;15:102–4.

[173] Smith TC, Gray GC, Knoke JD. Is systematic lupus erythematosus, amyotropic lateral sclerosis, or fibromyalgia associated with Persian Gulf War service: an examination of Department of Defense hospitalization data. Am J Epidemiol 2000;151(11):1053–9.

[174] Gresham LS, Molgaard CA, Golbeck AL, et al. Amyotropic lateral sclerosis and occupational heavy metal exposure: a case-control study. Neuroepidemiology 1986;5: 29–38.

[175] Barohn RJ, Rowland LP. Neurology and Gulf War veterans. Neurology 2002;59:1484–5.

[176] Horner RD, Kamins KG, Feussner JR, et al. Occurrence of amyotropic lateral sclerosis among Gulf War veterans. Neurology 2003;61(6):742–9.

[177] Jamal G, Hansen S, Apartoloulos F, et al. The "Gulf War syndrome:" is there evidence of dysfunction in the nervous system? J Neurol Neurosurg Psychiatry 1996;60:449–51.

[178] Sharief MK, Pridden J, Delamont RS, et al. Neurophysiologic analysis of neuromuscular symptoms in UK Gulf War veterans. Neurology 2002;59:1518–25.

[179] Gray GC, Reed RJ, Kaiser KS, et al. Self-reported symptoms and medical conditions among 11,868 Gulf War-era veterans. Am J Epidemiol 2002;155:1033–44.

[180] Haley RW. Excess incidence of ALS in young Gulf War veterans. Neurology 2003;61: 750–6.

[181] Rose MR. Gulf War service is an uncertain trigger for ALS. Neurology 2003;61:730–1.

[182] Armon C. Occurrence of amyotropic lateral sclerosis among Gulf War veterans. Neurology 2004;62(6):1027.

[183] Perry T, Bergeron C, Biro A, et al. B-N-Methylamino-L-alanine: chronic oral administration is not neurotoxic to mice. J Neurol Sci 1989;94:173–80.

[184] Kurland L, Hirano A, Malamus N, et al. Parkinsonism-dementia complex, an endemic disease on the island of Guam. Trans Am Neurol Assoc 1961;86:115–20.

[185] Wiederholt W. Neuroepidemiologic research initiatives on Guam: past and present. Neuroepidemiology 1999;18:279–91.

[186] Morris H, Al-Sarraj S, Schwab C, et al. A clinical and pathological study of motor neurone disease on Guam. Brain 2001;124:2215–22.

[187] Pérez-Tur J, Buée L, Morris H, et al. Neurodegenerative diseases of Guam: analysis of TAU. Neurology 1999;53(2):411–3.

[188] Gellein K, Garruto RM, Syversen T, et al. Concentrations of Cd, Co, Cu, Fe, Mn, Rb, V, and Zn in formalin-fixed brain tissue in amyotropic lateral sclerosis and Parkinsonism-dementia complex of Guam determined by high-resolution ICP-MS. Biol Trace Elem Res 2003;96:39–60.

[189] Spencer P, Nunn P, Hugon J, et al. Motorneurone disease on Guam: possible role of food neurotoxin. Lancet 1986;1:965.

[190] Wilson J, Khabazian I, Wong M, et al. Behavioral and neurological correlates of ALS-parkinsonism dementia complex in adult mice fed washed cyad flour. Neuromolecular Med 2002;1(3):207–21.

[191] Armon C. Western pacific ALS/PDC and flying foxes: what's next? Neurology 2003;61:291.

[192] Khabazian I, Bains J, Williams D, et al. Isolation of various forms of sterol β-D-glucoside from the seed of Cyas circinalis: neurotoxicity and implications for ALS-parkinsonism dementia complex. J Neurochem 2002;82:516–28.

[193] Reed D, Labarthe D, Chen K, et al. A cohort study of amyotrophic lateral sclerosis and parkinsonism-dementia on Guam and Rota. Am J Epidemiol 1987;125:92–100.

[194] Cox P, Banack S, Murch S. Biomagnification of cyanobacterial neurotoxins and neurodegenerative disease among the Chamorro people of Guam. Proc Natl Acad Sci U S A 2003;100(23):13380–3.

[195] Cox P, Sacks O. Cyad neurotoxins, consumption of flying foxes, and ALS-PDC disease in Guam. Neurology 2002;58:956–9.

[196] Plato C, Garruto R, Galasko D, et al. Amyotrophic lateral sclerosis and parkinsonism-dementia complex of Guam: changing incidence rates during the past 60 years. Am J Epidemiol 2003;157(2):149–57.

[197] Spencer PS. Biological principles of chemical neurotoxicity. In: Spencer PS, Schaumburg HH, Ludolph AC, editors. Experimental and clinical neurotoxicology. 2nd edition. New York: Oxford University Press; 2000. p. 3–54.

[198] Schaumburg HH. Human neurotoxic disease. In: Spencer PS, Schaumburg HH, Ludolph AC, editors. Experimental and clinical neurotoxicology. 2nd edition. New York: Oxford University Press; 2000. p. 55–82.

[199] Morris JC. Evaluation of the demented patient. In: Morris JC, editor. Handbook of dementing illnesses. New York: Marcel Dekker, Inc.; 1994. p. 71–88.

NEUROLOGIC
CLINICS

ELSEVIER
SAUNDERS

Neurol Clin 23 (2005) 523–540

Gulf War Syndrome: A Toxic Exposure?
A Systematic Review

Gary S. Gronseth, MD

Department of Neurology, The University of Kansas Medical Center,
3599 Rainbow Boulevard, Mail Stop 2012, Kansas City, KS 66160

Some veterans serving in the first Persian Gulf War (1990–1991) reported unexplained symptoms during deployment or shortly after returning home [1]. Many of their symptoms were neurologic and included fatigue, muscle and joint pain, headaches, loss of memory, and poor sleep. This constellation of nonspecific symptoms has come to be known as Gulf War syndrome (GWS) [2].

Gulf War veterans (GWV) were exposed to unique, hazardous environmental conditions. Potential exposures included toxins—pyridostigmine bromide (used as a pretreatment to mitigate the effect of nerve agent exposure), nerve and mustard chemical weapons (potentially released by demolition of caches of stored chemical weapons), insecticides and insect repellants, depleted uranium (used in tank protective armor and in armor-piercing munitions), petroleum-based fuels, smoke from burning oil wells, and vaccinations. Veterans also were exposed to harsh physical conditions, including extreme temperatures, dusty conditions, and infectious diseases, such as leishmaniasis and sand fly fever. Also present was the psychologic stress invariably accompanying wartime operations.

Veterans groups, government agencies, and independent investigators naturally have attempted to link exposure to these wartime hazards and stressors causally to GWS. This article reviews the evidence addressing the potential links between these wartime hazards and GWS, with particular emphasis on the possible role of toxins in the development of GWS.

In preparing this article, the author used a modification of the evidence-based methodologies developed by the American Academy of Neurology (AAN). The use of this methodology in no way implies endorsement by the AAN of the findings or conclusions of this document.

E-mail address: gronseth@kumc.edu

0733-8619/05/$ - see front matter © 2005 Elsevier Inc. All rights reserved.
doi:10.1016/j.ncl.2004.12.011

Traditionally, a causal link between an exposure to an environmental hazard and an illness is considered established only after the following:

1. Formulation of a clear case definition of the illness that allows the accurate determination of the presence or absence of that illness;
2. Development of valid and reliable measures of exposure to the putative environmental hazard; and
3. Studies showing a consistent statistical association between the illness and hazard after controlling for potential confounders.

Defining Gulf War syndrome

Initial concerns about the presence of an unusual illness in GWV were prompted by reports from individual veterans and groups of veterans complaining of a constellation of similar but nonspecific symptoms [3]. More systematic surveys from several countries confirmed that GWV complained frequently of ill health manifested by a wide variety of symptoms [4–9]. Although the frequency of symptoms varied from survey to survey, common complaints included fatigue, joint and muscle pains, cognitive problems, and headaches. Because of the multisymptomatic nature of these complaints, prevalence estimates of GWS vary widely. Based on veterans' self reports, one study reports that 17% of British GWV believed they had GWS [10].

In-depth medical evaluations of GWV who had complaints have failed to identify an objectively definable, previously recognized disease to explain the symptoms in the majority of veterans [11–14]. Despite this, there is evidence that GWS has affected veterans' quality of life [15,16].

Given the heterogeneity of GWV symptoms, some investigators propose that GWS does not represent a single syndrome, but rather a group of syndromes. Several investigators have used multivariable statistical techniques, such as factor analysis, in an attempt to identify the underlying syndromes. In a study of 249 GWV, Haley et al [17] identified six syndrome factors, which he labeled impaired cognition, confusion-ataxia, arthromyoneuropathy, phobia-apraxia, fever-adenopathy, and weakness-incontinence. Several other investigators have challenged the validity of this technique, failed to replicate his results, or observed a similar clustering of symptoms in nonveterans and in veterans who did not have GWS [18–23].

Further complicating a coherent case definition is the apparent similarity between GWS and other medically unexplained conditions, such as chronic fatigue syndrome [8], fibromyalgia [6], and multiple chemical sensitivity [24]. Although case definitions for these conditions have been developed, their validity and usefulness is questioned [25–27]. Of particular importance is the similarity between GWS and the occurrence of medically unexplained illnesses after previous wars [28–30].

The combination of heterogeneous symptoms, the lack of an objective marker of disease, and the similarity to other medically unexplained illnesses makes the development of a reliable case definition of GWS difficult [31]. Further confounding formulation of a consistent case definition are reports of unreliable symptom reporting in GWV [32]. These difficulties complicate the design and execution of any study attempting to explore a causal link between toxic exposure and GWS.

Potential toxic exposures and their measurement

This section reviews some of the toxins considered potential causes of the GWS. In the subsequent section, the evidence attempting to link these toxins causally to GWS is reviewed.

Perhaps the most ubiquitous toxin exposure GWV experienced was the fine, dusty sand found throughout the eastern and central regions of the Arabian Peninsula. Investigators believed that acute respiratory symptoms in United States troops in the Al Eskan village region in 1991 were secondary to exposure to these airborne particulates [33]. These same investigators speculated that exposure to these fine particles, perhaps contaminated with low levels of nerve agents, somehow depleted the immune systems of the GWV and resulted in GWS [34].

The smoke from burning Kuwaiti oil well fires exposed some GWV to other particulate exposure toward the end of the war. This smoke, in combination with combustion products and organic compounds, is considered a possible cause of GWS [35]. One study found elevated levels of volatile organic compounds in 40 civilian fire fighters working in the burning oil fields [36]. The health implication of these elevations was not determined.

Although it is clear coalition troops were not exposed to large quantities of chemical warfare agents during the first Gulf War, low-level exposures to nerve agents released after demolition of several chemical weapons caches is strongly suspected [37]. Direct measurements of nerve agent levels resulting from demolition of these chemical weapons caches are unknown. Mathematical models, however, of potential exposures of GWV have been developed [38]. Nerve agents cause their acute effects by inhibiting acetylcholine esterase, thereby causing overstimulation of nicotinic and muscarinic receptors. The resulting depolarization blockade at skeletal muscles causes respiratory failure and death. Although the acute effects of nerve agents are well known, residual effects of acute exposure have been described only recently [39]. Even less is known about the long-term effects, if any, of low-level exposure.

GWV were supplied with several pesticides and insect repellants, including malathion, permethrin, and N,N-diethyl-meta-toluamide (DEET) [40]. Some GWV also wore pet flea collars to repel insects. Although the patterns of troop use of these chemicals was not measured systematically [41], some hypothesize that these agents, particularly in combination with heat exposure and exposures to other chemicals, contributed to the development of GWS [42]. Several laboratory studies have demonstrated that co-exposure to Gulf War–related chemicals and heat can affect toxin absorption [43,44]. The relevance of these findings to GWS is unknown.

Many United States troops took pyridostigmine bromide during the Gulf War as a protective measure against certain nerve agents that rapidly form irreversible covalent bonds with acetylcholine esterase [45]. Pyridostigmine is a carbamate that binds reversibly to the acetylcholinesterase, thereby protecting the enzyme from the nerve agent. In high doses, sometimes used in the treatment of myasthenia gravis, pyridostigmine can cause toxicity similar to that produced by nerve agents [46]. In lower doses, the drug usually is well tolerated. Common side effects usually are mild and limited to gastrointestinal symptoms caused by muscarinic overstimulation. Long-term effects of the use of pyridostigmine in patients who had myasthenia gravis have not been described. Many investigators consider GWS the chronic sequelae of pyridostigmine use during the war [47].

Lending further credence to the hypothetic role of organophosphates to the development of GWS, several studies show that some GWV who had GWS had decreased activity of the enzyme paraoxonase [48,49], an enzyme present in human serum that detoxifies organophosphates [50]. These findings suggest that GWV who had GWS may have been predisposed to long-term consequences of low-level organophosphate exposure from insecticides or nerve agents because of a relative enzyme deficiency. Complicating this interpretation is the finding that paraoxonase activity was decreased equally in GWV who had or did not have symptoms of GWS [51].

Depleted uranium, used during the Gulf War in armor and armor-piercing munitions, also has been a proposed toxin responsible for GWS [52]. Because it is less radioactive than naturally occurring uranium, its potential toxicity relates primarily to its chemical properties and possible renal toxicity. In general, exposures of GWV to depleted uranium were not measurably higher than exposure to naturally occurring uranium [53,54]. An important exception was GWV who were victims of friendly fire incidents and who had elevated levels of urinary uranium [55]. Detailed medical evaluations performed on 50 United States GWV documented elevated levels of urinary uranium.

One of the major challenges in any study attempting to find an association between a Gulf War–related toxic exposure and GWS is a valid and reliable method for measuring the level of exposure. Many studies have resorted to GWV self-reports to determine the level of exposure [56]. Unfortunately, such self-reported exposures in GWV have been shown to be unreliable and over-reported [57,58].

Associations between exposure and Gulf War syndrome

Process

To find studies attempting to measure a statistical association between GWS and various exposures, the author searched the National Library of Medicine's MEDLINE database from 1990 to August 2004 using the MeSH heading, "Gulf War syndrome," and the text words, "gulf war illness" and "gulf war." Identified titles and abstracts for articles were screened for those that measured potential associations between exposures and GWS. Only articles published in English were considered. To identify articles missed by the initial search strategy, references in the identified articles were reviewed. Four hundred seventy-five articles were identified with the initial search strategy; 78 of these were considered potentially relevant to the question of causation.

Non–Gulf War syndrome health outcomes

Many of the studies identified dealt with health outcomes in GWV other than the development of GWS. Authors report small but statistically significant excess mortality rates from unintentional injuries (eg, motor vehicle accidents) in GWV compared with non-GWV [59–62]. The increases in accidental death rates occurred during and after deployment to the Persian Gulf.

Other studies address hospitalization rates in GWV. Several studies show increased rates of postwar hospitalizations in GWV compared with other veterans, possibly explained by participation in GWV health registry [63,64]. Also potentially explained by participation in the GWV health registry are reported increased rates of hospitalization for unexplained illnesses in GWV [65]. Two studies measured no association between postwar hospitalization rates in GWV and modeled exposures to oil well fire smoke [66] or potential low-level nerve agent vapors after munitions demolition [64].

The risk of birth defects and other health problems among children of GWV were studied after anecdotal reports of increased birth defects in GWV. Increased rates of birth defects were not found in several epidemiologic studies [67–70]. GWV postwar conceptions, however, were found at increased risk for ectopic pregnancies and spontaneous abortions compared with nondeployed female veterans [71].

Finally, there are some reports of a small but statistically significant increase in the risk of specific illnesses in GWV. Most notable among these are reports of an increased risk of amyotrophic lateral sclerosis [72,73] in GWV. Whether or not this increased risk is related to toxin exposure remains unknown.

These studies of mortality, hospitalization, birth defects, and specific previously recognized disease are of extreme importance. Because they do not address GWS specifically, however, they are not directly relevant to the scope of this article and are not discussed further.

Studies addressing Gulf War syndrome

To identify articles pertinent to the question of causation of GWS, the 78 articles identified after the MEDLINE search were reviewed and considered eligible for inclusion if they met these criteria: inclusion of at least 10 subjects; inclusion of persons who did and did not have GWS; inclusion of persons who had varying exposures to the putative causal factor (deployment to the Gulf War theater of operations being one potential causal factor); explicitly providing a definition of GWS; and explicitly stating the method used for measuring exposures to the putative casual factor. Twenty studies, published from 1995 to 2002, met these prespecified inclusion criteria [4,5,9,19,24,56,74–87]; they are listed in Table 1. Although not always stated explicitly in these reports, it is likely that several studies are from the same investigators or institutions that studied the same cohorts.

Sample sizes varied widely, from 41 subjects to more than 18,000. Two studies used a case-control design, recruiting subjects based on whether or not they had GWS [56,84]. The remaining studies used a cross-sectional design. Data regarding the presence of GWS and exposures was obtained using a questionnaire. The questionnaires were completed variably via telephone interview, in-person interview, or personally by the subject. Reported response rates to survey varied form 41% to 100%.

The presence of GWS always was determined by subject-reported symptoms. Most studies used the number of symptoms from a standardized symptom checklist as the primary outcome variable. Others required a predefined number of symptoms from several domains to define GWS [5,77,82,85–87]. A few studies used case definitions from other conditions, such as chronic fatigue or multiple chemical sensitivity syndrome, to define GWS [24,76,84]. One study used factor-analysis–defined syndromes as the outcome [74]. Another study used unexplained gastrointestinal symptoms as the major outcome [80].

The most common risk factor studied was deployment to the Persian Gulf area during or near the time of the Gulf War. Most investigators also studied the association between GWS and exposures to pesticides, insect repellants (including flea collars), smoke from burning oil fires, and perceived exposure to chemical warfare agents. A few studies attempted to determine if the time of deployment relative to the war (before, during, or after) was associated with GWS [77,86]. Exposures were determined completely based on subject self-report.

Based on these methodologic characteristics, the studies were graded using the classification-of-evidence schemes listed in Box 1 This scheme is a modification of one undergoing development by the AAN. Briefly, the scheme rates a study on a quality scale of I to IV based on an assessment of

Table 1
Methodologic characteristics of studies measuring the association between risk factors and Gulf War syndrome

Author	Year	Setting	Design	% Resp	N	GWS case definition	Exposures measured	Associations	Class[a]
Stretch	1995	Congressionally mandated study of service members from Hawaii and Pennsylvania serving during Operation Desert Storm	CS	NS	4000	Physical health symptoms	Deployment to PG	Deployed veterans reported more physical health symptoms than nondeployed veterans	III
Anonymous	1997	Telephone interview survey of PGW and non-PGW military personnel in Iowa	CS	76	3695	Self-reported symptoms	Deployment of PG	GWV with a higher self-reported prevalence of medical and psychiatric conditions	II
Haley	1997	Selected GMV from a Naval construction battalion	CS	100	249	Factor analysis–derived syndromes	Self-reported: wearing flea collars; adverse effects of pyridostigmine; belief in chemical weapons exposure; DEET	"Impaired-cognition" with flea collars; "confusion-ataxia" with pyridostigmine; "artho-myo-neuropathy" with DEET	IV
Pierce	1997	Stratified sample of United State Air Force women	CS	NS	525	Reported health problems	Deployment to PG	Deployed reported significantly more general and gender-specific health problems	III

(continued on next page)

Table 1 (continued)

Author	Year	Setting	Design	% Resp	N	GWS case definition	Exposures measured	Associations	Class[a]
Bell	1998	Telephone survey of 100 randomly selected veterans	CS	41	41	Sensitivity to chemicals	Deployment to PG; self-reported exposure to wartime pesticides and insect repellants	More chemical sensitivity in deployed and those with wartime chemical exposures	III
Fukuda	1998	Questionnaire administered to current active-duty Air Force members	CS	NS	3723	1+ symptoms from 2 of 3 categories (fatigue, mood cognition, and musculoskeletal	Deployment to GW; time of deployment; duties during war	Multiple symptoms with deployment; symptoms not associated with time of deployment	III
Kroenke	1998	GWV with health concerns evaluated in the Department of Defense Comprehensive Clinical Evaluation Program	CS	100	18,495	Individual symptoms	Self-reported exposures; types of combat experience	No associations with individual symptoms	IV
Gray	1999	Questionnaire administered to 14 Seabee command	CS	NS	1497	List of 41 symptoms	Deployment; self-reported exposures	GWV with higher prevalence of 35 of 41 symptoms; multiple symptom exposure-associations	III

Ishoy	1999	Questionnaire on gastrointestinal symptoms administered to Danish GMV and age/gender/profession-matched controls	CS	NS	943	Gastrointestinal symptoms	Deployment; 24 physical. Chemical, or biological exposures self-reported	Increased prevalence of symptoms associated with deployment burning of waste, and insecticides	III
Proctor	1999	Stratified, random samples of GWV and nondeployed Gulf-era veterans from New England and New Orleans	CS	NS	341	Symptoms on a 52-item health symptom checklist	Deployment; self-reported exposures to pesticides, debris from Scuds, chemical warfare agents, smoke from tent heaters	Deployment associated with symptoms; self-reported exposures associated with body-system symptom score	III
Suadicani	1999	Questionnaire on neuropsychologic symptoms administered to Danish GWV and age/gender/profession-matched controls	CS	NS	943	3+ symptoms: cognitive problems, dizziness, fatigue, insomnia	Deployment; 24 physical, chemical or biological exposures self-reported	Symptoms associated with deployment and multiple physicochemical exposures	III
Unwin	1999	Random sample United Kingdom GMV and other veterans	CS	65	1274	4-symptom and illness checklist	Deployment; self reported exposures, including vaccination	GMV reported symptoms more frequently than other control; all self-reported exposures associated with all symptoms	III

(continued on next page)

Table 1 (*continued*)

Author	Year	Setting	Design	% Resp	N	GWS case definition	Exposures measured	Associations	Class[a]
Doebbeling	2000	Population-based sample of GMV and other Gulf War-era controls	CS	76	3695	Symptom checklist	Deployment	Every symptom associated with deployment	II
Fiedler	2000	Questionnaire administered to GMV with and without CFS	CC	100	103	CFS	Self-reported combat and chemical exposures	Combat and all exposures associated with CFS	III
Nisenbaum	2000	Self-administered questionnaire from GMV of four Air Force units	CS	NS	1002	Illness characterized by a combination of fatigue, mood-cognition, and musculoskeletal symptoms	Self-reports of pyridostigmine; insect repellants and belief in exposure to chemical weapons	Symptoms associated with all self-reported exposures	III
Steele	2000	Survey of Kansas GMV and non-GWV	CS	NS	2030	Chronic symptoms in 3 of 6 domains	Deployment; vaccination; time of deployment	Symptoms associated with deployment leaving theater in June or July of 1991	III
Cherry	2001	Questionnaire administered 7+ years after the war to United Kingdom GMV	CS	85	7971	Health indices from symptom questionnaire	Self-reports of 14 exposures	Handling pesticides, vaccinations and exposure to smoke associated with symptoms	IV
Reid	2001	Survey of UK GMV and nondeployed veterans	CS	65	8177	MCS; CFS	Deployment; self-reports of exposures to pesticides and other chemicals	CFS, and MCS associated with deployment. MCS associated with pesticides.	III

Study	Year	Description	Design	Resp.	N	Outcome	Exposure	Findings	Risk of bias[a]
Spencer	2001	Analysis of risk factors in GMV who had unexplained illness and healthy controls	CC	100	354	Unexplained illness	Self-report combat conditions; heat stress; pyridostigmine, insecticides, repellants	Illness associated only with heat and combat	IV
Wolfe	2002	Survey mailed to members of the Ft. Devens cohort	CS	44	1290	Symptoms from at least two of three symptom categories	Self-reported use of pyridostigmine, anthrax vaccination, tent heaters, exposures to smoke, chemical odors	All factors associated with symptoms in logistic regressions	IV

Abbreviations: CC, case control; CFS, chronic fatigue syndrome; CS, cross sectional; MCS, multiple chemical sensitivity; NS, not stated; PGW, Persian Gulf War. Resp, percentage of sample for which outcome and exposure data obtained.

[a] Risk of bias relative to a causal link between deployment and GWS.

Box 1. Definitions for strength of evidence for causation

Class I. A prospective cohort survey of persons who have
varying exposures to the putative causative factor. Exposure to
the factor is determined by a valid and reliable measure. The
outcome of interest is determined in most (greater than 85%)
persons after a sufficiently long period of time. The
association between the putative causal factor and outcome
is adjusted for potential confounders. The outcome, if not
objective, is measured in a fashion that is masked to the
exposure.

Class II. A cohort survey or cross-sectional study of persons who
have varying exposures to the putative causative factor.
Exposure to the factor is determined by a valid and reliable
measure. The outcome of interest is determined in most
(greater than 70%) persons. The association between the
putative causal factor and outcome is adjusted for potential
confounders. The outcome, if not objective, is measured in
a fashion that is masked to the exposure.

Class III. A cohort survey or cross-sectional or case-control study
of persons who have varying exposures to the putative
causative factor. Exposure to the factor is determined by
a valid and reliable measure. The outcome of interest is
determined in many persons. The outcome, if not objective,
is measured in a fashion that is independent of the exposure.

Class IV. Any study not meeting the criteria in class I, II, or III.

---

the risk of bias using several empirically validated domains. Studies graded
class I are judged to have a low risk of bias. Studies graded class IV are
judged to have a high risk of bias.

Regarding the question of a causal relationship between exposure to
chemical toxins and the development of GWS, most studies measure a strong
association between all toxin exposures and GWS, regardless of how GWS
was defined. All 20 studies meeting the prespecified inclusion criteria are
assessed as having a high risk of bias (class IV). All studies potentially are
biased by reliance on subject self-reported exposure to chemical exposures.
As stated previously, such self-reports cannot be considered reliable or
valid [57].

For the purpose of grading the risk of bias in the studies pertaining to the
question of a causal relationship between deployment to the Persian Gulf
during the war and the development of GWS, the self-report of deployment
was considered a valid measure of exposure. Investigators easily were able to
confirm deployment to the Persian Gulf. Five studies were graded class IV

Box 2. Definitions for strength of conclusions

Level A. Established as causal; requires that two or more distinct class I studies demonstrate a consistent association between the putative causal factor and the outcome.

Level B. Probably causal; requires that a single class I study demonstrates an association between the putative causal factor and the outcome or that two or more distinct class II studies demonstrate a consistent association between the putative causal factor and the outcome.

Level C. Possibly causal; requires that a single class II study demonstrates an association between the putative causal factor and the outcome or that two or more distinct class III studies demonstrate a consistent association between the putative causal factor and the outcome.

Level U. Data inadequate or conflicting. Given current knowledge, the causal relationship is unproved and conclusions cannot be made.

---

because they did not compare outcomes in GWV to controls (these studies were designed to address the question of toxin exposure, not deployment) [5,56,74,78,87].

Virtually all studies designed to do so measured strong associations between deployment to the Persian Gulf during the war and GWS. Twelve studies were judged to have a moderately high risk of bias (class III) because of a case-control design or low (or unstated) survey response rates. Two studies were judged to have a moderate risk of bias (class II). These were cross-sectional studies with greater than 70% survey response rates [4,19].

Summary

Using the strength-of-conclusion scheme enumerated in Box 2, based on two class II studies, there is probably a causal link between deployment to the Persian Gulf theater of operation and the development of the poorly defined multisymptom illness known as GWS (level B).

Based on class IV studies, there is insufficient evidence to determine if exposure to toxins encountered during the Persian Gulf war caused GWS (level U).

A major limitation of the literature regarding the GWS is the reliance on self-reporting to measure exposure to putative causal toxins [57]. Although objective measures of toxin exposure in GWV generally is unavailable, modeling techniques to estimate exposure levels to low-level nerve agents and smoke from oil well fires have been developed [38,64,66]. It would be useful to determine if exposure levels determined by these techniques are associated with GWS.

The lack of a clear case definition GWS also hampers research. Some go even further, claiming that the absence of such a definition renders the condition illegitimate. Although an objective marker to GWS would be useful for studies, the absence of such a marker does not make the syndrome any less legitimate. In essence, GWS merely is a convenient descriptive term that describes a phenomenon: GWV reporting suffering from medically unexplained health-related symptoms. In this sense, it shares much with the other medically unexplained syndromes encountered in practice.

The real debate surrounding medically unexplained conditions is not whether or not they exist, but defining their cause. In this regard, investigators fall into two camps. One camp insists that the conditions are caused by a yet-to-be-discovered medical problem, rejecting out of hand the possibility of a psychologic origin. The other camp insists the conditions are fundamentally psychogenic rejecting the possibility of an undiscovered medical condition. The evidence shows, however, that the conditions exist, the suffering is real, and the causes are unknown.

References

[1] Gavaghan H. NIH panel rejects Persian Gulf syndrome. Nature 1994;369:5.
[2] Mathews J. Panel urges further research on Gulf war illness, possible increased cancer risks in veterans. J Natl Cancer Inst 1994;86:820–2.
[3] Greene S. Push for Gulf syndrome research. Nature 1993;364:19.
[4] Anonymous. Self-reported illness and health status among Gulf War veterans. A population-based study. The Iowa Persian Gulf Study Group [comment]. JAMA 1997;277:238–45.
[5] Cherry N, Creed F, Silman A, et al. Health and exposures of United Kingdom Gulf war veterans. Part II: the relation of health to exposure [comment]. Occup Environ Med 2001;58: 299–306.
[6] Escalante A, Fischbach M. Musculoskeletal manifestations, pain, and quality of life in Persian Gulf War veterans referred for rheumatologic evaluation [comment]. J Rheumatol 1998;25:2228–35.
[7] Kipen HM, Hallman W, Kang H, et al. Prevalence of chronic fatigue and chemical sensitivities in Gulf Registry Veterans [comment]. Arch Environ Health 1999;54:313–8.
[8] McCauley LA, Joos SK, Barkhuizen A, et al. Chronic fatigue in a population-based study of Gulf War veterans. Arch Environ Health 2002;57:340–8.
[9] Stretch RH, Bliese PD, Marlowe DH, et al. Physical health symptomatology of Gulf War-era service personnel from the states of Pennsylvania and Hawaii. Mil Med 1995;160:131–6.
[10] Chalder T, Hotoph M, Unwin C, et al. Prevalence of Gulf war veterans who believe they have Gulf war syndrome: questionnaire study. BMJ 2001;323:473–6.
[11] Stuart JA, Murray KM, Ursano RJ, et al. The Department of Defense's Persian Gulf War registry year 2000: an examination of veterans' health status. Mil Med 2002;167:121–8.
[12] Sharief MK, Pridden J, Delamont RS, et al. Neurophysiologic analysis of neuromuscular symptoms in UK Gulf War veterans: a controlled study [comment]. Neurology 2002;59: 1518–25.
[13] Barohn RJ, Rowland LP. Neurology and Gulf War veterans [comment]. Neurology 2002;59: 1484–5.

[14] Amato AA, McVey A, Cha C, et al. Evaluation of neuromuscular symptoms in veterans of the Persian Gulf War. Neurology 1997;48:4–12.

[15] Haley RW, Maddrey AM, Gershenfeld HK. Severely reduced functional status in veterans fitting a case definition of Gulf War syndrome. Am J Public Health 2002;92:46–7.

[16] Voelker MD, Saag KG, Schwartz DA, et al. Health-related quality of life in Gulf War era military personnel. Am J Epidemiol 2002;155:899–907.

[17] Haley RW, Kurt TL, Hom J. Is there a Gulf War Syndrome? Searching for syndromes by factor analysis of symptoms [comment]. JAMA 1997;277:215–22 [erratum: JAMA 1997;278: 388].

[18] Ismail K, Everitt B, Blatchley N, et al. Is there a Gulf War syndrome? [comment]. Lancet 1999;353:179–82.

[19] Doebbeling BN, et al. Is there a Persian Gulf War syndrome? Evidence from a large population-based survey of veterans and nondeployed controls [comment]. Am J Med 2000; 108:695–704.

[20] Knoke JD, Smith TC, Gray GC, et al. Factor analysis of self-reported symptoms: does it identify a Gulf War syndrome? [comment]. Am J Epidemiol 2000;152:379–88.

[21] Bourdette DN, McCauley LA, Barkhuizen A, et al. Symptom factor analysis, clinical findings, and functional status in a population-based case control study of Gulf War unexplained illness. J Occup Environ Med 2001;43:1026–40.

[22] Everitt B, Ismail K, David AS, et al. Searching for a Gulf War syndrome using cluster analysis [comment]. Psychol Med 2002;32:1371–8.

[23] Shapiro SE, Lasarev MR, McCauley L. Factor analysis of Gulf War illness: what does it add to our understanding of possible health effects of deployment? Am J Epidemiol 2002;156: 578–85.

[24] Reid S, Hotopf M, Hull L, et al. Multiple chemical sensitivity and chronic fatigue syndrome in British Gulf War veterans. Am J Epidemiol 2001;153:604–9.

[25] Kennedy G, Abbot NC, Spence V, et al. The specificity of the CDC-1994 criteria for chronic fatigue syndrome: comparison of health status in three groups of patients who fulfill the criteria. Ann Epidemiol 2004;14:95–100.

[26] Kipen HM, Fiedler N. Environmental factors in medically unexplained symptoms and related syndromes: the evidence and the challenge. Environ Health Perspect 2002;4:597–9.

[27] Hyams KC. Developing case definitions for symptom-based conditions: the problem of specificity. Epidemiol Rev 1998;20:148–56.

[28] Clauw DJ, Engel CC Jr, Aronowitz R, et al. Unexplained symptoms after terrorism and war: an expert consensus statement. J Occup Environ Med 2003;45:1040–8.

[29] Jones E, Hodgins-Vermaas R, McCartney H, et al. Post-combat syndromes from the Boer war to the Gulf war: a cluster analysis of their nature and attribution. BMJ 2002;324:321–4 [erratum: 397].

[30] Soetekouw PM, de Vries M, van Bergen L, et al. Somatic hypotheses of war syndromes [comment]. Eur J Clin Invest 2000;30(7):630–41.

[31] Ferrari R, Russell AS. The problem of Gulf War syndrome. Med Hypotheses 2001;56: 697–701.

[32] McCauley LA, Joos SK, Lasarer MR, et al. Gulf War unexplained illnesses: persistence and unexplained nature of self-reported symptoms. Environ Res 1999;81:215–23.

[33] Korenyi-Both AL, Juncer DJ. Al Eskan disease: Persian Gulf syndrome [comment]. Mil Med 1997;162:1–13.

[34] Korenyi-Both AL, Sved L, Korenyi-Both GE, et al. The role of the sand in chemical warfare agent exposure among Persian Gulf War veterans: Al Eskan disease and "dirty dust" [comment]. Mil Med 2000;165:321–36.

[35] Schmidt CW. Soldiers and oil well smoke. Respiratory connection remains hazy [comment]. Environ Health Perspect 2002;110:690.

[36] Etzel RA, Ashley DL. Volatile organic compounds in the blood of persons in Kuwait Oil Fires. Int Arch Environ Occup Health 1994;66:125–6.

[37] Gray GC, Smith TC, Knoke JD, et al. The postwar hospitalization experience of Gulf War Veterans possibly exposed to chemical munitions destruction at Khamisiyah, Iraq. Am J Epidemiol 1999;150:532–40.

[38] Smith TC, Gray GC, Weir JC, et al. Gulf War veterans and Iraqi nerve agents at Khamisiyah: postwar hospitalization data revisited. Am J Epidemiol 2003;158:457–67.

[39] Abu-Qare AW, Abou-Donia MB. Sarin: health effects, metabolism, and methods of analysis. Food Chem Toxicol 2002;40:1327–33.

[40] Pennisi E. Chemicals behind Gulf War syndrome? Science 1996;272:479–80.

[41] Plapp FW Jr. Permethrin and the Gulf War Syndrome. Arch Environ Health 1999;54:312.

[42] Ferguson E, Cassaday HJ. The Gulf War and illness by association. Br J Psychol 1999;90: 459–75.

[43] Wester RC, Quan D, Maibach HI. In vitro percutaneous absorption of model compounds glyphosate and malathion from cotton fabric into and through human skin. Food Chem Toxicol 1996;34:731–5.

[44] Baynes RE, Monteiro-Riviere NA, Riviere JE. Pyridostigmine bromide modulates the dermal disposition of [14C] permethrin. Toxicol Appl Pharmacol 2002;181:164–73.

[45] Schumm WR, Reppert EJ, Jurich AP, et al. Pyridostigmine bromide and the long-term subjective health status of a sample of over 700 male Reserve Component Gulf War era veterans. Psychol Rep 2002;90:707–21.

[46] Karczmar A. Invited review: anticholinesterases: dramatic aspects of their use and misuse. Neurochem Int 1998;32:401–11.

[47] Shen ZX. Pyridostigmine bromide and Gulf War syndrome. Med Hypotheses 1998;51:235–7.

[48] Mackness B, Durrington PN, Mackness MI. Low paraoxonase in Persian Gulf War Veterans self-reporting Gulf War Syndrome. Biochem Biophys Res Commun 2000;276: 729–33.

[49] Haley RW, Billecke S, La Du BN. Association of low PON1 type Q (type A) arylesterase activity with neurologic symptom complexes in Gulf War veterans. Toxicol Appl Pharmacol 1999;157:227–33.

[50] Mackness B, Mackness MI, Arrol S, et al. Effect of the molecular polymorphisms of human paraoxonase (PON1) on the rate of hydrolysis of paraoxon. Br J Pharmacol 1997;122:265–8.

[51] Hotopf M, Mackness MI, Nikolaou V, et al. Paraoxonase in Persian Gulf War veterans. J Occup Environ Med 2003;45:668–75.

[52] Bolton JP, Foster CR. Battlefield use of depleted uranium and the health of veterans. J R Army Med Corps 2002;148:221–9.

[53] Bem H, Bou-Rabee F. Environmental and health consequences of depleted uranium use in the 1991 Gulf War. Environ Int 2004;30:123–34.

[54] Bleise A, Danesi PT, Burkart W. Properties, use and health effects of depleted uranium (DU): a general overview. J Environ Radioactivity 2003;64:93–112.

[55] McDiarmid MA, Squibb K, Engelhardt S, et al. Surveillance of depleted uranium exposed Gulf War veterans: health effects observed in an enlarged "friendly fire" cohort. J Occup Environ Med 2001;43:991–1000.

[56] Spencer PS, McCauley LA, Lapidus JA, et al. Self-reported exposures and their association with unexplained illness in a population-based case-control study of Gulf War veterans. J Occup Environ Med 2001;43:1041–56.

[57] McCauley LA, Joos SK, Spencer PS, et al. Strategies to assess validity of self-reported exposures during the Persian Gulf War. Portland Environmental Hazards Research Center. Environ Res 1999;81:195–205.

[58] Mahan CM, Kang HK, Dalager NA, et al. Anthrax vaccination and self-reported symptoms, functional status, and medical conditions in the National Health Survey of Gulf War Era Veterans and their families. Ann Epidemiol 2004;14:81–8.

[59] Kang HK, Bullman TA. Mortality among US veterans of the Persian Gulf war. N Engl J Med 1996;335:1498–504.

[60] Writer JV, DeFraites RF, Brundage JF. Comparative mortality among US military personnel in the Persian Gulf region and worldwide during Operations Desert Shield and Desert Storm. JAMA 1996;275:118–21.

[61] Macfarlane GJ, Thomas E, Cherry N. Mortality among UK Gulf War veterans. Lancet 2000;356:17–21.

[62] Kang HK, Bullman T. Counterpoint: negligible "healthy-warrior effect" on Gulf War veterans' mortality [comment]. Am J Epidemiol 1998;148:324–5.

[63] Gray GC, Smith TC, Kang HK, et al. Are Gulf War veterans suffering war-related illnesses? Federal and civilian hospitalizations examined, June 1991 to December 1994. Am J Epidemiol 2000;151:63–71.

[64] Gray GC, Coate BD, Anderson CM, et al. The postwar hospitalization experience of US veterans of the Persian Gulf war. N Engl J Med 1996;335:1505–13.

[65] Knoke JD, Gray GC. Hospitalizations for unexplained illnesses among US veterans of the Persian Gulf War [comment]. Emerg Infect Dis 1998;4:211–9.

[66] Smith TC, Heller JM, Hooper TI, et al. Are Gulf War veterans experiencing illness due to exposure to smoke from Kuwaiti oil well fires? Examination of Department of Defense hospitalization data. Am J Epidemiol 2002;155:908–17.

[67] Aranata MR, Moore CA, Olney RS, et al. Goldenhar syndrome among infants born in military hospitals to Gulf War veterans. Teratol 1997;56:244–51.

[68] Cowan DN, DeFraites RF, Gray GC, et al. The risk of birth defects among children of Persian Gulf War veterans. N Engl J Med 1997;336:1650–6.

[69] Cowan DN, Gray GC, DeFraites RF. Counterpoint: responding to inadequate critique of birth defects paper [comment]. Am J Epidemiol 1998;148:326–7.

[70] Penman AD, Tarver RS, Currier MM. No evidence of increase in birth defects and health problems among children born to Persian Gulf War Veterans in Mississippi. Mil Med 1996; 161:1–6.

[71] Araneta MR, Kamens DR, Zau AC, et al. Conception and pregnancy during the Persian Gulf War: the risk to women veterans. Ann Epidemiol 2004;14:109–16.

[72] Horner RD, Kamins KG, Feussner JR, et al. Occurrence of amyotrophic lateral sclerosis among Gulf War veterans [comment]. Neurology 2003;61:742–9.

[73] Haley RW. Excess incidence of ALS in young Gulf War veterans [comment]. Neurology 2003;61:750–6.

[74] Haley RW, Kurt TL. Self-reported exposure to neurotoxic chemical combinations in the Gulf War. A cross-sectional epidemiologic study [comment]. JAMA 1997;277:231–7.

[75] Pierce PF. Physical and emotional health of Gulf War veteran women. Aviat Space Environ Med 1997;68:317–21.

[76] Bell IR, Warg-Damiani L, Baldwin CM, et al. Self-reported chemical sensitivity and wartime chemical exposures in Gulf War veterans with and without decreased global health ratings. Mil Med 1998;163:725–32.

[77] Fukuda K, Nisenbaum R, Stewart G, et al. Chronic multisymptom illness affecting Air Force veterans of the Gulf War [comment]. JAMA 1998;280:981–8.

[78] Kroenke K, Koslowe P, Roy M. Symptoms in 18,495 Persian Gulf War veterans. Latency of onset and lack of association with self-reported exposures [comment]. J Occup Environ Med 1998;40:520–8.

[79] Gray GC, Kaiser KS, Hawksworth AW, et al. Increased postwar symptoms and psychological morbidity among US Navy Gulf War veterans. Am J Trop Med Hyg 1999; 60:758–66.

[80] Ishoy T, Suadicani P, Guldager B, et al. Risk factors for gastrointestinal symptoms. The Danish Gulf War Study. Dan Med Bull 1999;46:420–3.

[81] Proctor SP, Heeren T, White RF, et al. Health status of Persian Gulf War veterans: self-reported symptoms, environmental exposures and the effect of stress. Int J Epidemiol 1999; 27:1000–10.

[82] Suadicani P, Ishoy T, Guldager B, et al. Determinants of long-term neuropsychological symptoms. The Danish Gulf War Study. Dan Med Bull 1999;46:423–7.

[83] Unwin C, Blatchley N, Coker W, et al. Health of UK servicemen who served in Persian Gulf War [comment]. Lancet 1999;353:169–78.

[84] Fiedler N, Lange G, Tiersky L, et al. Stressors, personality traits, and coping of Gulf War veterans with chronic fatigue. J Psychosom Res 2000;48:525–35.

[85] Nisenbaum R, Barrett DH, Reyes M, et al. Deployment stressors and a chronic multisymptom illness among Gulf War veterans. J Nerv Ment Dis 2000;188:259–66.

[86] Steele L. Prevalence and patterns of Gulf War illness in Kansas veterans: association of symptoms with characteristics of person, place, and time of military service. Am J Epidemiol 2000;152:992–1002.

[87] Wolfe J, Proctor SP, Erickson DJ, et al. Risk factors for multisymptom illness in US Army veterans of the Gulf War. J Occup Environ Med 2002;44:271–81.

ELSEVIER
SAUNDERS

Neurol Clin 23 (2005) 541–552

NEUROLOGIC
CLINICS

The Neurology of Aviation, Underwater, and Space Environments

Lt Col Michael S. Jaffee, MD, USAF[a,b],*

[a]*Uniformed Services University of the Health Sciences, Bethesda, MD*
[b]*Wilford Hall Medical Center, 2200 Bergquist Drive, Suite 1/MMCN, Lackland
Air Force Base, TX 78236, USA*

Clinical neurology is the study of disease and dysfunction of the nervous system in our normal environment. Our normal environment is considered 1 atmosphere (atm) of pressure and has a gaseous composition of 21% oxygen and 78% nitrogen.

Aerospace and underwater neurology focus on the function of a normal nervous system exposed to environmental conditions other than those encountered in our normal standard conditions. Clinical considerations in these environments include the toxic effects of changes in atmospheric pressure and considerations of safety for aviators and scuba divers with neurologic disease. This article provides a brief overview of the environmental factors encountered in aviation, underwater, and space environments that are most implicated in neurologic dysfunction. A comprehensive review is beyond the scope of this venue.

Each of these environments has unique environmental factors related to neurologic dysfunction; there also are features shared between environments (Table 1). Environmental factors unique to the aviation environment are hypoxia and acceleration. Common environmental factors that affect the aviation and underwater environments are the effects of pressure and decompression. A unique factor of the underwater environment is the effect of gases at depth. The distinguishing feature of the space environment is microgravity.

* Wilford Hall Medical Center, 2200 Bergquist Drive, Suite 1/MMCN, Lackland Air Force Base, TX 78236.

E-mail address: michael.jaffee@lackland.af.mil

Table 1
Environmental factors related to neurologic dysfunction

	Environment		
Factor	Aviation	Underwater	Space
Hypoxia (gas at decreased pressure)	x		
Acceleration	x		
Pressure changes (gradual)	x	x	
Decompression (rapid change)	x	x	
Gases at depth (gases at increased pressure)		x	
Microgravity			x

Aviation environment

There are a number of different environmental factors that affect the nervous system at altitude in the aviation environment (Table 1). These factors include decreased oxygen, acceleration, mechanical vibration, and effects of motion on the vestibular system.

Hypoxia

Hypoxia is considered an oxygen deficiency at the tissue level. This deficiency may be caused by any number of abnormalities that affect uptake, transport, or use. The central nervous system (CNS) is thought to be particularly vulnerable to deficiencies in oxygenation. Four different types of hypoxia have been recognized: histotoxic, hyperemic, stagnant, and hypoxic [1].

Histotoxic hypoxia results from the inability of a cell to use delivered oxygen. This condition is usually due to dysfunction of the cytochrome oxidase system such as from the toxin cyanide. Hyperemic hypoxia is a decrease in oxygen use due to a reduction in oxygen carrying capacity such as in anemia. Carbon monoxide poisoning also causes this form of hypoxia due to its competitive blockade of hemoglobin oxygen binding sites and by shifting the oxygen dissociation curve to the left, making it more difficult to release peripheral oxygen to tissues. Stagnant hypoxia is decreased oxygen use due to inadequate blood flow systemically or locally. In normal environments, this type of hypoxia would be seen in clinical settings of shock. In the aviation environment, stagnant hypoxia can be a result of pooled blood from acceleration forces or seen as a complication of decompression sickness (DCS) [2].

Hypoxic hypoxia, the most common cause of hypoxia clinically and in the aviation environment, is a deficiency in alveolar oxygenation. In the normal clinical setting, this condition is most commonly due to a ventilation-perfusion mismatch. With increasing altitude, there are associated decreases in both air pressure and air density. With the decrease in pressure, there are associated decreases in partial pressures of the gases of our environment. At any altitude, the ratio of the gaseous components of air remains the same: 21% oxygen and 78% nitrogen. The total amount of oxygen we breathe is determined by the partial pressure of oxygen. Because the partial pressure of oxygen decreases with increasing altitude, the body and nervous system have less total oxygen available, which creates a risk of complications of decreased oxygen (hypoxia) [1].

In general, hypoxic hypoxia from altitude becomes clinically important whenever a human exceeds 10,000 feet in altitude. The CNS is usually the most sensitive organ to hypoxia and the first to manifest symptoms. Symptoms may include visual changes such as tunnel vision or blurred vision, fatigue, drowsiness, and headache. Clinical signs include confusion, behavioral changes, loss of coordination, and eventually, unconsciousness. An important consideration in aviation is the effect that hypoxia has on performance. There have been many studies documenting the decreased effective performance time of individuals exposed to hypoxic conditions. The onset of these symptoms is often so gradual and subtle that the aviator may not recognize his or her own decrease in cognitive performance. To enable pilots to understand their own signs and symptoms of hypoxia, they are often exposed to an altitude chamber and the condition of hypoxia during their training. This contingency must be considered because there is always a risk of mechanical failure at altitude [2].

"Time of useful consciousness" is the time from first exposure to an environment of decreased oxygen to when useful function is lost. It is not time to unconsciousness but is the time until the individual is incapable of taking proper corrective action. Time of useful consciousness becomes shorter with exertion and with increasing altitudes [1].

Treatment of hypoxic hypoxia is administration of 100% oxygen. If an oxygen system was already being used at the onset of symptoms, then a different source of oxygen should be used or the concentration should be increased. If the altitude is greater than 40,000 feet, then the oxygen must be administered under pressure. If the hypoxia cannot successfully be managed, then the aircraft should descend to an altitude of below 10,000 feet. Recovery of hypoxia symptoms is usually immediate with proper oxygenation, but symptoms such as headache and fatigue can persist [2].

Pressurized cabins are used on many aircraft to prevent hypoxia and the need for oxygen supplementation. Commercial aircraft cabins are usually pressurized to between 5000 and 7000 feet. Military cabins that are pressurized are usually maintained at 8000 feet. Pressurization to sea level is not cost effective. Pressurization is achieved by drawing in external air and delivering it, compressed, to the cabin. The outflow is controlled to maintain a positive ambient pressure [3].

Acceleration

Acceleration is the rate of change of velocity with time and occurs when the speed and/or direction of motion of a body alters [4]. Physiologic responses to acceleration are determined by its magnitude and by the duration and direction of its action. The magnitude is measured in multiples of the acceleration due to gravity (g) [5]. Duration is classified as being long or short, the time division between the two being arbitrarily set at 1 second [3]. The direction is defined by a system of anatomic axes. Pilots of civilian and military aircraft are exposed to $+gz$ at all times during G-force maneuvers because they sit upright in the flight deck. This notation refers to acceleration forces going from head to toe ("eyeballs down") [5].

The primary acute limitation to exposure to $+gz$ is the response of the CNS. The main symptoms are loss of vision and loss of consciousness due to decreased perfusion to the retina and brain as blood is forced toward the feet and away from the brain. The first vision lost is peripheral, followed by central vision, leading to a visual blackout. Loss of peripheral vision occurs when Pa is less than 50 mm Hg and blackout when Pa equals the intraocular pressure of approximately 20 mm Hg, which usually happens right before G-force–induced loss of consciousness (GLOC) [4].

Autoregulation controls cerebral blood flow during normal conditions. During G force, flow is maintained by a combination of autoregulation and the siphon effect. A pressure gradient is established between the afferent carotid arterial system and the efferent jugular venous system. This pressure differential is able to maintain cerebral blood flow with very low cerebral perfusion pressures by way of the siphon effect. Blood flow to the cerebellum and brainstem are maintained even when flow is diminished to higher cerebral centers [5].

GLOC results when blood flow to the nervous system is reduced below the critical level necessary to support conscious function. This result is a normal response to transient G-force–induced CNS ischemia. On average, there is an average total time of 15 seconds of unconsciousness, followed by a period of confusion and disorientation of 12 to 15 seconds [6]. Surveys by the US Air Force and the US Navy indicate that the pilot population of the fighter airframes report about a 12% to 14% incidence of GLOC [7].

There are often myoclonic jerks seen in association with GLOC. Centrifuge observational studies suggest that they occur in 70% of cases of GLOC. Research using EEG recordings demonstrates that during GLOC, delta activity but not epileptiform activity has been observed, even when GLOC is associated with myoclonic jerks [4].

Shared environmental stressors in aviation and underwater environments

Pressure

Human tissue is mostly composed of incompressible fluid. The gas-filled spaces of the body such as the lungs, sinuses, middle ear, and intestines are vulnerable to changes in pressure that can occur during ascent or descent. These gas-filled spaces of the body are governed by the gas laws: Boyle's, Dalton's, and Henry's [8].

Various forms of barotrauma occur when there is tissue damage when a gas-filled body space fails to equalize its internal pressure to accommodate changes in ambient pressure. These forms are governed primarily by Boyle's law, which states that at a constant temperature, the volume of a gas varies inversely with the applied pressure. Therefore, as pressure increases, volume decreases and conversely, when pressure decreases, volume expands [8,9]. There is a common pathophysiology to these "squeezes": engorgement of the mucosal lining, swelling, fluid build-up, and finally, hemorrhage into the space [3].

Problems when going from higher to lower pressures (increasing altitude in aviation and ascent to water surface when diving)
Middle ear. Middle ear barotrauma is the most common diving injury. These symptoms are prevented by repeated maneuvers such as the Valsalva or Frenzel that force exhalation against a pinched nose to keep the eustachian tube open to allow for pressure equalization of the middle ear [10].

Sinus block. On occasion, a branch of a cranial nerve can be affected. Maxillary sinus barotraumas of ascent have been associated with compression of the infraorbital branch of the trigeminal nerve, causing facial numbness [8].

Inner ear squeeze. Tinnitus, vertigo and decreased hearing are the typical symptoms of increased pressure affecting the inner ear (otic barotraumas). These symptoms may be indistinguishable from inner ear decompression sickness but the timing of symptoms and dive profile may help to clarify.

External ear squeeze. External ear pain can be associated with increasing pressures.

Problems when going from lower to higher pressure (decreasing altitude in aviation and diving deeper underwater)
Barodontalgia. Pain in a tooth can be a cause of facial pain. This pain is due to irritation of circulation in an already diseased pulp or to an increase in pressure in the air space behind a filling or deposit of caries [3].

Alternobaric vertigo. This form of vertigo arises when there is a sudden and unilateral pressure difference between the inner and middle ears. It usually arises after attempts are made at equalization with the Valsalva maneuver [10].

Pulmonary embolism and its sequelae include cerebral air embolism. Lungs expand in response to increased pressure, and when unable to vent, the pressure may be high enough to rupture alveoli and release air into the interstitial space. This air can go into one of four places: the mediastinum, subcutaneous tissue, the pleura of the lungs (pneumothorax), or the pulmonary veins through which the air bubbles can travel to the arterial circulation and cause an arterial gas embolism (AGE) that affects the cerebral or cardiac vasculature. An AGE that affects the cardiac vessels is known as AGE type I and accounts for 5% of cases. AGE accounts for 40% of the case load at active emergent dive centers in the United States. An AGE that affects the cerebral vasculature is known as AGE type II and accounts for 95% of cases. The differential diagnosis of cerebral AGE is decompression sickness (DCS) and the treatment is the same: hyperbaric recompression [8,11,12].

"Reverse" ear squeeze. In severe cases, the increase in middle ear pressure can cause reversible weakness of the facial nerve and Bell's palsy [11].

Expansion of gas in the intestine. Intestinal gas expansion can cause abdominal discomfort and increased flatulence.

Decompression sickness

DCS is a result of the release of inert gas bubbles into the bloodstream and tissues after a reduction in ambient pressure. The bubbles causing DCS are usually formed of nitrogen. When in an environment of increased pressure such as at altitude with aviation or diving at depth, the partial pressures of gases in a breathing mixture increase in proportion to the increase in ambient pressure in accordance with Dalton's law, which states that the total pressure equals the sum of partial pressures of each gas in the mixture. Oxygen is actively metabolized; however, nitrogen is inert and becomes dissolved until saturation. Henry's law relates this saturation to ambient pressure by stating that at a constant temperature, the amount of a given gas that will dissolve in a liquid is directly proportional to the partial pressure of that gas in contact with the liquid. During decompression, the increased level of nitrogen equilibrates by diffusing out of body tissues. The amount of dissolved nitrogen exceeds the body's ability to off-load the nitrogen, and the nitrogen comes out of solution as bubbles and enters the bloodstream and tissues [8,13].

Many factors affect nitrogen bubble formation. For scuba diving–related DCS, these factors include depth of the dive, length of time at depth, rate of ascent, and hypothermia. For aviation-related DCS, these factors include higher altitude (most commonly cited minimum altitude is 25,000 feet), time at altitude, faster rate of ascent, and exercise during altitude. Factors that increase the risk of DCS in aviation and diving environments include recent injury, age greater than 40 years, gender (women have a 3–4 times greater risk), and presence of a patent foramen ovale [14].

DCS symptoms have been classically grouped into type I DCS and type II DCS. Type I DCS includes joint pain and symptoms involving the skin and lymphatics. Type II DCS comprises serious symptoms or signs involving the nervous system (central or peripheral) or the cardiorespiratory system. Type II DCS usually requires rapid treatment [8].

The nitrogen bubbles cause neurologic dysfunction by mechanical effects that include nerve compression, vascular stenosis, or obstruction leading to distal ischemia. There are blood–bubble interface effects that include activation of inflammatory pathways and platelet aggregation produced by venous bubbles, with a release of vasoactive substances causing vasoconstriction [14].

Cerebral DCS most often involves the arterial circulation, whereas spinal cord DCS involves obstruction of venous drainage and the formation of bubbles within the parenchyma of the spinal cord [8].

Inner ear DCS presents with acute vertigo, nausea, emesis, nystagmus, and tinnitus. Spinal cord DCS usually presents with a partial myelopathy that localizes to the thoracic cord. Pathologic features within the cord include hemorrhagic infarcts, edema, bubble defects, axonal degeneration, and demyelination [13].

Cerebral DCS can present with an alteration in consciousness, weakness, headache, gait disturbance, fatigue, diplopia, or visual loss. The examination may show focal signs such as hemiparesis, aphasia, gait ataxia, or hemianopsia. The pathologic features of cerebral DCS are similar to those of spinal DCS, though usually not as pronounced. In addition, hyalinized vessels and lacune formation have been noted [8].

The diagnosis of neurologuic DCS is primarily clinical. MRI demonstrates abnormalities only 30% to 55% of the time. These abnormalities are best seen on T2-weighted images showing high signal lesions suggestive of ischemia, edema, and swelling. These lesions do not enhance with contrast [8].

Initial management consists of basic and advanced cardiac life support, 100% oxygen, hydration, and transport to a hyperbaric recompression facility. The definitive treatment is hyperbaric therapy using the USN Table 6 protocol. This consists of initial recompression to 60 feet with 100% oxygen for 60 minutes. The patient is then decompressed to 30 feet for two additional periods each of breathing pure oxygen and air. Hyperbaric recompression therapy reduces bubble size and increases the nitrogen gradient to expedite off-gassing. Most cases of neurologic DCS that receive prompt recompression therapy have a good recovery [13].

Differences between hypobaric (altitude) and hyperbaric (diving) DCS according to Stepanek [14] include (1) smaller nitrogen load with altitude exposure; (2) different bubble dynamics (slower release of bubbles with altitude exposure, even with the same pressure differential); (3) generally less severe symptomatology with altitude exposure; (4) different spectrum of clinical manifestations, even though there is significant overlap (altitude: cerebral > spinal; diving: spinal > cerebral); (5) inherent recompression with altitude exposure; and (6) gas density and composition (bigger role for water vapor, oxygen, and carbon dioxide at altitude).

Environmental issues in scuba diving

Effects of gas at pressures at depth

Gases taken to depth in a scuba tank remain unaffected. After gas is inhaled into the lungs, it has the same pressure as the surrounding water (ie, the ambient pressure). Because the total amount of a gas depends on the concentration and the pressure, as the ambient pressure increases, the total amount of gas exposure increases [10].

Nitrogen narcosis

Nitrogen narcosis results from a direct adverse effect of a high nitrogen pressure on nerve conduction. It causes an effect similar to alcohol or narcotics: giddiness, wooziness, disequilibrium, decreased coordination, and most important, impaired judgment. It has been known by more colorful names such as "rapture of the deep" and the "martini effect." It is always depth-related, and after it begins, it increases with increasing depth. It is said that each additional 50 feet is equivalent to another martini. The Professional Association of Diving Instructors states that nitrogen narcosis is a significant concern at any depth beyond 100 feet. The symptoms quickly resolve when the diver is brought to a more shallow depth [15].

Oxygen toxicity

Inhaled oxygen pressure that is too high can be toxic to the lungs and the CNS. Oxygen toxicity is why deep diving (greater than 170 feet) is conducted not with compressed air, with its 21% oxygen, but with a gas mixture that contains 10% oxygen (Nitrox). CNS symptoms of oxygen toxicity can be seen starting at 1.3 to 1.5 atm oxygen [16].

Symptoms of oxygen toxicity are variable and can include a generalized seizure. Other symptoms include twitching, vomiting, dizziness, vision or hearing abnormalities, anxiety, confusion, and irritability. In a 1966 review of 63 US Navy divers who had oxygen toxicity, generalized seizure was the first clinical manifestation in 25 (40%). Focal twitching was seen in 10 [17].

Possible mechanisms for how toxic levels of inspired oxygen affect the CNS include inactivation of enzymes containing sulphydryl groups (glyceraldehyde phosphate dehydrogenase, flavoprotein enzymes of the respiratory chain, and enzymes involved in oxidative phosphorylation), formation of free oxidizing radicals, and reduction in endogenous release of γ-aminobutyric acid [16].

Effects of other gases

There have been reports of carbon monoxide (CO) toxicity in divers. Symptoms range from headache to confusion and unconsciousness. Divers who are smokers are thought to be at greater risk. Cases of CO toxicity in divers are rare and have been ascribed to faulty air compressors used to fill a tank.

There are also concerns of carbon dioxide (CO_2) toxicity. This condition is more of a concern with the following circumstances: deep diving, heavy work, rapid shallow breathing, or "skip" breathing in which divers skip breaths in an effort to preserve air. Symptoms include shortness of breath, headache, confusion, and possibly, drowning [18].

Shallow-water blackout

Shallow-water blackout is a complication seen in breath-holding divers in the absence of scuba equipment or compressed air. It is sudden unconsciousness from lack of oxygen during a breath-hold dive [10].

Space neurology

The main aspects of the space environment that affect the nervous system are microgravity and various space hygiene issues (eg, radiation, toxicology, and life support) [19]. Gravity provides the CNS with a fundamental reference for estimating spatial orientation and coordinating movements in the terrestrial environment. Key developmental processes in mammals (eg, locomotion) require gravity stimuli [20].

Microgravity affects many systems of the body. Changes include redistribution of fluid and electrolytes, cardiac deconditioning, red blood cell alterations, immune system dysfunction, skeletal muscle atrophy, bone demineralization, and gastrointenstinal tract adaptations. The effect that is most relevant to neurology is the associated neurovestibular disturbances [21].

Neurovestibular disturbances

There are two main varieties of neurovestibular adaptation. The first includes vestibular reflex phenomena such as postural and movement illusions, sensations of rotation, nystagmus, vertigo, and dizziness [20].

The second form of neurovestibular adaptation is space motion sickness (SMS). SMS is due to the neurovestibular adaptation to microgravity. Symptoms that are similar to motion sickness include malaise, loss of appetite, and somnolence. There are differences between SMS and motion sickness, especially with autonomic symptoms. In SMS, there is rarely sweating, nausea, and pallor. Vomiting is usually episodic, sudden, and brief [21].

Onset of SMS ranges from minutes to hours after entering the microgravity environment and then usually resolves within 48 and 72 hours. There are two theories regarding the etiology of SMS. One is the fluid shift theory, in which SMS is caused by biochemical and biomechanical effects on the vestibular receptors. The prevailing theory involves sensory conflict that is a result of an adaptive increase in otoloth crystals and an increase in hair cells and synapses [22]. There is no correlation between SMS and prior motion sickness in astronauts.

Early literature quoted the incidence of SMS as being 40% to 50%. A more recent study reported that the incidence of SMS during a first shuttle flight was 67% [23]. Antiemetic injections have been the treatment of choice and are thought to produce a 50% reduction in symptoms. Future pharmacologic interventions may include anticonvulsants, CNS stimulants such as modafanil, 5HT3 agonists, and calcium channel blockers.

Just as adaptation occurs when going from $1g$ to a microgravity environment, there is more adaptation required when astronauts return to earth. This process involves going from a microgravity environment to being exposed to high G forces during re-entry and then a $1g$ environment. Symptoms include ataxia and decreased coordination [24]. These symptoms are thought to be due to changes in Purkinje cell morphology [25].

In addition, there have been reports of flashbacks of the vestibular symptoms experienced after return to Earth. These episodes have varied from 4 days to 2 months later [20].

Other neurology issues of space

The most common neurologic symptom reported by astronauts is headache, which has been reported by 67% of astronauts. Other neurologic consequences include impaired cognitive performance (ie, "space dementia") and impaired autonomic function. Neurologic complaints account for the most common reasons for taking medications in space. The most common reasons for taking medications in space are space motion sickness (30%), headache (20%), sleeplessness (15%), back pain (10%), and constipation (<10%) [21].

Back pain has been a chronic complaint of many astronauts. Although dull and localized to the low back, it is thought to have a different pathophysiology than the common back pain seen at $1g$. Back pain in microgravity is thought to be due to stretching of the anterior and posterior spinous ligaments, which results in approximately 7 cm of increased height at $0g$ [26].

Summary

It can be seen that aspects of different environments can have adverse effects on normal, healthy nervous systems. Aerospace and underwater neurology consultants are often required to evaluate aviators, divers, or astronauts who have a neurologic problem to determine whether they should be granted a waiver. In general, these considerations include course of the disorder (static, progressive, or paroxysmal), potential for sudden incapacitation that may compromise safety, predictability of course of the disorder, ability to monitor disease, and potential adverse effects of medications.

A background in the toxic effects of an abnormal environment on the nervous system can be used to make better clinical judgments when considering effects of exposing someone with an abnormal nervous system to such environmental stressors.

References

[1] Fisher P. High altitude respiratory physiology. In: O'Brien D, editor. USAF flight surgeons guide. 4th edition. San Antonio: USAF School of Aerospace Medicine; 1996.

[2] Pickard J. Atmosphere and respiration. In: DeHart R, Davis J, editors. Fundamentals of aerospace medicine. 3rd edition. Philadelphia: Lippincott Williams & Wilkins; 2002. p. 19–38.

[3] Harding R, Mills J. Aviation medicine. 2nd edition. BMJ 1988. p. 30–43.

[4] Burton R, Whinnery J. Biodynamics. In: DeHart R, Davis J, editors. Fundamentals of aerospace medicine. 3rd edition. Philadelphia: Lippincott Williams & Wilkins; 2002. p. 122–53.

[5] Eldridge L, Northrup S. Effects of acceleration. In: O'Brien D, editor. USAF flight surgeons guide. 4th edition. San Antonio: USAF School of Aerospace Medicine; 1996.

[6] Whinnery J, Whinnery A. Acceleration-induced loss of consciousness. Arch Neurol 1990;47: 764–76.

[7] Morrissette K, McGowan D. Further support for the concept of an GLOC syndrome: a survey of military high-performance aviators. Aviat Space Environ Med 2000;71: 496–9.

[8] Newton H. Neurologic complications of scuba diving. Am Fam Physician 2001;63:2211–8.

[9] Pennefather J. Physics and physiology. In: Edmond C, Lowry C, Pennefather J, et al, editors. Diving and subaquatic medicine. 4th edition. London: Arnold; 2002. p. 11–22.

[10] Martin L. Scuba diving explained. Questions and answers on physiology and medical aspects. Flagstaff (AZ): Best Publishing; 1997.

[11] Dick APK, Massey EW. Neurologic presentation of decompression sickness and air embolism in sport divers. Neurology 1985;35:667–71.

[12] Walker R. Pulmonary barotraumas. In: Edmonds C, Lowry C, Pennefather J, et al, editors. Diving and subaquatic medicine. 4th edition. London: Arnold; 2002. p. 137–50.

[13] Rudge F, Zwart B. Effects of decreased pressure: decompression sickness. In: O'Brien D, editor. USAF flight surgeons guide. 4th edition. San Antonio: USAF School of Aerospace Medicine; 1996.

[14] Stepanek J. Decompression sickness. In: DeHart R, Davis J, editors. Fundamentals of aerospace medicine. 3rd edition. Philadelphia: Lippincott Williams & Wilkins; 2002. p. 67–98.

[15] Richardson D, editor. Open water diver manual. Rancho Santa Margarita (CA): International PADI, Inc.; 1999.

[16] Cheshire W. Oxygen toxicity, nitrox diving, and seizures. American Academy of Neurology course. Annual meeting. Honolulu, HI, March 29–April 5, 2003.

[17] Gillen HW. Oxygen convulsions in man. Proceedings of the 3rd International Conference on Hyperbaric Medicine. Washington, DC: National Academy of Sciences; 1966.

[18] Clark J, Thorn S. Toxicity of oxygen, carbon dioxide, and carbon monoxide. In: Bove AA, editor. Diving medicine. 3rd edition. Philadelphia: W.B. Saunders Co.; 1997. p. 131–45.

[19] Locke J. Space environments. In: DeHart R, Davis J, editors. Fundamentals of aerospace medicine. 3rd edition. Philadelphia: Lippincott Williams & Wilkins; 2002. p. 245–70.

[20] Clark J. Neurological effects of space flight: adaptation, maladaptation, and readaptation. Presented at the 2004 Aerospace Medicine in Space Operations Course at USAF School of Aerospace Medicine. San Antonio, TX.

[21] Martin G. Space medicine. In: O'Brien D, editor. USAF flight surgeons guide. 4th edition. San Antonio: USAF School of Aerospace Medicine; 1996.

[22] Lackner J, Graybiel A. Etiological factors in space motion sickness. Aviat Space Environ Med 1983;54:675–81.

[23] Davis J, Vanderploeg JM, Santy PA, et al. Space motion sickness during 24 flights of the space shuttle. Aviat Space Environ Med 1988;59:1185–9.

[24] Paloski WH, Black FO, Reschke MF, et al. Vestibular ataxia following shuttle flights: effects of microgravity on otolith-mediated sebsorimotor control of posture. Am J Otol 1993;14: 9–17.

[25] Newberg A. Changes in the central nervous system and their clinical correlates during long-term spaceflight. Aviat Space Environ Med 1994;65:562–72.

[26] Wing PC, Tsang IK, Susak L, et al. Back pain and spinal changes in microgravity. Orthop Clin North Am 1991;22:255–62.

NEUROLOGIC
CLINICS

Neurol Clin 23 (2005) 553–570

Wilderness and Recreational Neurology

Ali R Malek, MD[a,b], Michael Hoffmann, MD[a,c],*

[a]Department of Neurology, University of South Florida, Tampa, FL, USA
[b]Neurocritical Care Unit, Tampa General Hospital, Tampa, FL, USA
[c]Stroke Program, Tampa General Hospital, Tampa, FL, USA

With increased access to once remote regions of the planet and renewed interest in exploring natural surroundings, previously geographically isolated and rare neurologic conditions can be encountered in any patient population. Rare envenomations and poisonings, once the purview of the tropical neurologist, now can be encountered by travelers to areas where creatures that have developed specialized defenses are endemic. Recognition, therefore, of the various potentially neurotoxic fauna and flora in these areas holds value, even for the urban neurologist. A distinction should be made between venom and poison: venom is a specialized toxic substance that a living creature can generate and deliver via biting or stinging, whereas a poison is a substance that, when consumed, is toxic.

Fauna

Although envenomations from bites and stings are rare in temperate climates, the morbidity and mortality of such events in tropical climates can be high. Despite the predilection of poisonous creatures for warmer climates, such animals are found in all animal classes, from unicellular protists to chordates, including the duck-billed platypus. The total number of species of venomous marine animals is estimated at 1200 [1], representatives of which inhabit every living ocean. Approximately 400 snake species dangerous to humans are known, and there are countless venomous arthropods found on every continent.

Reptiles

Of the approximately 3500 species of snakes, approximately 400 are sufficiently venomous to be a threat to humans. Of the lizards, only two

---

* Corresponding author. Department of Neurology, University of South Florida, 12901 Bruce B. Downs Boulevard, MDC 55, Tampa, FL 33612.
   E-mail address: mhoffman@hsc.usf.edu (M. Hoffmann).

0733-8619/05/$ - see front matter © 2005 Elsevier Inc. All rights reserved.
doi:10.1016/j.ncl.2004.12.002 *neurologic.theclinics.com*

species are venomous to humans; both are located in Mexico and the southwestern United States.

Snakes

The venomous species of snakes are the elapids: kraits, cobras, mambas, and coral snakes; the hydrophilic: true sea snakes, laticaudidae, sea kraits, and viperidae: the old world vipers and adders; and the crotalidae: rattlesnakes, copperheads, moccasins, and many others.

Snakes produce complex venoms composed of many substances, including peptides and polypeptides (many with enzymatic activity), inorganic substances, and metals. Most venomous snakes have neurotoxic and hemotoxic components; however, the proteroglyphs (snakes that have fixed fangs [eg, Elapidae, Hydrophiidae, Laticaudidae]) typically have more neurotoxic venoms and the solenoglyphs (snakes that have movable front fangs [eg, Crotalidae, Viperidae]) typically have predominantly hemotoxic venoms. The neurotoxic venoms, although diverse in formulation, result in essentially acetylcholine-mediated neuromuscular blockade, resulting in respiratory failure. Even those snakes notoriously lacking neurotoxins, such as the *Bothrops spp* of the *Viperidae*, however, can be of neurologic interest secondary to thrombin-like enzymes their venom may contain. These thrombin-like enzymes, seen in many species of the *Crotalidae* and *Viperidae*, may cause cerebrovascular infarctions and hemorrhages [2] and be the foundation of future medications used to treat acute ischemic events [3].

Lizards

There are only two venomous lizard species identified: the Gila monster, *Heloderma suspectum*, and the beaded lizard, *Heloderma horridum*. Their venom, containing high concentrations of serotonin, is transferred through saliva and is reported to cause hyperesthesia and dizziness without hypotension [4].

Amphibia

The class amphibia contains the anura (toads, frogs) and the urodela (salamanders, newts). Although many species within these groups are poisonous, only a few are of clinical significance to humans.

Toads and frogs

Within the anura, the toads of the family Bufonidae are of particular significance, in that in addition to many toads commonly secreting biogenic amines from their skin, they also produce the psychotomimetic idoalkylamines, bufotenin, bufotenidin, and bufotalin, which are described as causing hallucinations, vasoconstriction, and hypotension. Additionally, they secrete bufogenines, which affect smooth muscle contraction [5]. Of the frogs, the families Atelopodidae, Dendrobatidae, Discoglossidae, Hylidae,

Phyllomedusae, Pipidae, and Ranidae are of toxicologic significance. Tetrodotoxins, chiriquitoxin, zetekitoxins, all of which have significant neurotoxic effects, are found in species of the family Atelopodidae [6]. Batrachotoxin, one of the most potent neurotoxins known, is secreted by species of the Dendrobatidae family and is the main ingredient in the paralytic used in poison blowgun darts of the Noanamá Chocó and Emberá Chocó Indians of western Colombia [7]. Batrachotoxin modifies ion selectivity and voltage sensitivity in the sodium channels of the peripheral nerves, causing rapid paralysis [8]. The effects can be seen even when handling these particularly potent frogs.

Newts and salamanders

Tarichatoxin has been isolated from three species of newts of the genus *Taricha*: *T torosa, T rivularis,* and *T granulosa.* It later was identified as identical to tetrodotoxin, the same toxin as that from the puffer fish and that found in various species of frog and the blue-ringed octopus [9]. Samandarine, isolated from the skin of various salamanders, has a potent effect on the central nervous system (CNS), with anesthetic and hypertensive properties [10].

Marine animals

Toxic interactions with most of the approximately 1200 toxic marine animals are rare; there are, however, a few common sources of poisoning that have potentially serious implications for humans.

Protista

The protistans include approximately 80 species toxic to humans, with the most common representatives from the dinoflagellata order. Blooms of protistans are the cause of the phenomenon referred to as *red tide* and organisms normally considered edible, such as various mollusks and arthropods, become proportionally more toxic as they filter greater numbers of the toxic protists. Paralytic shellfish poison is a complex of poisons that includes saxitoxin and gonyautoxins, which can cause respiratory failure and death in patients who consume such organisms [11]. Within 30 minutes of ingestion, paresthesias that begin periorally and subsequently spread throughout the face, neck, and the distal extremities commonly are seen. Ataxia, incoherent speech, and aphonia are hallmarks of severe poisoning. Ciguatera also presents with a similar syndrome complex with associated gastrointestinal symptoms seen after ingestion of a reef fish that has concentrated levels of the dinoflagellate, *Gambierdiscus toxicus.* Excessive salivation and lacrimation, lethargy, respiratory distress, hypothermia, ataxia, hyporeflexia, perioral paresthesias, and dizziness are common neurologic findings. As most of the implicated fish species normally are edible, such poisonings are seen frequently in some parts of the world.

Enzyme-linked immunosorbent assay (ELISA) and radioimmunoassay can detect the toxin [12].

Porifera

Sponges are ubiquitous in the oceans and a potential cause of morbidity. Deposition of toxins through superficial abrasions caused by the sharp spicules can result in local trauma, which, although associated with malaise and joint pains, usually is not associated with severe systemic effects. Members of the Haliclonidae family, however, may contain neurotoxins, such as suberitine, that have the ability to block action potentials irreversibly [13].

Cnidaria

All cnidarians are venomous; however, their ability to produce morbidity or mortality in humans is directly proportional to the ability of their nematocysts, the specialized stinging cells they are equipped with, to penetrate the skin. There are three classes of cnidarians—the hydrozoa: hydromedusae and fire corals; the scyphozoa or true jellyfish; and the anthozoa: sea anemones, sea feathers, and alcyonarion corals. The toxic effects from encountering one of these creatures varies from local irritation to the Irukandji syndrome of delayed systemic effects, including backache, muscle pains, chest and abdominal pains, headache, nausea, vomiting, and restlessness, along with localized piloerection and sweating, tachycardia, and hypertension, to, as seen in the case of the sea wasp, *Chironex fleckeri*, death, sometimes within minutes [14]. Fortunately, of the more than 9000 species of cnidarians identified, fewer than 80 have been implicated in human injury.

Mollusca

Of the gastropods, the genus *Conus* contains species that can injure humans. *Conus geographicus*, the most toxic of the species, uses its venom apparatus as an offensive weapon to harpoon its piscine prey. If a human is stung, there is immediate localized pain followed initially by numbness around the wound and, subsequently, periorally and at the extremities. Within 30 minutes, tremor, muscle fasciculation, and ataxia may develop. In severe cases, progression to respiratory paralysis and death may occur.

The blue-ringed octopi, *Hapalochlaena lunulata* and *H maculosa*, are the deadliest of the cephalopods, with sufficient concentrations of tetrodotoxin in the saliva for a bite to result in respiratory paralysis and death [15].

Fish

The most common fish poisoning in humans is scombroid poisoning. There is considerable debate as to the actual offending agent; however, the accumulation of high dosages of histamine within tunas, bonitos, and other mackerel-like fish clearly is implicated. Also known as histamine fish poisoning, the decomposition by endogenous flora of the amino acid, histidine, liberating bioactive amines, predominantly histamine, results in nausea, vomiting, diarrhea, headache, burning of the throat, numbness, thirst, and generalized urticaria after consumption of the offending fish [16]. In cases of severe poisoning, muscular weakness may be seen.

The puffers contain high concentrations of tetrodotoxin, also known as fugu poison. The numbers of deaths from consumption of the puffer have decreased significantly since the Japanese requirement in 1958 for sushi chefs to be specially licensed to prepare tetchiri, the delicacy prepared from the puffer. It is, however, still used as an agent for suicide in Southeast Asia [17].

Hallucinatory fish poisoning is a self-limiting syndrome caused by the ingestion of certain species of mullet or goatfish. The syndrome consisting of dizziness, weakness, ataxia, hallucinations, and depression lasts less than 24 hours. Hallucinatory fish poisoning does not share a common cause with ciguatera and the offending agent is not well elucidated.

Venomous fish include the stingrays, scorpion fish (including the zebra fish and stone fish species), and weever fish. Their toxins predominantly are local and produce more pain and local injury than systemic effects; however, envenomation by types of scorpion fish can be associated with tremors, seizures, coma, and death. These agents commonly are thermally inactivated, and first aid involves high temperature immersion of the affected site [18].

Arthropods

The arthropods are responsible for more poisonings in humans than all other phyla combined, an amount, which, however, is inflated by the high incidence of anaphylactic reactions to bites and stings.

Spiders

Almost all of the 30,000 species of spider are venomous; however; only 200 are implicated in human morbidity. The widow spiders (*latrodectus* species) are found on all continents, with four species indigenous to the United States. Their venoms are complex; however, the neurotoxic component is identified as containing high amounts of leucine and isoleucine and a low amount of tyrosine [19]. Their bites typically are pinprick like, with subsequent aching pains of the large muscle groups. Fasciculations can be seen within 30 minutes. Rigidity of the abdomen, hyperreflexia, headache, dizziness, and high frequency tremor also can be seen. Severe hypertension may require the use of intravenous antihypertensive agents. Antivenin is reserved for severe cases of patients who are hypertensive or have significant cardiac disease; it also can be used during pregnancy and in children who have severe signs and symptoms of envenomation.

Brown spiders (*loxosceles* species) also are widespread throughout most of the world. Their venom causes significant damage to the vascular endothelium and can cause hemolysis and thrombocytopenia.

Bites from the funnel web spiders, family Hexathelidae, which are indigenous to parts of Australia, have resulted in human fatalities. The males typically have high concentrations of robustotoxin, which opens the sodium channels. Victims present with autonomic hyperactivity that can progress to coma and death. There are 13 recorded deaths from funnel web bites, but none have occurred since the introduction and local availability of antivenin.

Scorpions

Of the approximately 85 medically important scorpion species, the *Centruroides* genus is believed responsible for the majority of stings in the Americas. More than 70,000 stings a year have been reported in Mexico, with up to 100 deaths, mostly in infants. This number has been reduced tenfold with the introduction of antivenin. The clinical picture of a sting is different in children and in adults. In children, there is mild pain with localized tenderness followed by restlessness and random head and neck movements. Roving eye movements, nystagmos, and oculogyric movements commonly are described. An exaggerated startle response may be seen and tachycardia and hypertension precede the excessive salivation and respiratory failure that may occur [20]. In adults, the stings always are painful and the tachycardia occurs sooner. Ataxia may occur; however, symptoms tend to resolve within 12 to 24 hours.

Hymenoptera

The stings of hymenoptera (bees, wasps, hornets, ants) result in more deaths in the United States, as a result of anaphylactic reactions, than the bites and stings of all other venomous animals.

Ticks

Besides being vectors for numerous diseases, some species of ticks, notably *Dermacentor* and *Amblyomma*, can cause an ascending flaccid paralysis, particularly in children [21]. Generalized weakness and ataxia develop within 5 days of attachment of the tick and if it is not removed, bulbar and respiratory paralysis may ensue. It is imperative that the entire tick be removed so the capitulum does not remain in the wound. With the *Dermacentor sp*, symptom resolution is rapid after removal; however, the Australian *Ixodes holocyclus* induces paralysis that may linger for several days after removal [22].

Heat-related illnesses

The inability of humans to thermoregulate adequately in the face of extreme heat is reflected in the continuum of morbidity described as heat-related illness. Heat syncope refers to a fainting spell secondary to heat-induced orthostasis. Precipitating factors include volume depletion and prolonged standing or postural changes. A decrease in ambient temperature and placing the head down resolve this condition [23]. Heat cramps are seen on cessation of activity within a hot environment and are associated with depletion of electrolytes. Treatment involves supplementing electrolytes and fluids and decreasing temperature. Heat exhaustion is seen when hypovolemia and electrolyte depletion lead to cardiovascular insufficiency. Headache and encephalopathy can be seen, however; core temperature remains normal. If untreated, this illness may progress to heat stroke, which is characterized by hyperthermia with a core temperature above 105°F (40.6°C), anhidrosis, and encephalopathy. Predisposing factors to all heat-related illnesses include underlying medical conditions (eg, diabetes, Parkinson's disease, autonomic neuropathies), medications (eg, anticholinergics, diuretics, phenothiazines), and dehydration and alcohol use or abuse. Consequences of heat stroke include cerebral edema and petechial hemorrhages within the brain parenchyma. Recovery is dependent on how rapidly core temperature can be restored to a normal range.

Malaria and schistosomiasis

Malaria and schistosomiasis are the two most common zoonoses, ranking first and second in number of deaths worldwide. Malaria is discussed briefly in this article, as endemic areas are well known, travelers are forewarned, and prophylactic treatment and precautions known. Cerebral malaria, however, is appearing in medical centers in North America not accustomed to this condition, with approximately 1000 imported cases annually in the United States. *Plasomodium vivax*, *P malariae*, *P ovale*, and *P falciparum* constitute the four species transmitted to humans by the Anopheles mosquito. Induced malaria may occur by blood transfusions. The clinical syndrome comprising shaking chills (cold stage), fever (hot stage), diaphoresis, headache, dizziness, gastrointestinal symptoms, myalgias, arthralgias, and cough occurs in 4- to 6-hour attacks. Cerebral malaria is the most feared complication, occurring as a result of sequestration of parasitized red blood cells and vascular occlusion, causing headache, encephalopathy, coma, seizures, and stroke. Detection is achieved best by the buffy coat method in thick blood films.

Chorloquine is used for prophylaxis and mefloquine in drug-resistant areas, with alternates being malarone and doxycycline. Intravenous quinine dihydrochloride is used for severe malarial attacks and cerebral malaria. Cinchonism (toxicity), similar to the symptoms of cerebral malaria itself, needs monitoring and at times temporary discontinuation of therapy.

Schistosomiasis

Schistosomiasis is endemic to a large part of the world and is a major public health concern, second only to malaria in the tropics and subtropics.

In addition, inhabitants, contract workers, seasonal workers, and low-frequency events, such as water-based sporting events and recreational activities, pose a risk to individuals in South America, Africa, and Asia. Three schistosome species and several less prevalent species infect at least 200 million people in 74 countries worldwide. The estimated annual mortality from this hematogenous trematode fluke is approximately 200,000 people. Although the trematode is not native to North America, estimates indicate that more than 200,000 people infected with the trematode live in the United States (immigrants, contract workers, and sports enthusiasts) [24–27].

The life cycle of the digenic trematode involves the intermediate amphibious snail hosts (Biompheleria, Oncomelania) and humans. There is tropism in geographic distribution and human organ involvement among these species. *Schistosma mansoni* is found in South America (Brazil, Venezuela, and Surinam), several Caribbean islands, most of Africa, and the Middle East, with periportal fibrosis and portal hypertension the most important complications. *Schistosoma japonicum* is found in Southeast Asia (mainly China and the Philippines) with similar symptoms to *S mansoni*, but with a higher incidence of CNS involvement. *S hematobium* is extensive throughout Africa and the Middle East, with a predilection for the veins of the urinary tract, infrequently causing myelopathy [25].

Schistosomes reach the CNS at any time after the moment the worms have matured and the eggs have been laid. For this reason, CNS involvement may occur in all the clinical forms of schistosomal infection. The eggs in the CNS induce a cell-mediated periovular granulomatous reaction, sometimes inducing large necrotic-exudative granulomas, which, by virtue of mass effect, may cause increased intracranial pressure, focal neurologic signs, and rapidly progressing transverse myelitis (mostly lumbosacral). The random and sparse distribution of eggs in the CNS suggests that embolization of eggs from the portal mesenteric system to the brain and spinal cord is the main route of CNS invasion by schistosoma [28].

Biology and life cycle

Schistosome biology and life cycle are important to understand in the context of primary prevention and health hygiene measures. The schistosome life cycle is similar in all species with minor differences. Schistosomes even of the same species recently have been shown by restriction endonucleases to be genetically diverse and this is believed an important factor in the development of granulomas and fibrosis [29]. The life cycle commences with the eggs deposited in fresh water; a short-lived (8–12 hours), free-swimming miracidium hatches from an egg and infects the appropriate intermediate snail host. An amplification process then occurs, wherein the miracidium multiplies through a first- and then second-stage sporocyst to produce many cercariae (usually thousands from one miracidium), which also are released into the water, this time targeting the human or other vertebrate host. These cercariae are viable for only approximately 48 hours, after which they no longer are infectious. Once a cercaria penetrates the host, it is called a schistosomula. A journey through several organs then occurs, from the skin to the peripheral lymphatic and venous vessels, in approximately 2 days, to the right side of the heart and lung within a week, and thereafter via an intravascular route to the liver portal vessels, feeding on the blood and eventually developing into adult worm, producing 20 to 290 eggs per day (*S japonicum* produces 3500 eggs per day). These sexually mature worms leave the liver after they mate and migrate to the mesenteric plexus (in the case of *S mansoni*) or the vesical plexus (in the case of *S hematobium*). The female worms pass the eggs through the bladder or bowel, excreting them via the urine or feces. People inhabiting and frequenting rivers and waterways thus are able to complete the schistosome life cycle, with their excreta finding their way back into the water [27].

Pathophysiology

The clinical manifestations of the pathophysiologic response to schistosomiasis infections vary throughout the different stages of the schistosome life cycle and its intersection with a human host.

1. Initial invasion: termed *cercarial dermatitis* or *swimmer's itch*, it is caused by penetration into the skin by cercariae of human and non-human schistosomes.
2. Maturation stage: acute schistosomiasis or Katayama fever is an allergic response to a developing antigenic mass of ova and worms presenting as a serum sickness or an acute febrile illness with pyrexia, urticaria, pulmonary and liver involvement, and lymphadenopathy.
3. Chronic schistosomiasis: host immune reaction to the eggs in organs with the formation of edema, granulation tissue, fibrosis, vascular obstruction, and calcification.

In areas where schistosomiasis is endemic, initial infection mostly is unnoticed. Factors responsible for this include age of first exposure, nature of exposure, transfer of antigens, antibodies and anti-idiotypes from the mother. Visitors to endemic areas, alternatively, may suffer an acute febrile illness as a manifestation of the immune response to the eggs and worms (Katayama fever). Such people have an elevated eosinophil count and immune complexes that react vigorously to schistosome antigens. The immune response may be measured by lymphocyte blastogenesis. The inflammatory and fibrotic response of host tissue determines the severity of an individual's disease. Although protective immunity has been demonstrated in experimental animals, it has not been documented adequately in humans. The immune response that an individual may mount to schistosomal infection includes antibodies, eosinophils, neutrophils, macrophages, and complement. The schistosomule is relatively susceptible to an immune attack in the first few days after infection, gradually becoming resistant with maturity. Several mechanisms are responsible, including schistosomules coating their tegument with host proteins to evade recognition by the host's immune surveillance system. The egg antigen–induced granulomatous response by the host is T-cell mediated, which, after initially causing growth of the granuloma, subsequently diminishes with continuing infection resulting from the recruitment of suppressor T cells. Eggs and granulomas release fibroblast proliferation factors with eventual end-stage portal fibrosis in the liver, with S mansoni and glomerulonephritis from systemically circulating immune complexes.

The CNS disease involvement is rare (3% to 5%) and occurs as a result of aberrant deposition of eggs in nervous tissue, either by migration of adult worms or transport of eggs into nervous system circulation by collateral veins [30].

Clinical syndromes: systemic and neurologic

Systemic

Acute schistosomiasis. Usually occurring in visitors and rarely found in endemic populations, acute schistosomiasis is most common with S mansoni and S japonicum (rarely S hematobium). Initial itching of the skin where the cercariae penetrate may be followed by weeks of systemic illness (pyrexia, weight loss, angioedema, cough, and headache), called Katayama fever and is not diagnosed easily, especially when presenting in North America and, consequently, forms part of the differential of pyrexia of unknown origin and pyrexia with protracted course. Diagnosis is established by considering possible exposure, a marked eosinophilia, increased immune complexes, antibodies to adult schistosome gut antigens, and eggs in the stool or eggs seen on microscopy from rectal biopsy.

Hepatic fibrosis: Symmers' fibrosis. Globally, the most significant complication of schistosomiasis infections (S mansoni, S japonicum, S mekongi) classically is the left lobe of the liver affected with macroscopic pipe stem fibrosis, progressive disease resulting in portal hypertension, hepatosplenomegaly, esophageal and gastric varices, and hematemesis. Pulmonary hypertension may complicate hepatic periportal fibrosis and portal hypertension and is likely the result of the obliteration of pulmonary arterioles by granulomatous inflammation secondary to embolization of schistosome eggs. Periportal fibrosis is diagnosed best by ultrasonography and liver biopsies.

Glomerulonephritis. This is a rare complication resulting from immune complex disease, as in pulmonary hypertension, that occurs almost exclusively in people who have periportal fibrosis in any of its three major forms (*S mansoni, S hematobium, S japonicum*).

Anemia. Protein-losing enteropathy results from inflammatory polyps that develop in the large intestine from deposition of eggs causing the formation of an exudative granulomatous process, inflammatory cells, and fibrosis. A dysentery-like illness may develop. Salmonella infections are not infrequent in patients who have *S hematobium* infections and it is postulated that a type of symbiosis may exist between salmonella and schistosomiasis, the salmonella being protected from the host immune system by either co-existence either within the schistosome or attachment to it. This has clinical importance in that both require treatment.

Central nervous system involvement

CNS involvement was first reported in 1889 in Japan by Yamagiwa, who described intracerebral granulomas with *S japonicum* ova. Overall, CNS complications from schistosomiasis has been reported as rare, but from postmortem and recent clinical studies, it is apparent that nervous system involvement occurs in many more patients than is suggested by clinical symptomotology. Involvement occurs with *S mansoni, S hematobium*, and *S japonicum*, the former two species causing mainly spinal cord involvement and the latter cerebral lesions (up to 3% of infections).

The mechanism of central nervous system invasion. Ectopic egg deposition is responsible for nervous system involvement; the usual sites of infection and subsequent organ damage are the splenohepatic system and urinary tract and bladder. The route by which eggs are deposited remains speculative and unproven. A valveless plexus of veins, named after Batson, connects the deep iliac veins and inferior vena cava with the veins of the brain and spinal cord. It is postulated that during episodes of increased intra-abdominal pressure (coughing, defecation, valsalva, constipation, urinary retention), the abdominal venous flow can become reversed and the eggs that are deposited normally in the portacaval system can enter the spinal cord and subsequently cerebral veins. Other mechanisms include embolization to the brain via portal-pulmonary arteriovenous anastomosis and direct oviposition by adult worms residing adjacent to the cerebral veins or vertebral venous veins. It also is postulated that the smaller egg size of *S japonicum* and the far greater daily egg production accounts for the more frequent cerebral involvement by this species [29–34].

Spinal schistosomiasis. Spinal schistosomiasis is the most common form of CNS involvement, with *S mansoni* and *S hematobium* displaying a predilection for the lower spinal cord. All the forms discussed later arise from ectopic schistosome ova deposition with host inflammatory responses and tissue damage afterwards. Schistosomal spinal cord disease is the result almost solely of *S hematobium* and *S mansoni* and in endemic areas is a common cause of myelopathy of nontraumatic cause, as pointed out recently by Haribhai et al [32].

Intrathecal granuloma formation. Granulomatous mass lesions nearly always are low lumbar and sacral, with the most common level of involvement the T12-L1, conus, and cauda equina regions. The clinical presentation is a radicular syndrome with flaccid, often asymmetric paraparesis with hyporeflexia or areflexia associated with sphincter dysfunction, low back pain, and dermatomal sensory impairment attributed to lesions affecting the sacral, lumbar, and, at times, lower thoracic segments. Rarely, the paraparesis or plegia is associated with velocity-dependent increased hypertonicity. The presentation of the myelopathy is acute to subacute over days to a few weeks.

Transverse myelitis. Temporally, either an acute or subacute presentation constitutes the most common form of spinal cord involvement. As with the intrathecal granuloma form of affliction, the predilection is for the lower cord, unlike other forms of myelitis, which more commonly infect the midthoracic cord. The pathophysiology in this form is postulated to be vasculitis of the spinal vessels with myelonecrosis following. Clinical presentation is with symmetric or asymmetric flaccid paraparesis, sensory impairment, sphincter incontinence, and back and limb pain. It is a diagnosis of exclusion.

Radiculitis. This clinical presentation, radiculitis, occurs when the granulomas impinge on a nerve root, with accompanying host reaction and inflammation and tissue fibrosis. Multiple nerve root involvement may occur and eventually lead to a spinal arachnoiditis diagnosed from circumstantial evidence, myelography, CT myelography, or MRI.

Radiculomyelitis. The various forms of spinal cord involvement denote merely anatomic variations of the infections and extent. Clinical signs of upper and lower motor neuron involvement in the lower spinal cord along with the necessary cerebrospinal fluid (CSF) pleocytosis, peripheral blood eosinophilia, radiology, and serologic tests for schistosomiasis are required for a diagnosis of radiculomyelitis.

Vascular events. This is the rarest form of spinal involvement possibly underreported with a differential diagnosis of acute anterior spinal artery occlusion. A recent prospective study from Brazil reported on 63 patients who had schistosomal myeloradiculopathy and were treated treated with corticosteroid and praziquantel. The most frequent radiographic findings included enlargement of the medullary cone and of the roots of the cauda equina. Prognosis was favorable in 38 (60.3%) patients and improvement usually started usually within the first 48 hours after commencing on steroids [34].

Spinal schistosomiasis presents the clinician with a differential diagnosis of nontraumatic myelopathy, including:

1. Parasitic infections (schistosomiasis, neurocysticercosis, gnathostomiasis, paragonomiasis)
2. Fungal infections (cryptococcosis, echinococcosis)
3. Bacterial infections (neurosyphilis, tuberculosis)
4. Viral infections (HTLV-1 myelopathy, HIV-myelopathy, Epstein-Barr myelopathy, cytomegalovirus myelopathy, hepatitis-associated myelopathy)
5. Demyelinating conditions (multiple sclerosis, Devic's disease)
6. Deficiency diseases (subacute combined-degeneration, vitamin B_{12}-deficiency)
7. Tumors (ependymomas, Burkitt's lymphoma)

Cerebral schistosomiasis

Focal deficits: mass lesions. The frequency of infection with *S japonicum* ranges from 2% to 5%, but no systematic studies are available. Almost any presentation consistent with mass lesions in the cortex, subcortical regions, basal nuclei, and white matter can occur with long tract signs and even isolated headache may occur. An encephalopathic presentation may occur with *S hematobium* and *S mansoni* and with *S japonicum*. Anatomic brain imaging with MRI brain scanning usually is diagnostic with appropriate clinical, laboratory evidence, and electroencephalogram in the diagnosis of the encephalopathic forms [24,27].

Epilepsy. This may present as generalized or focal jacksonian seizure types. Paroxysmal theta and delta slowing, asymmetric background rhythms, and spikes and sharp waves are reported by electroencephalographers.

Encephalitis/encephalomyelitis and meningitis. These occur as fulminating illness with spiking fever; behavioral changes and long tract signs of motor, sensory, and visual tract deficits; coma; meningeal irritation; and papilledema signifying raised intracranial pressure. The interval between exposure and first cerebral symptoms ranges from 6 weeks to 6 months.

Cerebrovascular events. These events are rare, but egg embolism and border zone infarctions resulting from microembolism with multiple distal border zone ischemic strokes associated with hypereosinophilia due to acute *S mansoni* infestation are two reported mechanisms [35].

Diagnosis and treatment. Given a history of exposure and an appropriate clinical syndrome, laboratory diagnosis is important, as the differential diagnosis of infective disorders affecting the brain and spinal cord is wide (Box 1). A peripheral eosinophilia (absolute count > 700/μL) is invariable, and stool and urine specimens are important to test for the ova, bearing in mind that with *S hematobium*, mid-day urine specimens most likely yield eggs in patients harboring them. Rectal mucosal biopsy is useful if urine and stool specimens are negative and suspicion remains high. In endemic populations, urine, stool specimens, and rectal biopsies frequently are positive for ova in entirely asymptomatic persons.

Haribhai et al [32] used serodiagnostic tests in a comprehensive prospective myelopathy protocol, finding that CSF–ELISA was moderately sensitive but not absolutely specific. Evengard's study [32a] compared the total IgE, total eosinophil counts, ELISA, and indirect immunofluorescence and found the specificity and sensitivity of the ELISA best at 95% and 96%, respectively.

Another test is the indirect hemagglutination test, with relatively low sensitivity. To date, the ELISA test has been the most reliable, with egg antigens giving better results than worm antigens. The polymerase chain reaction is the most sensitive method for detecting DNA and already has been applied to the diagnosis of toxoplasmosis, falciparum malaria, and Chagas' disease and may be a future tool for schistosomiasis testing.

CSF testing is important for diagnosis and for excluding other spinal infections. The findings are relatively nonspecific and include a pleocytosis of approximately 100 cells per μL, with a lymphocyte and, less commonly, a neutrophil predominance and at times eosinophilia. The latter is highly suggestive of parasitic diseases in general. Protein elevation is the rule, as are normal to slightly depressed glucose levels. CSF–ELISA levels and

---

Box 1. Classification of schistosomal central nervous system involvement

1. Spinal schistosomiasis
   Granulomatous medullary compressive type: conus and
     cauda equina
   Acute and subacute transverse myelitic
   Radicular type
   Radiculomyelitic type
   Vascular
2. Cerebral schistosomiasis
   Mass lesions: focal deficits
   Epilepsy
   Vascular: border zone and embolic
3. Encephalitis/encephalomyelitis and meningitis

intrathecal antibody production are useful diagnostic measurements that decrease after appropriate praziquantel therapy.

Radiology. Most studies to date have used myelography and CT myelography, with characteristic features being an expanded lower spinal cord or conus medullaris in the granulomatous cord mass lesions. Myelography on its own classically shows a partial or at times complete block of approximately one vertebral body vertical extent. Myelography is relatively insensitive and a normal myelogram does not exclude the diagnosis, being superseded by MRI. MRI changes include an irregularly enlarged conus or lower spinal cord with heterogeneous enhancement. With more advanced or longstanding disease, cord atrophy may be noted with CT or MRI scanning. In schistosomal transverse myelitis, early studies with CT myelography usually are normal with MRI scanning sometimes showing changes, none of which are specific.

Management and treatment

Control of schistosomiasis

Health education measures include the curbing of indiscriminate urination and defecation into streams and rivers. Intermediate host control involves the use of molluscicides or destroying the snail habitat. Such drastic measures, however, need to be assessed in terms of environmental impact and ecosystem homeostasis. Currently, management is restricted to the chemotherapy of infected or symptomatic individuals.

Chemotherapy

The mainstay treatment of all forms of schistosomiasis, either systemic or involving the nervous system, is praziquantel, given in an oral dosage of 40 mg/kg immediately. Oxamniquine 15 mg/kg in a single oral dosage with food is similarly effective. Metrifonate has advantages of low cost but an inconvenient dosing of 7.5 to 10 mg/kg administered biweekly for three dosages [36–39].

Steroids

The use of steroids is controversial, but because of the inflammatory component of granulomatous and necrotic myelitis lesions, they are used in conjunction with praziquantel, especially in severe infections. Rapid resolution of clinical symptoms has been documented many times using steroids alone. A commonly used dosage is 60 mg/d for 2 weeks [32,36,37].

Topical treatment

N,N-diethyl-meta-toluamide (DEET) was studied as a schistosomiasis prophylactic in vivo for the use in individuals who had limited exposure.

Application of 50% DEET to skin after exposure to lake water is promising after a limited recent study in Malawi [40].

Surgery

Laminectomy may be required in patients presenting with acute paraplegia, incontinence, and spinal granulomatous mass lesions on radiologic imaging.

Vaccination

Despite almost 40 years of effort, there still is no effective vaccine against schistosomiasis, although a single vaccine candidate currently is undergoing clinical trials. Although the schistosome parasites cause little in the way of disease, the trapped eggs in the tissues of the host elicit powerful and damaging immune responses responsible for the pathology. The problems remain in the identification of appropriate protective antigens that elicit immune responses that attack the parasite without cross-reacting with egg antigens, which increase the chance of developing severe chronic disease in infected individuals [41].

Prognosis

The majority of patients improve dramatically with chemotherapy, especially if treated early in the course of disease. Improvement occurs within days to weeks after treatment with steroids and with praziquantel. With clinical improvement, concomitant normalization of the CSF glucose, protein, cells, ELISA titers, and spinal cord conus shrinkage (in those who have documented swelling) can be expected, as shown by Haribhai et al in their prospective myelopathy study [32]. Scrimgeour et al report a mortality decrease from 72% before 1965 to 11.5% or less in 1985 in patients who had confirmed schistosomal myelopathy [30]. With MRI and more accurate serodiagnostic techniques, this figure may be lower at the time of this writing. The current trend in treatment in patients who have a schistosomal syndrome is early use of praziquantel, using steroids in selected cases. Depending on circumstances, treatment based on circumstantial evidence alone is to administer effective therapy to affected persons using drugs that have minimal side effects.

From a more global perspective, the failure of a vaccine to date has prompted multinational consensus on primary prevention [42]. Prospects remain, however, for specific treatment with the advent of the S mansoni genome project [43] and newer chemotherapeutic agents [44].

References

[1] Russel FE. Marine toxins and venomous and poisonous marine animals. In: Blaxter JHS, Russell FS, Yonge CM, editors. Advances in marine biology. London: Academic Press; 1984. p. 60.

[2] Mosquera A, Idrovo LA, Tafur A, et al. Stroke following Bothrops spp. snakebite. Neurology 2003;60:1577–80.

[3] Sherman DG. Antithrombotic and hypofibrinogenetic therapy in acute ischemic stroke: what is the next step? Cerebrovasc Dis 2004;17(Suppl 1):138–43.

[4] Strimple PD, Tomassoni AJ, Otten EJ, et al. Report on envenomation by a Gila monster (Heloderma suspectum) with a discussion of venom apparatus, clinical findings, and treatment. Wilderness Environ Med 1997;8:111–6.

[5] Maciel NM, Schwartz CA, Rodrigues Pires O Jr, et al. Composition of indolealkylamines of Bufo rubescens cutaneous secretions compared to six other Brazilian bufonids with phylogenetic implications. Comparative Biochemistry & Physiology. Part B. Biochem Mol Biol 2003;134:641–9.

[6] Yotsu-Yamashita M, Kim YH, Dudley SC Jr, et al. The structure of zetekitoxin AB, a saxitoxin analog from the Panamanian golden frog Atelopus zeteki: a potent sodium-channel blocker. Proc Natl Acad Sci USA 2004;101:4346–51.

[7] Myers CW, Daly JW, Malkin B. A dangerously toxic new frog. Bull Am Museum Natural History 1978;161.

[8] Catterall WA. Neurotoxins that act on voltage-sensitive sodium channels in excitable membranes. Annu Rev Pharmacol Toxicol 1980;20:15–43.

[9] Fuhrman FA. Tetrodotoxin, tarichatoxin, and chiriquitoxin: historical perspectives. Ann N Y Acad Sci 1986;479:1–14.

[10] Daly JW, Myers CW, Whittaker N. Further classification of skin alkaloids from neotropical poison frogs (Dendrobatidae), with a general survey of toxic/noxious substances in the amphibia. Toxicon 1987;25:1023–95.

[11] Garcia C, del Carmen Bravo M, Lagos M, et al. Paralytic shellfish poisoning: post-mortem analysis of tissue and body fluid samples from human victims in the Patagonia fjords. Toxicon 2004;43:149–58.

[12] Matta J, Navas J, Milad M, et al. A pilot study for the detection of acute ciguatera intoxication in human blood. J Toxicol Clin Toxicol 2002;40:49–57.

[13] Cariello L, Tosti E, Zanetti L. The hemolytic activity of suberitine. Comp Biochem Physiol [C] 1982;73:91–3.

[14] Harrison SL, Leggat PA, Fenner PJ, et al. Reported knowledge, perceptions, and behavior of tourists and North Queensland residents at risk of contact with jellyfish that cause the "Irukandji syndrome." Wilderness Environ Med 2004;15:4–10.

[15] Walker DG. Survival after severe envenomation by the blue-ringed octopus (Hapalochlaena maculosa). Med J Australia 1983;2:663–5.

[16] Hall M. Something fishy: six patients with an unusual cause of food poisoning! Emerg Med 2003;15:293–5.

[17] Matsui T, Ohtsuka Y, Sakai K. [Recent advances in tetrodotoxin research] [Japanese]. Yakugaku Zasshi 2000;120:825–37.

[18] Perkins RA, Morgan SS. Poisoning, envenomation, and trauma from marine creatures. Am Fam Physician 2004;69:885–90.

[19] Grishin EV. Neurotoxin from black widow spider venom. Structure and function. Adv Exp Med Biol 1996;391:231–6.

[20] Osnaya-Romero N, de Jesus Medina-Hernandez T, Flores-Hernandez SS, et al. Clinical symptoms observed in children envenomated by scorpion stings, at the children's hospital from the State of Morelos, Mexico. Toxicon 2001;39:781–5.

[21] Greenstein P. Tick paralysis. Med Clin North Am 2002;86:441–6 [Mar.].

[22] Grattan-Smith PJ, Morris JG, Johnston HM, et al. Clinical and neurophysiological features of tick paralysis. Brain 1997;120(Pt 11):1975–87.

[23] Lugo-Amador NM, Rothenhaus T, Moyer P. Heat-related illness. Emerg Med Clin North Am 2004;22:315–27.

[24] Blansjaar BA. Schistosomiasis. In: Vinken PJ, Bruyn GW, editors. Handbook of clinical neurology. Amsterdam: North Holland; 1988. p. 535–43.

[25] Savioli L, Renganathan E, Montresor A, et al. Control of schistosomiasis—a global picture. Parasitol Today 1997;13:444–8.

[26] Mahmoud AAF, Wahab MFA. Schistosomiasis. In: Warren KS, Mahmoud AAF, editors. Tropical and the geographic medicine. 2nd edition. New York: McGraw-Hill; 1990. p. 458–73.

[27] Nash TE, Cheever AW, Ottesen EA, et al. Schistosome infections in humans: perspectives and recent findings. Ann Intern Med 1982;97:740–54.

[28] Pittella JE. Neuroschistosomiasis. Brain Pathol 1997;7:649–62.

[29] Capron A, Dessaint JP. Immunologic aspects of schistosomiasis. Annu Rev Med 1992;43: 209–18.

[30] Scrimgeour EM, Gajdusek DC. Involvement of the central nervous system in Schistosoma mansoni and S hematobium infection. Brain 1985;108:1023–38.

[31] Cosnett JE, Van DJ. Schistosomiasis (Bilharzia) of the spinal cord: case reports and clinical profile. Q J Med 1985;61:1131–9.

[32] Haribhai HC, Bhigjee AI, Bill PL, et al. Spinal cord schistosomiasis. A clinical, laboratory and radiological study, with a note on therapeutic aspects. Brain 1991;114:709–26.

[32a] Evengard B. Diagnostic and clinical aspects of schistosomiasis in 182 patients treated at a Swedish ward for tropical diseases during a 10-year period. Scandinavian Journal of Infectious Diseases 1990;22(5):585–94.

[33] Case records of the Massachusetts General Hospital. Weekly clinicopathologic exercises. Case 21–195. A 21 year old man with fever, diarrhea and weakness of the legs during a sojourn in Kenya. N Engl J Med 1985;312:1376–83.

[34] Carod Artal FJ, Vargas AP, Horan TA, et al. Schistosoma mansoni myelopathy: clinical and pathologic findings. Neurology 2004;63:388–91.

[35] Ferrari TC, Moreira PR, Cunha A, et al. Spinal cord schistosomiasis: a prospective study of 63 cases emphasizing clinical and therapeutic aspects. J Clin Neurosci 2004;11:246–53.

[36] King CH, Mahmoud AAF. Drugs five years later. Praziquantel. Ann Intern Med 1989;110: 290–6.

[37] Molyneux ME, Galatius-Jensen F. Successful drug treatment of schistosomal myelopathy: a case report. S Afr Med J 1978;54:871–2.

[38] Watt G, Adapon B, Long GW, et al. Praziquantel in treatment of cerebral schistosomiasis. Lancet 1986;2:529–32.

[39] Hagan P, Appleton CC, Coles GC, et al. Schistosomiasis control: keep taking the tablets. Trends Parasitol 2004;20:92–7.

[40] Jackson F, Doherty JF, Behrens RH. Schistosomiasis prophylaxis in vivo using N, N-diethyl-m-toluamide (DEET). Trans R Soc Trop Med Hyg 2003;97:449–50.

[41] Lebens M, Sun JB, Czerkinsky C, et al. Current status and future prospects for a vaccine against schistosomiasis. Expert Rev Vaccines 2004;3:315–28.

[42] Schistosomiasis Control in Sub-Saharan Africa. Proceedings of a round table, Lisbon, Portugal, September 9, 2002. Bull Soc Pathol Exot 2004;97:3–63.

[43] LoVerde PT, Hirai H, Merrick JM, et al. Schistosoma mansoni genome project: an update. Parasitol Int 2004;53:183–92.

[44] Bonn D. Schistosomiasis: a new target for calcium channel blockers. Lancet Infect Dis 2004;4:190.

ELSEVIER
SAUNDERS

NEUROLOGIC
CLINICS

Neurol Clin 23 (2005) 571–597

Radiation as a Nervous System Toxin

L. Cameron Pimperl, Lt Col, USAF, MC

*Department of Radiation Oncology, Wilford Hall Medical Center, 2200 Bergquist Drive,
Suite 1/MMCN, Lackland Air Force Base, TX 78236, USA*

The neurotoxic effects of radiation can be characterized best by the study of a broad range of radiation exposures from various sources. These sources include radiation used therapeutically in the medical field, low-level exposures from various sources, and higher level exposures from nuclear accidents or intentional exposures in the atomic bomb survivors.

Although there are substantial coherent data among people exposed to higher doses of radiation from medical exposures, radiologic accidents, and the atomic bomb survivors, there is a great deal of controversy and an enormous body of literature over the effects of low-level exposures. Much of the available data at all levels of exposure exhibit what is referred to as a "dose response" for adverse effects, meaning that the likelihood of the event occurring or the severity of the effect increases with increasing radiation dose. Much effort is expended in the literature to attempt to characterize the doses involved and to attempt to correlate outcomes with dose levels. Where small numbers of adverse events occur, a pattern of clustering of these events among the individuals with the highest levels of exposures can lend support to radiation as a causal factor. Although this article alludes to the dose data to some extent, they are presented in a broad conceptual context, and the reader is referred to the references themselves for more detail.

The impact of exposure of living cells to radiation

Radiation exposure may or may not damage living cells, causing death in some, and modifying others. Considerable numbers of cells can be lost from most tissues or organs without substantial effect, but if the number lost is

---

The views expressed in this article are those of the author and do not reflect the official policy of the Department of Defense or other Departments of the United States Government.

E-mail address: loyd.pimperl@lackland.af.mil

significant enough, clinically apparent harm or even death can result. Even in cells that do not die, modifications caused by irradiation can develop. These modifications are usually repaired; however, when they are not completely repaired, they may be transferred to the cell's progeny and occasionally produce a cancer cell. If germ cells are modified in this way, potentially hereditable abnormalities may be produced that are transmitted to the offspring of the exposed individual [1,2].

The cancer-causing potential of radiation exposure can be statistically significant when large populations are studied, although in absolute terms the impact may be rather small. For example, of the 86,500 survivors of the bombings of Hiroshima and Nagasaki, there have been more than 440 solid cancer deaths caused by radiation exposure (excluding leukemia), although further follow-up of still-living survivors is necessary to determine the total impact [3]. Cases of known excess cancer deaths caused by solid tumors thus far represent 0.5% of that population.

Radiation effects other than carcinogenesis vary depending on the tissue type studied. Considerable variability exists between the radiosensitivity of various organs and tissues, with the most affected tissues generally being those that have greater reproductive activity and greater cell turnover. Within the nervous system, the effects of radiation can produce functional aberrations that are a combination of the direct toxic effects on the neurons themselves, combined with the adverse impact on neuronal function that results from injury to the broad range of supporting cells and tissues.

Pathophysiology of radiation neurotoxicity

Response of the nervous system to radiation injury is similar to the response elsewhere in the body. High doses of brain irradiation can lead to rapid death because of neuronal cell injury. Nonlethal doses of radiation can lead to varying degrees of gliosis similar to the fibrotic response elsewhere in the body. Injury to oligodendroglia can produce demyelination and resulting impairment of nerve impulse transmission. Damage to the blood-brain barrier can produce cerebral edema. Vascular injury can produce impairment of circulation with resulting ischemic injury. Secondary neoplasms can be produced. These injuries can occur in the peripheral nervous system to a lesser extent—and generally at higher doses—than in the central nervous system (CNS), with brachial plexopathy being one of the more common examples [4].

From autopsies on humans treated with radiation for malignancies of the nervous system or for other malignancies nearby, various pathologic changes after irradiation have been categorized as early (before 6 months), intermediate (from 6–9 months), and delayed (more than 12 months). Early injury to the brain may produce shallow sulci and flattened convolutions, and tonsillar herniation may be present. Evidence of focal demyelination and edema may be appreciated histologically. Blood vessels may be dilated, and platelet-fibrin thrombi may be present with perivascular collections of mononuclear cells [4].

The delayed pathologic findings may include a small brain with wide sulci and dilated ventricles. Brain necrosis may be found, usually only in the white matter and usually soft and waxy on the cut surface, but older lesions may be more contracted and circumscribed. Microscopically, myelin destruction accompanied by vascular changes can be seen with hemorrhagic exudates and occlusion of capillaries. A loss of endothelial cells occurs, and severe cases can result in vasogenic edema [5–7]. Calcifications sometimes occur, presumably representing lesions of mineralizing microangiopathy [8]. Plaques of demyelination may be found in white matter. Ischemic infarcts may be seen but are much less common than necrosis or plaques [4].

The pathogenesis of delayed lesions is multifactorial. Vascular injuries with loss of microvasculature and large blood vessel injury produce various degrees of ischemia. Necrosis can develop and is possibly related to vascular injury caused by the predominant occurrence in less well-vascularized white matter. Plaques of demyelination may be the result of either altered function or reduction in number of oligodendrocytes. Endothelial cell responses also may play a role, and certain cytokines and free radicals produced by injured cells may contribute to the injury [4].

Acute radiation syndrome

Acute radiation syndromes occur with single whole-body exposures in excess of 1 to 2 Gy. Exposure is characterized by severe effects on the CNS at higher doses of more than 50 Gy, with death occurring within 10 to 36 hours after exposure. Postmortem studies reveal extensive endothelial cell injury with perivascular edema and hemorrhage, and in the CNS, cerebral edema is common. With doses higher than 1000 Gy, direct neuronal injury can be seen [9].

Sources of nervous system exposure to radiation

Sources of radiation exposure include natural and man-made sources. Natural sources include radioactive substances that exist within the earth and cosmic rays that project through the atmosphere. Human activities, such as mining, increase exposure to naturally occurring sources. Man-made sources include nuclear weapons programs and nuclear power plants. Other man-made sources are related to radiation use in industry and medical fields [1]. All of these sources may contribute to human injury in varying degrees, which are generally recognized to be relative to the level of the exposure in the individual. Low levels of exposure seem to generate small risks of adverse effects, and there is controversy over whether a threshold exists below which there is no adverse effect. Some controversial evidence even exists to support the idea that low doses may provide a beneficial effect of radiation exposure on the organism as a whole [10]. Analysis of the atomic bomb survivors has suggested a simple linear dose response with continued risk of carcinogenesis down to zero dose [11].

Levels of radiation exposure

Exposure to varying levels of radiation produces varying levels of absorbed dose (energy absorbed per unit mass) within the body, the standard unit being the gray (Gy), and commonly expressed as $1/100^{th}$ of a gray, the centigray (cGy). To take into account varying biologic effects of different types of radiation, an entity called the effective dose is used, and the standard unit is the sievert (Sv). For the purposes of this article, 1 Sv can be assumed to reflect 1 Gy.

The amount of radiation dose that results from exposure to natural sources averages 2.4 mSv across the planet, with a typical range of 1 to 10 mSv. The doses that result from man-made sources globally vary substantially. The calculated average dose caused by atmospheric nuclear weapons testing indicates a peak annual exposure of 150 μSv in 1963, which diminished to 5 μSv in 2000. Additional exposures near nuclear weapons installations have occurred, but monitoring of the levels has been limited. Nuclear power reactors produce small contributions of less than 0.2 μSv per year as an average per person exposure worldwide. Some industrial processes that use radionuclides result in local exposures of at most 100 μSv, with 1 to 10 μSv being more common [1].

Medically related radiation exposures produce doses in individual patients typically in the 0.1- to 10-mSv range for diagnostic procedures and much higher targeted doses of approximately 0.7 to 80 Gy for therapeutic procedures. Occupational exposures to man-made sources in individuals exposed in mining, defense, medical, and industrial activities produce an average dose of 0.6 mSv, and enhanced exposures to natural sources in individuals in air travel, mining, and other monitored occupations average 1.8 mSv.

Nuclear accidents and the bombing of Hiroshima and Nagasaki with atomic weapons have produced much higher levels of exposure to local populations, which has resulted in a higher incidence of radiation-related adverse events. These populations provide the bulk of the data on the potential adverse effects of radiation. In the Chernobyl accident, recovery operation workers received an average of 100 mSv, evacuated individuals received 30 mSv, and individuals who remained in contaminated areas for the following decade received 10 mSv. Much higher exposures occurred in individuals who lived nearby and persons involved locally in managing the accident [1,12].

Historical experiences of nervous system exposure to radiation above background

Radiation carcinogenesis in the nervous system

Radium dial painters

More than 40 years ago, workers ingested radium while shaping the painting brushes for radium dials. The bone-seeking characteristic of radium produced prolonged exposures in bone, which produced bone necrosis, osteomyelitis, neoplasms, and exposure to nearby tissues. The main secondary neoplasms noted were osteosarcomas and carcinomas of the paranasal sinuses and mastoids. Increased neural tumors outside the brain were reported [13].

Patients with ankylosing spondylitis

Approximately 2000 Germans were treated with intravenous (IV) injections of radium for treating ankylosing spondylitis and other diseases. They experienced marked increases in bone sarcomas. In a large study from the United kingdom, patients with ankylosing spondylitis who were treated with external radiation showed increased risks for leukemia, non-Hodgkin's lymphoma, multiple myeloma, and cancers of esophagus, colon, pancreas, lung, bones, soft tissue, prostate, kidney, and bladder. Increased neural tumors were not reported [14–16].

Thorotrast

Thorotrast was a radioactive IV contrast medium used in the 1930s through 1940s. It was phagocytosed and localized in the liver, spleen, bone marrow, and bone and less so in the regional lymph nodes, kidneys, and lungs [17]. Increased incidence of hepatic malignancies has been reported, with latency ranges from 16 to more than 40 years. No increased incidence of CNS malignancy was noted in a series of patients who underwent cerebral arteriography with thorotrast [18]. Thorotrast also was injected into the paranasal sinuses, with subsequent cancers in the paranasal sinuses being reported [19,20].

Underground miners

Miners have had reportedly increased rates of mortality from carcinoma of the lung. Reported studies on some of these groups of miners have been confounded by other factors, such as the presence of arsenic and cigarette smoking and uncertainties regarding accurate dose estimation [17].

Dental procedures

For patients exposed to radiation during dental procedures, some studies have [21–24] and some have not [25–27] supported increased risks of developing CNS tumors.

Therapeutic irradiation

Patients with tinea capitis represent a large cohort of approximately 200,000 patients treated worldwide with scalp irradiation during the first half of the twentieth century. A report of 18,030 patients who had skin hemangiomata, some of whom were treated with radiation, showed no increased risk for CNS tumors [28].

In one study of patients irradiated for tinea capitis in childhood, 60 neural tumors arose in 10,834 patients evaluated, with the mean dose to neural tissue estimated at 1.5 Gy. A control population of the same number of patients produced a total of eight occurrences of neural tumors; a relative risk of 6.9 for the irradiated subjects was reported. There was a relative risk of 8.4 for tumors in the head and neck, ranging from 33 for neurilemomas to 9.5 for meningiomas to 2.6 for gliomas [29]. Of note, the total of 60 neural tumors in this large population yields an incidence of 0.6% as compared with the control population/baseline rate of 0.07%. Other studies that supported increased risks associated with irradiation during childhood included other studies of irradiation for tinea capitis [30], hemangioma [31], inflamed tonsils [32,33], and enlarged thymus gland [34]. The absolute risk associated with those exposures was small, however.

CNS tumors that resulted from childhood cancer treatment have been reported. A report on 4400 childhood cancer survivors in Europe indicated elevated risks of CNS tumors in patients treated with radiation, with significantly more benign tumors induced as compared with malignant tumors [35]. A study of 9720 patients treated on Children's Cancer Study Group protocols revealed 24 CNS tumors, which was reported as a 22-fold excess when compared with SEER (Surveillance, Epidemiology, and End Reporting; a program of the National Cancer Institute) data [36]. Notably, these 24 cases represent 0.2% of the study population.

A small excess of brain cancers 15 to 20 years after nasopharyngeal radium treatments in children has been reported after estimated brain doses of less than 44 to 177 cGy. Three brain tumors were detected in 904 patients, 2 of which were confirmed histologically as astrocytomas [37]. A group of 5379 children treated for various benign conditions of the head and neck yielded 66 cases of neural tumors [32].

For adults, reports indicate an increased risk after fractionated radiotherapy for pituitary adenoma [38,39], with a cumulative risk of 1.9% over 20 years in 334 patients given a median dose of 45 Gy [39]. Modern techniques of radiotherapy may be increasing the risk of second malignancies [40,41].

The effects of combined exposure to radiation and other harmful agents have been studied. For radiation-induced carcinogenesis, simple additive effects are predicted when exposure to other potentially harmful agents occurs along with exposure to radiation. Evidence exists to support more than simple additive effects in individuals exposed to cigarette smoke and radiation, however, as seen in the radon miner studies [1], although in the atomic bomb survivors simple additivity has been suggested for lung cancer risk among smokers [42]. This evidence has not been studied as closely for the nervous system specifically.

Accidental exposures

Residents of the Marshall Islands were inadvertently exposed to radioactive fallout when prevailing winds shifted during a test detonation in the south Pacific. They were not evacuated until 2 days after detonation, so they suffered significant exposure, with whole-body estimates ranging from 0.11 to 1.9 Gy. Some of the residents developed acute radiation sickness. Subsequent follow-up has been performed carefully, with several comparison groups used. Medical problems have included thyroid adenomas and nodules with associated hypothyroidism and papillary thyroid cancer. Growth retardation observed in the children is most probably related to hypothyroidism. There was a single case of acute myelogenous leukemia and stomach cancer.

Increased risks of death caused by leukemia have been noted among military members associated with nuclear testing in Nevada but are not statistically significant. Excess mortality caused by solid tumors has not been appreciated [43]. Residents of southwestern Utah exposed to fallout from these tests also have not shown increased risk of death from solid tumors [44]. Residents of the former Soviet Union exposed to the nuclear facility discharges near the Mayak nuclear plant have not shown significant risks of solid tumors [45]. The Chernobyl accident in 1986 was marked by substantial exposures, especially radioactive iodine and cesium, which produced dramatic increases in carcinoma of the thyroid for individuals exposed in childhood (approximately 1800 persons in the severely contaminated areas) [1]. Concern over exposure across Europe from the Chernobyl incident has led to some estimates that up to 21,000 Europeans will die of cancer over the next 50 years as a result of the radiation effects [17]. Because of its short latency interval, leukemia would be the first radiation-induced malignancy expected to appear. There has been no increase in leukemia to date, and there is no evidence yet of other nonmalignant disorders related to ionizing radiation [1,12]. Multiple other radiation accidents worldwide since 1945 have as-yet unknown delayed consequences [17].

Atomic bomb survivors

One would expect substantial acute radiation injury data to be derived from the survivors of the atomic bomb blasts at Hiroshima and Nagasaki, yet because of the chaos and massive mechanical and fire injury associated with the blasts, little acute injury information was gleaned. The Japanese National census of 1950 estimated that 283,500 surviving Japanese residents were exposed to the atomic bombs. Many of these survivors were located significant distances away, with 90% of them exposed to less than 10 cGy. In these bomb survivors, no increased incidence of brain tumors has been seen, although some excess of nervous system tumors outside the brain has been reported [46]. A dose response was seen for the development of nervous system tumors as a combined group and independently for schwannomas, which suggests radiation as a possible cause for some of these tumors [47].

Occupational nuclear workers

Some evidence exists to support [48] and deny [49] a relationship between increased cancer risk among radiation workers at the nuclear facility at Portsmouth Naval Shipyard. In other nuclear worker studies, there is some evidence of a slight excess risk of solid cancers, although this evidence is statistically weak [17]. In a study of workers at the Oak Ridge facility, evidence has suggested increases in cancer mortality, particularly leukemia [50]. Two other studies of radiation workers show weak but positive correlations with exposure and cancer, but only for leukemias and multiple myeloma [51,52]. Other exposure factors in these large populations also could play a role in the outcomes [53]. Other studies of radiation workers have suggested no increased risks of brain cancer [54–56].

Radiologists

Radiologists in the first half of the twentieth century showed an increased incidence of malignancies, including skin cancers, leukemia, lymphoma, multiple myeloma, and cancer of the lung and pancreas, after roughly estimated whole-body doses of 1 to 5 Gy over a career. Either reports on relative causes of death in reports on these populations do not report CNS tumor-related death or the numbers are too small to conclude increased risk compared with control populations [57–59].

Carcinogenesis in prenatally exposed individuals

Radiation-induced cancer among individuals exposed in utero in the atomic bombings has not been demonstrated clearly, and longer follow-up is needed [1,60,61]. In the Oxford Survey Report, a relative risk for CNS tumors of 1.42 was reported in patients who had been exposed prenatally during obstetric radiography [62]. An increased risk for malignancy in this report has been questioned by some researchers [63], but others support an increased risk in these patients [64,65]. A small case control study on children in one area of Australia who were diagnosed with brain tumors showed no increased risk caused by prenatal irradiation [26]. Although intentional exposure of the developing fetus should be avoided if at all possible, some researchers conclude that circumstances exist in which even therapeutic irradiation to a pregnant patient might be considered after careful analysis of the known risks and benefits [66].

Clinical manifestations of therapeutic irradiation

Studies on patients treated with radiation for brain tumors and for prophylactic therapy to prevent the clinical development of malignancy involving the CNS have produced substantial documentation of the effects of CNS irradiation at therapeutic doses.

Radiation necrosis

Doses of 50 to 60 Gy produced reported rates of necrosis of 0.1% to 5% after doses of 50 to 60 Gy fractionated over 5 to 6 weeks [5–7]. These data are limited by uncertainty in the actual number of individuals at risk and by the frequent lack of tissue examination to confirm the diagnosis. Symptoms are primarily caused by mass effect, but severe focal neurologic abnormalities also can occur related to the location of the lesion. Abnormal electroencephalographic findings also may be observed [5]. Surgical debulking may be required if steroid therapy is inadequate to control symptoms.

Necrotizing leukoencephalopathy

Multiple areas of white matter injury may occur because of loss of myelin and oligodendrocytes. Cerebral atrophy can be appreciated, and mineralizing microangiopathy can produce areas of intracerebral calcification detected on imaging [67–70]. Symptoms can include seizures, spasticity, ataxia, lethargy, and motor deficits. The risk increases when IV or intrathecal methotrexate is used in conjunction with cranial irradiation, and it seems to be substantially worse in children with leukemia that involves the CNS, as opposed to children treated in the prophylactic setting [71].

Neuropsychological and cognitive effects

Patients who undergo central nervous system irradiation as children

The process of normal nervous system development in children produces more vulnerability to the effects of irradiation of the nervous system. The brain develops postnatally by increasing the size but not the number of neurons. Growth of axons and formation of dendritic arborizations occur with the development of complex synaptic connections within the first several years of life, but growth occurs most rapidly during the first 3 years [72]. Myelination continues through puberty [73].

Numerous reports support an adverse impact on cognitive function in patients who undergo cranial irradiation [67,68,74–76]. Although the analysis of adverse outcomes can be complicated by the use of neurotoxic chemotherapy, surgery, and neurotoxic manifestations of the disease process itself, evidence exists to support a generally modest but clear adverse impact on IQ in children who are treated prophylactically for acute lymphoblastic leukemia (ALL) with cranial irradiation. This typically results in children being at the lower end of the normal range [77–79], although some children exhibit severe impairment and some subgroups are at greater risk for impairment than others (see later discussion).

The large database of patients treated with scalp irradiation for tinea capitis also has demonstrated slightly abnormal results in several neuro-cognitive-related parameters. One large study of approximately 11,000 children who were irradiated in Israel from 1950 through 1960 as part of a campaign to eradicate tinea capitis demonstrated trends in lower examination scores on scholastic aptitude, IQ, and psychological tests, more frequent mental hospital admissions, and the completion of fewer school grades when compared with control populations [80]. Many of the differences did not reach statistical significance, and even in instances in which statistical significance was observed, the absolute differences were small, possibly related to the relatively low doses involved. For example, on a high school aptitude test, the mean score for irradiated patients was 59.4 compared with 61.2 in the matched general population control group. Matched analysis of the differences in the scores in the two groups reached statistical significance. For this test, there was no significant difference when comparing the irradiated population against a sibling control group. A phantom study was performed to determine the expected typical radiation dose given to the brain, skull, and thyroid gland under typical conditions in these patients [81]. The study estimated that during a typical course of treatment, the surface of the brain received between 121 and 139 cGy and that 2.5 cm deep in the brain the dose was 95 to 121 cGy. Adjustments to these data to account for patients treated more than once and to account for each patient's head size based on age have been reported, with a mean of the estimated doses to neural tissue of 150 cGy [82].

Another series of patients irradiated for tinea capitis also showed increases in mental illness as compared with a nonirradiated control group. A control population of 1413 nonirradiated patients with tinea capitis was compared with the study population of 2043 irradiated patients with tinea capitis. Statistical significance was reached with respect to differences between the two groups, but the absolute differences were small. For example, the incidence of a combination of mental disorders was 3.2% in the irradiated group versus 1.3% in the nonirradiated group, with a relative risk of 2.5 [83]. A follow-up study on the same group of patients updated these rates to 8.1% and 6.4%, respectively, which eliminated the statistical significance of the relative difference except in a subset analysis of white patients only [30]. Dose estimates with phantom measurements by this group indicated brain doses typically of 140 cGy [84]. A later phantom study estimated pituitary doses at 49 ± 6 cGy [85], which could also provide an indication of the doses to the deepest portions of the brain caused by anatomic proximity.

Considerably higher doses are involved in treating known malignancy in the CNS or providing prophylaxis to prevent spread to the CNS of a known malignancy that arises elsewhere, with typical doses in the range of 1200 cGy to 6000 cGy. Generally lower doses—in the 1200 cGy to 2400 cGy range—are used for prophylactic treatment for leukemia, with higher doses required for brain tumors. There is a stronger indication of neurocognitive impairment in patients with brain tumors, as discussed later, which is likely caused by the higher radiation often involved and the mechanical impact of surgery and the disease process itself. The volume irradiated also plays a crucial role, with more adverse neurocognitive outcome associated with larger volumes of the CNS being irradiated.

Children treated prophylactically to the central nervous system for acute lymphoblastic leukemia

A large amount of data exists concerning the adverse impact of cranial irradiation given to treat brain tumors or provide prophylactic treatment for ALL. Factors other than radiation play a role, but there is adverse neurocognitive impact in some patients. Multivariate analysis of a group of patients with ALL randomized to 18 Gy versus 24 Gy—some of whom were randomized to low- versus high-dose IV methotrexate—showed IQs in the normal range. This analysis was independent of radiotherapy dose if patients who received high-dose methotrexate were excluded. IQs were lower in the group given high-dose methotrexate [86]. In a later study of patients treated with and without 18-Gy radiotherapy and randomized to conventional or high-dose methotrexate, impairments were noted with the combination of high-dose methotrexate, radiotherapy, and female gender, but radiotherapy alone was not independently associated with adverse cognitive outcomes [87].

Another report indicated a possible adverse impact on memory with the combination of intrathecal methotrexate and high-dose IV methotrexate without radiotherapy [88] Hal. One report suggested that neuropsychological deficits with IV methotrexate were comparable to those seen with 1800 cGy cranial irradiation [89]. Williams and Davis [90] reviewed 28 studies and were unable to determine clearly whether one form of CNS prophylaxis was worse than another for cognitive deficits. In contrast, another review of 41 studies indicated that patients who received cranial radiotherapy had lower scores than (1) patients who received chemotherapy only, (2) the general population, (3) healthy siblings, and (4) cancer patients who did not receive CNS therapy of any type [91]. Other reports supported no adverse effect on intelligence, memory, or academic achievement in patients treated with intrathecal chemotherapy and no radiation [92,93]. One report of monozygotic twins, both of whom were treated with 2400 cGy whole-brain irradiation for ALL, produced nearly identical IQ patterns with subtle differences in other studied neurocognitive parameters [94].

Whether deficits require cranial irradiation and intrathecal methotrexate has been considered. Mulhern et al [79] reported on patients treated with intrathecal methotrexate and cranial irradiation versus high-dose methotrexate and found that IQs were within normal limits, but they reported declines in 22% to 30% of children regardless of treatment. A CALGB (Cancer and Leukemia Group B) protocol that produced data on 110 patients with ALL who were treated with different forms of CNS prophylaxis noted poorer academic achievement, greater psychological stress, and poorer self-image in the irradiated patients [95].

Learning problems in these patients can include memory deficits (often short-term memory being the most affected), diminished speed of mental processing, and difficulty acquiring new knowledge [96]. The effects are more severe in children who are irradiated at younger ages and possibly in female patients [67,79,86,90,91,97,98].

Some evidence supports the idea that cranial irradiation in children with ALL is more likely to impact on nonverbal cognitive processing skills as opposed to verbal skills [91,92,99,100]. Many researchers have theorized that underlying attention or processing deficits are to blame [101–103].

Children treated to the central nervous system for brain tumors

Data in children treated for CNS tumors also indicate substantial evidence of IQ deterioration after radiotherapy [76,102–106]. These studies show that 17% to 31% of the children have IQs below 70 and that only 12% to 56% have IQs above 90 [104,107,108]. Lower IQs have been demonstrated in patients treated with radiation as opposed to chemotherapy or surgery for brain tumors [76,109], although cognitive impairment has been noted in patients treated with surgery alone [110]. Younger children experience greater impact when large volumes are irradiated [96]. In children who are irradiated at 3 years of age or younger, the adverse impact of radiation therapy to the brain can be particularly dramatic [75,96,102–104]; for example, one report indicated an overall rate of disability of 58% in surviving children [95].

Evidence supports the fact that cognitive declines in children treated with radiation therapy to the brain for medulloblastoma are the result of the inability to acquire new skills and process new information rather than the loss of information or skills acquired previously [111].

There are indications that late neurocognitive effects are improving with new strategies of reduced doses of radiotherapy and more selective use of radiotherapy for CNS prophylaxis in leukemia [112,113]. There is controversy regarding whether 18 Gy causes fewer problems than 24 Gy [77,79,86,88,97]. Some researchers have suggested that the lower dose may result simply in a delay in the appearance of neuropsychological sequelae [109].

Reduced doses for radiation therapy for childhood brain tumors also have shown signs of improved intellectual outcomes [114]. Efforts have continued to reduce doses wherever possible [115]. In a comparison of 48 children treated with whole-brain radiation at three dose levels of 36 Gy, 24 Gy, and 18 Gy, patients who received lower doses showed improved IQ scores. Patients treated at younger ages fared more poorly in IQ scores, and the results were believed to be independent of the underlying disease type (24 patients had ALL and 24 patients had medulloblastoma or primitive neuroectodermal tumor) [116]. It is widely accepted that delaying radiation as long as possible in young children improves neuropsychological outcome, but even with delayed therapy provided by chemotherapy, patients with medulloblastoma require irradiation and develop substantial neuropsychological deficits when irradiated at younger than 5 years of age [117]. Attempts to decrease volumes receiving higher doses unnecessarily has resulted in potential technical improvements, but concerns also have been expressed that recent technologic developments in high-precision radiotherapy may increase the risk of second malignancies caused by the exposure of larger areas of the body to lower doses [40,41].

Efforts to attempt to treat or prevent neurocognitive impairment in survivors of childhood brain tumors have demonstrated opportunities in cognitive remediation approaches, pharmacologic therapy, and environmental optimization [102,103].

Patients who undergo central nervous system irradiation as adults

Neuropsychological impairment has been noted in adult patients treated with prophylactic cranial irradiation for lung cancer, most commonly small-cell lung cancer [118–121]. Some reports include high dose per fraction regimens, such as 4 Gy × 5 fractions or 3 Gy × 10 fractions. Even in these cases, the impairment is often judged to be borderline, and many patients demonstrate pretreatment baseline neurocognitive impairment [122]. Whether there is net neurocognitive benefit by preventing neurologic impairment caused by metastatic disease versus the neurologic impairment that results from the treatment itself is the subject of lively debate [119,123–128].

Adult patients treated for primary brain tumors also have demonstrated neurocognitive impairment. In one report, 28 patients at a mean follow-up interval of 7 years were alive for analysis out of a group of 101 patients treated with postoperative radiotherapy for low-grade glioma [129]. These 28 patients were compared with a group of 23 patients who were treated with surgery alone at a mean follow-up interval of 10 years. The patients who were treated with radiation therapy had significantly poorer cognitive function on statistical analysis. Some of the performance parameters studied were not different between the two groups (eg, verbal IQ scores). Other studies of the impact on neurocognitive function in adult patients irradiated for primary brain tumors have generally shorter follow-up intervals, with mixed results on whether neurocognitive impairment occurs in these patients and in particular if impairment primarily is caused by the disease itself [130–136]. A larger study of 101 patients with low-grade glioma who were alive at a median follow-up of 7.4 years after radiotherapy was performed using Mini Mental Status Exam only, without more in-depth neuropsychological testing [137]. In these patients, there was improvement in cognitive abilities in patients with an abnormal baseline Mini Mental Status Exam, and only 5% of the patients tested at 5 years had a decrease of more than three points from baseline Mini Mental Status Exam score. In another cohort of patients with high-grade glioma followed by Mini Mental Status Exam, there was no clear trend to cognitive worsening in patients evaluated up to 24 months after treatment [138].

Adult patients treated for brain metastases treated with whole-brain radiation often have limited survival, and limited data are available on the incidence of neuropsychological impairment produced by radiation in this setting. One study that used unusually high radiation dose per fraction documented substantial dementia in 12 total patients representing 1.9% to 5.1% of patients in two cohorts [139]. Many patients with brain metastases have poor neurologic function as the result of the disease process, and improvement from baseline Mini Mental Status Exam was reported in a group of patients with brain metastasis after whole-brain irradiation [140]. The presence of declining scores was associated strongly with an approaching terminal event in this group. The adverse impacts of uncontrolled metastatic disease on neuropsychological function have been reported by others [141–143]. Whether whole-brain radiation has a net beneficial or adverse effect in these patients is still somewhat controversial [142,144], and the conclusion that the net effect is adverse is often indicated as justification for using only local therapies, such as radiosurgery [145–147].

The somnolence syndrome

The somnolence syndrome has been reported in children who receive radiation to the brain, with onset occurring 1 to 2 months after radiotherapy. Typical drowsiness, anorexia, irritability, nausea, apathy, and dizziness can be seen in as many as 40% to 60% of children [7,67,148] and generally resolves spontaneously. There are conflicting reports regarding whether children who experience somnolence syndrome are more likely to develop cognitive deficits [91].

Imaging correlates of radiation injury to the nervous system

Many characteristic imaging findings are associated with various forms of radiation injury. Imaging correlations in one small study of 21 patients treated with 18 to 24 Gy cranial irradiation plus intrathecal methotrexate showed that intracerebral calcifications correlated with the number of intrathecal methotrexate doses and with lower IQ scores [98]. Radiographic findings of the extent of periventricular low-density lesions have been correlated with neuropsychological impairment in patients treated with prophylactic cranial irradiation for small-cell lung cancer [122]. A gradient of increasing severity of neuropsychological impairment was correlated with

CT scan findings that ranged from normal to cortical atrophy to intracerebral calcifications in a group of children with ALL who were treated with cranial irradiation and methotrexate [149]. In an attempt to correlate magnetic resonance spectroscopy abnormalities after cranial irradiation with neurocognitive outcomes, some have reported magnetic resonance spectroscopy abnormalities [150,151], but Davidson et al [152] did not.

Magnetic resonance spectroscopy has been used for numerous other applications in the brain, including the differentiation of recurrent tumor from radionecrosis [153]. Positron emission tomography also has been useful in this regard [154]. Magnetic resonance correlates of a group of 41 patients irradiated with various techniques indicated ventricular abnormalities or sulci enlargement in 50% of the subjects, with higher grade MR lesions being seen in patients receiving higher doses to larger volumes [70]. Lacunar infarcts have been noted on MRI evaluation of asymptomatic children previously treated for brain tumors and are more common in patients irradiated at younger than 5 years of age [155]. In this study, IQ results for patients with these lesions did not differ from matched controls. The number of incidentally discovered MR abnormalities after childhood irradiation for ALL was high enough in one study to suggest that screening may be advisable [156].

A psychophysiologic study of patients treated with prophylactic cranial irradiation for lung cancer demonstrated no change between the pretreatment and immediate posttreatment results of a battery of auditory event-related potentials during a short memory test [157].

The effect of prenatal exposure to radiation

The impact of prenatal radiation exposure on the developing nervous system has been studied to some extent in animals. Rat data show that irradiation at day 16 produces distortions of the gyri in the cerebellum and deficiencies in the granular and molecular layers of the cerebellum. If irradiated between day 19 and 21, disordered neuronal migration is common [158–160].

Mental retardation and small head size have been reported in survivors of the atomic bombs who were exposed prenatally. An increased frequency of unprovoked seizures and reduced intelligence scores and school performance also were reported. Out of 1544 cases studied that were prenatally exposed, 30 cases of severe mental retardation were found (1.9%). Three of these cases had Down syndrome, 1 had encephalitis in infancy, and 1 had a retarded sibling. Among these 5 cases, retardation may not be radiation related (resulting in a 1.6% rate). Careful study of the incidence of subsequent mental retardation as a function of developmental age at exposure indicates no apparent increased risk before postovulatory week 8 or after week 25. Fetuses exposed between 8 and 15 weeks' gestation at doses of 1 Gy or more represent the highest risk group. In 26 of these 30 cases studied in terms of head size, 15 had small heads, as defined by two standard deviations below the mean for that age and sex group. In a study group of 1473 cases, 62 had small head sizes (4.2%). Researchers have questioned whether the assumption is accurate that small head size is the result of fewer surviving neurons [161].

It is worth noting that in a normally distributed general population, 2.5% of individuals would be classified as having a "small head" by these criteria. In another study that attempted to estimate the excess caused by radiation in the previously mentioned cases, many of the instances of small head size were shown to be likely related to generalized growth impairment [162], which indicated that the increased numbers of small head sizes in this population could be caused only by generalized growth impairment, particularly if there was no coexisting mental retardation [162,163].

Studies on IQ scores have shown no evidence of radiation-related effects on intelligence among individuals exposed at 0 to 7 weeks or more than 26 weeks after ovulation. The mean test scores decline with increasing estimated dose in the 8- to 25-week group [164]. Similar results are seen for school performance [165]. The estimated clinically lowest dose to produce severe mental retardation from these studies is 0.61 Gy [166].

Increased incidence of seizure activity similarly has been shown to be related to 8- to 15-week postovulatory age at exposure, and it increases with the level of exposure [167].

Limited opportunity for pathologic evaluation of individuals with possible radiation-related mental retardation includes the autopsies of four patients exposed prenatally and followed in the atomic bomb survivor studies. Two of the four patients were mentally retarded. One patient, who was exposed at the developmental age of 20 weeks' gestation to a dose estimated to be less than 1 cGy, died at 9 years because of leukemia. Autopsy findings indicated extensive brain hemorrhages. His brain was of normal weight and architecture. The second patient died at 29 years from cardiac insufficiency after exposure of less than 1 cGy in postovulatory week 24. The patient had normal brain weight and architecture. The third patient had brain weight lower than normal, was mentally retarded, and died at 20 years after exposure of less than 1 cGy in postovulatory week 31. On examination, however, her brain demonstrated normal patterns of gray and white matter. The fourth patient, who died at 16 years from meningitis, probably was exposed at postovulatory week 8 or 9, which was adjusted to account for likely premature birth. The estimated dose to the mother's uterus was 1.2 Gy. Multiple pathologic abnormalities were described. His brain weighed 840 g, and he was bilaterally micro-ophthalmic, with microcorneae and bilateral hypoplasia of the retina, which was most noticeable in the macular area. Massive heterotopic gray matter was seen around the lateral ventricles, and within these areas histologically abnormal arrangements of nerve cells were appreciated. Both mamillary bodies were missing, and the relationship of these structures to the limbic system is interesting because the boy was known to be severely emotionally disturbed. The cerebellum and hippocampi were histologically normal [168–171]. Ectopic gray matter commonly has been appreciated in rodents exposed to ionizing radiation [172].

MRI was performed on five Hiroshima survivors with severe mental retardation who were exposed at 8 to 15 weeks' gestation. Impaired development with ectopic gray matter was noted in two individuals exposed at 12 to 13 weeks' gestation, which possibly indicated abnormal neuronal migration [166]. The mamillary bodies were of normal size. In another two individuals exposed at 12 to 13 weeks after ovulation, no areas of ectopic gray matter were noted, but other abnormalities were noted, including enlargement of the gyri and cisterna magna. In one of the two patients, there was a markedly small corpus callosum and a poorly developed cingulate gyrus. Patients exposed at 15 weeks after ovulation showed no abnormalities in brain architecture on MRI [171].

Notably, neuronal migration disorders have been reported under other conditions. An autopsy study of 58 Japanese patients with cerebral palsy included 19 individuals who underwent microscopic analysis, 4 of whom had heterotopic gray matter [173]. Heterotopic gray matter has been noted in patients with epilepsy without history of prior irradiation [174]. Other cases of mental retardation with no known exposure to radiation also have demonstrated ectopic gray matter. Differences may exist in the pattern of the ectopia [171].

Hereditary effects of radiation exposure

In children of atomic bomb survivors conceived after the bombings, there has not yet been a demonstration that cancer risk is increased as a result of gonadal irradiation in the atomic bomb survivors [61]. Occupational workers studied for leukemia risk in offspring likewise have not demonstrated a causal relationship [175]. Researchers recently estimated the impact of radiation exposure on mutations known to be associated with specific genetic alterations in humans. The United Nations Scientific Committee on the Effects of Atomic Radiation estimated the total hereditary risk to be 0.3% to 0.5% per gray to the first generation after radiation exposure. Neurologic diseases, such as Huntingdon's disease and neurofibromatosis, were part of the model [2].

Radiation neurotoxicity of the spinal cord

The spinal cord is often irradiated during radiation therapy courses to various nearby body sites and organs. Early radiation injury can include areas of demyelination and areas of spongiform change. Vascular changes can be present 4 to 5 months after irradiation, with fibrin thrombi, endothelial cell proliferation, and perivascular edema. Delayed injury can include areas of cord necrosis with glial proliferation at the margins. Microvascular injury and direct parenchymal cell injury play a role in the pathogenesis of these lesions [4]. The tolerance doses clinically used in radiation therapy practice are generally 45 Gy at 1.8 to 2 Gy per fraction, which predicts for incidence of myelopathy of approximately 0.2% [176].

Radiation myelopathy presents clinically with spasticity, paresis, gait changes, and, less likely, Brown-Sequard syndrome, incontinence, and pain. The functional deficit corresponds to the spinal cord level injured. Symptoms usually appear more than 5 to 6 months after irradiation. The dramatic nature of the clinical outcome drives the highly conservative choice of tolerance dose in practice, even sometimes producing inadequate tumor control probability of the targeted lesion [177]. A transient radiation myelopathy associated with a Lhermitte's sign occurs in some patients whose spinal cord has been irradiated. The symptoms consist of an electric shock sensation down the spine and extremities and are believed to be secondary to transient demyelination [178]. The symptoms resolve generally within a few months, and there are no known long-term sequelae.

Radiation-induced malignancy of the spinal cord and peripheral nerves has been reported in the ankylosing spondylitis experience [15,179].

Radiation neurotoxicity of the peripheral nerves

Peripheral nerves are generally accepted to be more tolerant of radiation injury than the CNS. Neuropathies have been reported after irradiation to the lumbosacral plexus, the brachial plexus, and other peripheral nerves, however [180–184]. On pathologic study, irradiated peripheral nerves may adhere to adjacent tissues. Fibrosis can be seen microscopically within nerve trunks, and blood vessel changes, as discussed in reference to the spinal cord, may be seen. Schwann cell loss or injury results in areas of demyelination [4].

Radiation doses more than 60 Gy, in 1.8- to 2-Gy fractions, causes increased incidence of neuropathy, and 54 Gy, in 1.8-Gy fractions, has been reported as associated with a 1% incidence of neuropathy. Increasing total dose and increasing fraction size result in increased risk [184]. The clinical presentation of radiation-induced neuropathy can include varying degrees of pain, anesthesia, and muscle weakness [180,183,184]. These symptoms appear from 6 months to many years after irradiation.

Summary

Neurotoxicity from radiation can range widely and produce effects that may include (1) small absolute increases in cancer risks, (2) subtle effects on higher level functioning in some individuals, (3) severe cognitive impairment in some individuals, (4) severe focal injury that may include necrosis or irreversible loss of function, and (5) overwhelming and rapidly fatal diffuse injury associated with high-dose, whole-body exposures. An understanding of the implications of nervous system exposure to radiation can guide efforts in radiation protection and aid in the optimization of the medical uses of radiation.

Acknowledgments

The author wishes to thank Mary Hollaway for assistance in preparing the manuscript.

References

[1] United Nations Scientific Committee on the Effects of Atomic Radiation. 2000 report. New York: United Nations; 2000. p. 2–17.

[2] United Nations Scientific Committee on the Effects of Atomic Radiation. 2001 report. New York: United Nations; 2001. p. 1–160.

[3] Preston D, Shimizu Y, Pierce D, et al. Studies of mortality of atomic bomb survivors: report 13. Solid cancer and non-cancer disease mortality: 1950–1997. Radiat Res 2003;160(4): 381–407.

[4] Fajardo LF, Berthrong M, Anderson RE. Nervous system. In: Radiation pathology. New York: Oxford University Press; 2001. p. 351–63.

[5] Martins A, Johnston J, Henry J, et al. Delayed radiation necrosis of the brain. J Neurosurg 1977;47:336–45.

[6] Marks J, Wong J. The risk of cerebral radionecrosis in relation to dose, time and fractionation: a follow-up study. Prog Exp Tumor Res 1985;29:210–8.

[7] Anscher M, Green D, Kneece S, et al. Radiation injury of the brain and spinal cord. In: Wilkins R, Rengachary S, editors. Neurosurgery update II: vascular, spinal, pediatric, and function neurosurgery. New York: McGraw-Hill; 1991. p. 42–9.

[8] Price R, Birdwell D. The central nervous system in childhood leukemia. III: mineralizing microangiopathy and dystrophic calcification. Cancer 1978;42(2):717–28.

[9] Fajardo LF, Berthrong M, Anderson RE. Acute radiation syndrome. In: Radiation pathology. New York: Oxford University Press; 2001. p. 43–51.

[10] Luckey T. Radiation hormesis overview. RSO Magazine 2002;8(4):22–41.

[11] Preston D, Pierce D, Shimizu Y, et al. Dose response and temporal patterns of radiation-associated solid cancer risks. Health Phys 2003;85(1):43–6.

[12] United Nations Scientific Committee on the Effects of Atomic Radiation. 2000 Annex J. New York: United Nations; 2000. p. 451–566.

[13] Rowland R, Lucas H. Radium-dial workers. In: Boice JD Jr, Fraumeni JF Jr, editors. Radiation carcinogenesis: epidemiology and biological significance. New York: Raven Press; 1984. p. 231–40.

[14] Weiss H, Darby S, Doll R. Cancer mortality following x-ray treatment for ankylosing spondylitis. Int J Cancer 1994;59(3):327–38.

[15] Darby S, Doll R, Gill S, et al. Long term mortality after a single treatment course with x-rays in patients treated for ankylosing spondylitis. Br J Cancer 1987;55(2):179–90.

[16] Lewis C, Smith P, Stratton I, et al. Estimated radiation doses to different organs among patients treated for ankylosing spondylitis with a single course of x-rays. Br J Radiol 1988; 61(723):212–20.

[17] Fajardo LF, Berthrong M, Anderson RE. Exposures of human populations to ionizing radiation. In: Radiation pathology. New York: Oxford University Press; 2001. p. 19–42.

[18] Andersson M, Carstensen B, Storm H. Mortality and cancer incidence after cerebral arteriography with or without thorotrast. Radiat Res 1995;142:305–20.

[19] Fabrikantn J, Dickson R, Fetter B. Mechanism of radiation carcinogenesis at the clinical level. Br J Cancer 1964;18:459–77.

[20] Rankow R, Conley J, Fodor P. Carcinoma of the maxillary sinus following thorotrast instillation. J Maxillofac Surg 1974;2(2–3):119–26.

[21] Preston-Martin S, Mack W, Henderson B. Risk factors for gliomas and meningiomas in males in Los Angeles County. Cancer Res 1989;49(21):6137–43.

[22] Preston-Martin S, Yu M, Henderson B, et al. Risk factors for meningiomas in men in Los Angeles County. J Natl Cancer Inst 1983;70(5):863–6.

[23] Preston-Martin S, Yu M, Benton B, et al. N-nitroso compounds and childhood brain tumors: a case-control study. Cancer Res 1982;42(12):5340–5.

[24] Preston-Martin S, Paganini-Hill A, Henderson B, et al. Case-control study of intracranial meningiomas in women in Los Angeles County, California. J Natl Cancer Inst 1980;65(1):67–73.

[25] Kuijten R, Bunin G, Nass C, et al. Gestational and familial risk factors for childhood astrocytoma: results of a case-control study. Cancer Res 1990;50(9):2608–12.

[26] McCredie M, Maisonneuve P, Boyle P. Antenatal risk factors for malignant brain tumours in New South Wales children. Int J Cancer 1994;56(1):6–10.

[27] Ryan P, Lee M, North B, et al. Amalgam fillings, diagnostic dental x-rays and tumours of the brain and meninges. Eur J Cancer B Oral Oncol 1992;28B(2):91–5.

[28] Fürst C, Lundell M, Holm L, et al. Cancer incidence after radiotherapy for skin hemangioma: a retrospective cohort study in Sweden. J Natl Cancer Inst 1988;80(17):1387–92.

[29] Ron E, Modan B, Boice J, et al. Tumors of the brain and nervous system after radiotherapy in childhood. N Engl J Med 1988;319(16):1033–9.

[30] Shore R, Albert R, Pasternack B. Follow-up study of patients treated by x-ray epilation for tinea capitis: resurvey of post-treatment illness and mortality experience. Arch Environ Health 1976;31:21–8.

[31] Karlsson P, Holmberg E, Lundell M, et al. Intracranial tumors after exposure to ionizing radiation during infancy: a pooled analysis of two Swedish cohorts of 28,008 infants with skin hemangioma. Radiat Res 1998;150(3):357–64.

[32] Schneider A, Shore-Freedman E, Bekerman C, et al. Radiation-induced tumors of the head and neck following childhood irradiation. Medicine (Baltimore) 1985;64(1):1–15.

[33] Sznajder L, Abrahams C, Parry D, et al. Multiple schwannomas and meningiomas associated with irradiation in childhood. Arch Intern Med 1996;156(16):1873–8.

[34] Hildreth N, Shore R, Hempelmann L, et al. Risk of extra-thyroid tumors following radiation treatment in infancy for thymic enlargement. Radiat Res 1985;102:378–91.

[35] Little M, de Vathaire F, Shamsaldin A, et al. Risks of brain tumour following treatment for cancer in childhood: modification by genetic factors, radiotherapy and chemotherapy. Int J Cancer 1998;78(3):269–75.

[36] Neglia J, Meadows A, Robison L, et al. Second neoplasms after acute lymphoblastic leukemia in childhood. N Engl J Med 1991;325(19):1330–6.

[37] Sandler D, Comstock G, Matanoski G. Neoplasms following childhood radium irradiation of the nasopharynx. J Natl Cancer Inst 1982;68(1):3–8.

[38] Tsang R, Laperriere N, Simpson W, et al. Glioma arising after radiation therapy for pituitary adenoma: a report of four patients and estimation of risk. Cancer 1993;72:2227–33.

[39] Brada M, Ford D, Ashley S, et al. Risk of second brain tumour after conservative surgery and radiotherapy for pituitary adenoma. BMJ 1992;304:1343–51.

[40] Hall E, Wuu C. Radiation-induced second cancers: the impact of 3D-CRT and IMRT. Int J Radiat Oncol Biol Phys 2003;56(1):83–8.

[41] Hall E, Henry S. Kaplan Distinguished Scientist Award 2003: The Crooked Shall Be Made Straight. Dose-response relationships for carcinogenesis. Int J Radiat Biol Phys 2004;80(5): 327–37.

[42] Pierce D, Sharp G, Mavuchi K. Joint effects of radiation and smoking on lung cancer risk among atomic bomb survivors. Radiat Res 2003;159(4):511–20.

[43] Thaul S, Page W, Crawford H, et al. Summary. In: The five series study: mortality of military participants in US nuclear weapons tests. Washington DC: National Academy Press; 2000. p. 1–4.

[44] Machado S, Land C, McKay F. Cancer mortality and radioactive fallout in Southwestern Utah. Am J Epidemiol 1987;125(1):44–61.

[45] United Nations Scientific Committee on the Effects of Atomic Radiation Annex A: sources and effects of ionizing radiation. New York: United Nations; 1994. p. 11–183.

[46] Pierce D, Shimizu Y, Preston D, et al. Studies of the mortality of atomic bomb survivors. Report 12, Part 1. Cancer: 1950–1990. Radiat Res 1996;146(1):1–27.

[47] Preston D, Ron E, Yonehara S, et al. Rumors of the nervous system and pituitary gland associated with atomic bomb radiation exposure. J Natl Cancer Inst 2002;94(20): 1555–63.

[48] Najarian T, Colton T. Mortality from leukaemia and cancer in shipyard nuclear workers. Lancet 1978;1(8072):1018–20.

[49] Rinsky R, Zumwalde R, Waxweiler R, et al. Cancer mortality at a naval nuclear shipyard. Lancet 1981;1(8214):231–5.

[50] Wing S, Shy C, Wood J, et al. Mortality among workers at Oak Ridge National Laboratory: evidence of radiation effects in follow-up through 1984. JAMA 1991;265(11): 1397–402.

[51] Kendall G, Muirhead C, MacGibbon B, et al. Mortality and occupational exposure to radiation: first analysis of the National Registry for Radiation Workers. BMJ 1992; 304(6821):220–5.

[52] Gilbert E, Fry S, Wiggs L, et al. Analysis of combined mortality data on workers at the Hanford Site, Oak Ridge National Laboratory, and Rocky Flats Nuclear Weapons Plant. Radiat Res 1989;120(1):19–35.

[53] Schull WJ. Epilogue. In: Effects of atomic radiation. New York: Wiley-Liss; 1995. p. 274–96.

[54] Cardis E, Gilbert E, Carpenter L, et al. Effects of low doses and low dose rates of external ionizing radiation: cancer mortality among nuclear industry workers in three countries. Radiat Res 1995;142(2):117–32.

[55] Muirhead C, Goodill A, Haylock R, et al. Occupational radiation exposure and mortality: second analysis of the National Registry for Radiation Workers. J Radiol Prot 1999;19(1): 3–26.

[56] Wang J, Inskep P, Boice J, et al. Cancer incidence among medical diagnostic x-ray workers in China, 1950–1985. Int J Cancer 1990;45(5):889–95.

[57] Smith P, Doll R. Mortality from cancer and all causes among British radiologists. Br J Radiol 1981;54:187–94.

[58] Matanoski G, Seltser R, Sartwell P, et al. The current mortality rates of radiologists and other physician specialists: specific causes of death. Am J Epidemiol 1975;101(3): 199–210.

[59] Court Brown W, Doll R. Expectation of life and mortality from cancer among British radiologists. BMJ 1958;34(5090):181–7.

[60] Yoshimoto Y, Kato H, Schull W. Risk of cancer among children exposed in utero to A-bomb radiations, 1950–84. Lancet 1988;2(8612):665–9.

[61] Yoshimoto Y. Cancer risk among children of atomic bomb survivors. JAMA 1990;264(5): 596–600.

[62] Bithell J, Stewart A. Pre-natal irradiation and childhood malignancy: a review of British data from the Oxford survey. Br J Cancer 1975;31:271–87.

[63] Miller R, Boice J. Cancer after intrauterine exposure to the atomic bomb. Radiat Res 1997; 147(3):396–7.

[64] Wakeford R, Little M. Risk coefficients for childhood cancer after intrauterine irradiation: a review. Int J Radiat Biol Phys 2003;79(5):293–309.

[65] Doll R, Wakeford R. Risk of childhood cancer from fetal irradiation. Br J Radiol 1997;70: 130–9.

[66] Greskovich J, Macklis R. Radiation therapy in pregnancy: risk calculation and risk minimization. Semin Oncol 2000;27(6):633–45.

[67] Dropcho E. Central nervous system injury by therapeutic irradiation. Neurol Clin 1991; 9(4):969–88.

[68] Duffner P, Cohen M. Long-term consequences of CNS treatment for childhood cancer. Part II: clinical consequences. Pediatr Neurol 1991;7(4):237–42.

[69] Cohen M, Duffner P. Long-term consequences of CNS treatment for childhood cancer. Part I: pathologic consequences and potential for oncogenesis. Pediatr Neurol 1991;7(3): 157–63.

[70] Constine L, Konski A, Ekholm S, et al. Adverse effects of brain irradiation correlated with MR and CT imaging. Int J Radiat Oncol Biol Phys 1988;15(2):319–30.

[71] Halperin EC, Constine LS, Tarbell NJ, et al. Late effects of cancer treatment. In: Pediatric radiation oncology. Philadelphia: Lippincott Williams and Wilkins; 1999. p. 457–537.

[72] Packer R, Sposto R, Atkins T, et al. Quality of life in children with primitive neuroecto-dermal tumors (medulloblastoma) of the posterior fossa. Pediatr Neurosci 1987;13(4): 169–75.

[73] Dobbing J, Sands J. The quantitative growth and development of the human brain. Arch Dis Child 1963;48:757–67.

[74] Duffner P, Cohen M. The long-term effects of central nervous system therapy on children with brain tumors. Neurol Clin 1991;9(2):479–95.

[75] Jannoun L. Are cognitive and educational development affected by age at which prophylactic therapy is given in acute lymphoblastic leukaemia? Arch Dis Child 1983;58: 953–8.

[76] Kun L, Mulhern R, Crisco J. Quality of life in children treated for brain tumors: intellectual, emotional, and academic function. J Neurosurg 1983;58:1–6.

[77] Halberg F, Kramer J, Moore I, et al. Prophylactic cranial irradiation dose effects on late cognitive function in children treated for acute lymphoblastic leukemia. Int J Radiat Oncol Biol Phys 1991;22(1):13–6.

[78] Rowland J, Glidewell O, Sibley R, et al. Effects of different forms of central nervous system prophylaxis on neuropsychologic function in childhood leukemia. J Clin Oncol 1984;2(12): 1327–34.

[79] Mulhern R, Fairclough D, Ochs J. A prospective comparison of neuropsychologic performance of children surviving leukemia who received 18-Gy, 24-Gy, or no cranial irradiation. J Clin Oncol 1991;9(8):1348–56.

[80] Ron E, Modan B, Floro S, et al. Mental function following scalp irradiation during childhood. Am J Epidemiol 1982;116(1):149–60.

[81] Werner A, Modan B, Davidoff D. Doses to brain, skull and thyroid following x-ray therapy for tinea capitis. Phys Med Biol 1968;13(2):247–58.

[82] Ron E, Modan B, Boice J Jr. Mortality after radiotherapy for ringworm of the scalp. Am J Epidemiol 1988;127(4):713–25.

[83] Albert R, Omran A. Follow-up study of patients treated by x-ray epilation for tinea capitis. Arch Environ Health 1968;17:899–918.

[84] Schulz R, Albert R. Doses to organs of the head from the x-ray treatment of tinea capitis. Arch Environ Health 1968;17:935–50.

[85] Harley N, Albert R, Shore R, et al. Follow-up study of patients treated by x-ray epilation for tinea capitis: estimation of the dose to the thyroid and pituitary glands and other structures of the head and neck. Phys Med Biol 1976;21(4):631–42.

[86] Waber D, Tarbell N, Kahn C, et al. The relationship of sex and treatment modality to neuropsychologic outcome in childhood acute lymphoblastic leukemia. J Clin Oncol 1992; 10(5):810–7.

[87] Waber D, Tarbell N, Fairclough D, et al. Cognitive sequelae of treatment in childhood acute lymphoblastic leukemia: cranial radiation requires an accomplice. J Clin Oncol 1995; 13(10):2490–6.

[88] Mulhern R, Wasserman A, Fairclough D, et al. Memory function in disease-free survivors of childhood acute lymphocytic leukemia given CNS prophylaxis with or without 1,800 cGy cranial irradiation. J Clin Oncol 1988;6(2):315–20.

[89] Ochs J, Mulhern R, Fairclough D, et al. Comparison of neuropsychologic functioning and clinical indicators of neurotoxicity in long-term survivors of childhood leukemia given cranial radiation or parenteral methotrexate: a prospective study. J Clin Oncol 1991;9(1): 145–51.

[90] Williams J, Davis K. Central nervous system prophylactic treatment for childhood leukemia. neuropsychological outcome studies. Cancer Treat Rev 1986;13(2):113–27.

[91] Fletcher J, Copeland D. Neurobehavioral effects of central nervous system prophylactic treatment of cancer in children. J Clin Exp Neuropsychol 1988;10(4):495–538.

[92] Copeland D, Fletcher J, Pfefferbaum-Levine B, et al. Neuropsychological sequelae of childhood cancer in long-term survivors. Pediatrics 1985;75(4):745–53.

[93] Copeland D, Moore B, Francis D, et al. Central and peripheral nervous system effects of cancer treatment on children: a longitudinal study [abstract]. J Clin Exp Neuropsychol 1990;12:77.

[94] Prince M, Souheaver G, Berry D. Neuropsychological effects of irradiation and chemotherapy treatments upon children with acute lymphoblastic leukemia: a case study of monozygotic twins. Neurotoxicology 1988;9(3):341–50.

[95] Syndikus I, Tait D, Ashley S, et al. Long-term follow-up of young children with brain tumors after irradiation. Int J Radiat Oncol Biol Phys 1994;30(4):781–7.

[96] Mulhern R, Hancock J, Fairclough D, et al. Neuropsychological status of children treated for brain tumors: a critical review and integrative analysis. Med Pediatr Oncol 1992;20: 181–91.

[97] Meadows A, Massari D, Fergusson J, et al. Declines in IQ scores and cognitive dysfunctions in children with acute lymphocytic leukaemia treated with cranial irradiation. Lancet 1980; 2(8254):1015–8.

[98] Iuvone L, Mariotti P, Colosimo C, et al. Long-term cognitive outcome, brain computed tomography scan, and magnetic resonance imaging in children cured for acute lymphoblastic leukemia. Cancer 2002;95(12):2562–70.

[99] Peckham V, Meadows A, Bertel N, et al. Educational late effects in long-term survivors of childhood acute lymphocytic leukemia. Pediatrics 1988;81(1):127–33.

[100] Tamaroff M, Salwen R, Miller D, et al. Comparison of neuropsychologic performance in children treated for acute lymphoblastic leukemia with 1800 rads cranial radiation plus intrathecal methotrexate or intrathecal methotrexate alone [abstract]. Proceedings of the American Society of Clinical Oncology 1984;3:198.

[101] Brouwers P, Poplack D. Memory and learning sequelae in long-term survivors of acute lymphoblastic leukemia: association with attention deficits. J Pediatr Hematol Oncol 1990; 12(2):174–81.

[102] Mulhern R, Butler R. Neurocognitive sequelae of childhood cancers and their treatment. Pediatr Rehabil 2004;7(1):1–14.

[103] Mulhern R, Merchant T, Gajjar A, et al. Late neurocognitive sequelae in survivors of brain tumours in childhood. Lancet Oncol 2004;5(7):1–15.

[104] Danoff B, Cowchock S, Marquette C, et al. Assessment of the long-term effects of primary radiation therapy for brain tumors in children. Cancer 1982;49(8):1580–6.

[105] Spiegler B, Bouffet E, Greenberg M, et al. Change in neurocognitive functioning after treatment with cranial radiation in childhood. J Clin Oncol 2004;22(4):706–13.

[106] Reddick W, White H, Glass J, et al. Developmental model relating white matter volume to neurocognitive deficits in pediatric brain tumor survivors. Cancer 2003;97(10):2512–9.

[107] Spunberg J, Chang C, Goldman M, et al. Quality of long-term survival following irradiation for intracranial tumors in children under the age of two. Int J Radiat Oncol Biol Phys 1981;7(6):727–36.

[108] Packer RJ, Sposto R, Atkins TE, et al. Prospective evaluation of neuropsychological function in children treated for medulloblastoma. In: Green DM, D'Angio GJ, editors. Late effects of treatment for childhood cancer. New York: Wiley-Liss, Inc.; 1992. p. 41–8.

[109] Moore I, Dramer J, Wara W, et al. Cognitive function in children with leukemia: effect of radiation dose and time since irradiation. Cancer 1991;68(9):1913–7.

[110] Levisohn L, Cronin-Golomv A, Schmahmann J. Neurophychological consequences of cerebellar tumour resection in children: cerebellar cognitive affective syndrome in a paediatric population. Brain 2000;123:1041–50.

[111] Palmer S, Goloubeva O, Reddick W, et al. Patterns of intellectual development among survivors of pediatric medulloblastoma: a longitudinal analysis. J Clin Oncol 2001;19(8): 2302–8.

[112] Waber D. More good news about neuropsychological late effects in long-term survivors of acute lymphoblastic leukemia [guest commentary]. J Pediatr Hematol Oncol 2002;24(2): 86–7.

[113] Waber D, Shapiro B, Carpentieri S, et al. Excellent therapeutic efficacy and minimal late neurotoxicity in children treated with 18 grays of cranial radiation therapy for high-risk acute lymphoblastic leukemia. Cancer 2001;92(1):15–22.

[114] Ris M, Packer R, Goldwein J, et al. Intellectual outcome after reduced-dose radiation therapy plus adjuvant chemotherapy for medulloblastomas: a children's cancer group study. J Clin Oncol 2001;19(15):3470–6.

[115] Packer R, Goldwein J, Nicholson H, et al. Treatment of children with medulloblastomas with reduced-dose craniospinal radiation therapy and adjuvant chemotherapy: a children's cancer group study. J Clin Oncol 1999;17(7):2127–36.

[116] Silber J, Radcliffe J, Peckham V, et al. Whole-brain irradiation and decline in intelligence: the influence of dose and age on IQ scores. J Clin Oncol 1992;10(9):1390–6.

[117] Walter A, Mulhern R, Gajjar A, et al. Survival and neurodevelopmental outcome of young children with medulloblastoma at St Jude Children's Research Hospital. J Clin Oncol 1999;17(12):3720–8.

[118] Ahles T, Silberfarb P, Herndon J, et al. Psychologic and neuropsychologic functioning of patients with limited small-cell lung cancer treated with chemotherapy and radiation therapy with or without warfarin: a study by the cancer and leukemia group B. J Clin Oncol 1998;16(5):1954–60.

[119] Einhorn L. The case against prophylactic cranial irradiation in limited small cell lung cancer. Semin Radiat Oncol 1995;5(1):57–60.

[120] Crossen J, Garwood D, Glatstein E, et al. Neurobehavioral sequelae of cranial irradiation in adults: a review of radiation-induced encephalopathy. J Clin Oncol 1994; 12(3):627–42.

[121] Senzer N. Rationale for a phase III study of erythropoietin as a neurocognitive protectant in patients with lung cancer receiving prophylactic cranial irradiation. Semin Oncol 2002; 29(6 Suppl 19):47–52.

[122] Laukkanen E, Klonoff H, Allan B, et al. The role of prophylactic brain irradiation in limited stage small cell lung cancer: clinical, neuropsychologic, and CT sequelae. Int J Radiat Oncol Biol Phys 1988;14(6):1109–17.

[123] Turrisi A. Prophylactic cranial irradiation in small-cell lung cancer: is it still controversial or is it a no-brainer? Oncologist 2000;5:299–310.

[124] Hovenden A. Prophylactic cranial irradiation in small-cell lung cancer: is it still controversial or is it a no-brainer? Oncologist 2000;5(6):520.

[125] Gore E. Prophylactic cranial irradiation for patients with locally advanced non-small-cell lung cancer. Oncology 2003;17(6):775–9.

[126] Kotalik J, Yu E, Markman B, et al. Practice guideline on prophylactic cranial irradiation in small-cell lung cancer. Int J Radiat Oncol Biol Phys 2001;50(2):309–16.

[127] Pottgen C, Eberhardt W, Stuschke M. Prophylactic cranial irradiation in lung cancer. Curr Treat Options Oncol 2004;5(1):43–50.

[128] Gregor A, Cull A, Stephens R, et al. Prophylactic cranial irradiation is indicated following complete response to induction therapy in small cell lung cancer: results of a multicentre randomised trial. Eur J Cancer 1997;33(11):1752–8.

[129] Surma-aho O, Niemelä M, Vilkki J, et al. Adverse long-term effects of brain radiotherapy in adult low-grade glioma patients. Neurology 2001;56:1285–90.

[130] Glosser G, McManus P, Munzenrider J, et al. Neuropsycological function in adults after high dose fractionated radiation therapy of skull base tumors. Int J Radiat Oncol Biol Phys 1997;38:231–9.

[131] Vigliani M, Sichez N, Poisson M, et al. A prospective study of cognitive functions following conventional radiotherapy for supratentorial gliomas in young adults: 4-year results. Int J Radiat Oncol Biol Phys 1996;35:527–33.

[132] Armstrong C, Ruffer J, Corn B, et al. Biphasic patterns of memory deficits following moderate-dose partial-brain irradiation: neuropsychologic outcome and proposed mechanisms. J Clin Oncol 1995;13:2263–71.

[133] Gregor A, Cull A, Traynot E, et al. Neuropsychometric evaluation of long-term survivors of adult brain tumors: relationship with tumor and treatment parameters. Radiother Oncol 1996;41:55–9.

[134] Taphoorn M, Schiphorst A, Snoek F, et al. Cognitive functions and quality of life in patients with low-grade gliomas: the impact of radiotherapy. Ann Neurol 1994;36: 48–54.

[135] Kleinberg L, Wallner K, Malkin M. Good performance status of long-term disease-free survivors of intracranial gliomas. Int J Radiat Oncol Biol Phys 1993;26:129–33.

[136] Imperato J, Paleologos N, Vick N. Effects of treatment on long-term survivors with malignant astrocytomas. Ann Neurol 1990;28:818–22.

[137] Brown P, Buckner J, O'Fallon J, et al. Effects of radiotherapy on cognitive function in patients with low-grade glioma measured by the Folstein mini-mental state examination. J Clin Oncol 2003;21(13):2519–24.

[138] Taylor B, Buckner J, Cascino R, et al. Effects of radiation and chemotherapy on cognitive function in patients with high grade glioma. J Clin Oncol 1998;16(6):2195–201.

[139] DeAngelis L, Delattre J, Posner J. Radiation-induced dementia in patients cured of brain metastases. Neurology 1989;39:789–96.

[140] Murray K, Scott C, Zachariah B, et al. Importance of the mini-mental status examination in the treatment of patients with brain metastases: a report from the radiation therapy oncology group protocol 91–04. Int J Radiat Oncol Biol Phys 2000;48(1):59–64.

[141] Regine W, Scott C, Murray K, et al. Neurocognitive outcome in brain metastases patients treated with accelerated-fractionation vs. accelerated-hyperfractionated radiotherapy: an analysis for radiation therapy oncology group study 91–04. Int J Radiat Oncol Biol Phys 2001;51(3):711–7.

[142] Patchell R, Regine W. The rationale for adjuvant whole brain radiation therapy with radiosurgery in the treatment of single brain metastases. Technol Cancer Res Treat 2003; 2(2):111–5.

[143] Armstrong C, Gyato K, Awadalla A, et al. A critical review of the clinical effects of therapeutic irradiation damage to the brain: the roots of controversy. Neuropsychol Rev 2004;14(1):65–86.

[144] Regine W. The radiation oncologist's perspective on stereotactic radiosurgery. Technol Cancer Res Treat 2002;1(1):43–9.

[145] Sneed P, Lamborn K, Forstner J, et al. Radiosurgery for brain metastases: is whole brain radiotherapy necessary? Int J Radiat Oncol Biol Phys 1999;43(3):549–58.

[146] Amendola B, Wolf A, Coy S, et al. Gamma knife radiosurgery in the treatment of patients with single and multiple brain metastases from carcinoma of the breast. Cancer J 2000;6(2): 88–92.

[147] Flickinger J. Radiotherapy and radiosurgical management of brain metastases. Curr Oncol Rep 2001;3(6):484–9.

[148] Eiser C. Intellectual abilities among survivors of childhood leukaemia as a function of CNS irradiation. Arch Dis Child 1978;54(5):391–5.

[149] Brouwers P, Riccardi R, Fedio P, et al. Long-term neuropsychologic sequelae of childhood leukemia: correlation with CT brain scan abnormalities. J Pediatr 1985;106(5):723–7.

[150] Chan Y, Roebuck D, Yuen M, et al. Long-term cerebral metabolite changes on proton magnetic resonance spectroscopy in patients cured of acute lymphoblastic leukemia with previous intrathecal methotrexate and cranial irradiation prophylaxis. Int J Radiat Oncol Biol Phys 2001;50(3):759–63.

[151] Virta A, Patronas N, Raman R, et al. Spectroscopic imaging of radiation-induced effects in the white matter of glioma patients. Magn Reson Imaging 2000;18(7):851–7.

[152] Davidson A, Tait D, Payne G, et al. Magnetic resonance spectroscopy in the evaluation of neurotoxicity following cranial irradiation for childhood cancer. Br J Radiol 2000;73: 421–4.

[153] Rock J, Scarpace L, Hearshen D, et al. Associations among magnetic resonance spectroscopy, apparent diffusion coefficients, and image-guided histopathology with special attention to radiation necrosis. Neurosurgery 2004;54(5):1111–7; discussion 1117–9.

[154] Chao S, Suh J, Raja S, et al. The sensitivity and specificity of FDG PET in distinguishing recurrent brain tumor from radionecrosis in patients treated with stereotactic radiosurgery. Int J Cancer 2001;96(3):191–7.

[155] Fouladi M, Langston J, Mulhern R, et al. Silent lacunar lesions detected by magnetic resonance imaging of children with brain tumors: a late sequela of therapy. J Clin Oncol 2000;18(4):824–31.

[156] Laitt R, Chambers E, Goddard P, et al. Magnetic resonance imaging and magnetic resonance angiography in long term survivors of acute lymphoblastic leukemia treated with cranial irradiation. Cancer 1995;76(10):1846–52.

[157] Parageorgiou C, Dardoufas C, Kouloulias V, et al. Psychophysiological evaluation of short-term neurotoxicity after prophylactic brain irradiation in patients with small cell lung cancer: a study of event related potentials. J Neurooncol 2000;50(3):275–85.

[158] Cowen D, Geller L. Long-term pathological effects of prenatal X: irradiation on the central nervous system of the rat. J Neuropathol Exp Neurol 1960;19:488–527.

[159] Hicks S, Schaufus C, Williams A, et al. Some effects of ionizing radiation and metabolic inhibition of the developing mammalian nervous system. J Pediatr 1952;40:489–513.

[160] Hicks S. Developmental malformations produced by radiation: a time table of their development. AJR Am J Roentgenol 1953;69:272–93.

[161] Otake M, Yoshimaru H, Schull W. Severe mental retardation among the prenatally exposed survivors of the atomic bombing of Hiroshima and Nagasake: a comparison of the T65DR and DS86 dosimetry systems. Hiroshima: Radiation Effects Research Foundation; 1987. TR 16–87.

[162] Otake M, Fujikoshi Y, Schull W, et al. A longitudinal study of growth and development of stature among prenatally exposed atomic bomb survivors. Radiat Res 1993;134(1): 94–101.

[163] Schull W. Cognitive function and prenatal exposure to ionizing radiation. Teratology 1999; 59(4):222–6.

[164] Schull W, Otake M, Yoshimaru H. Effect on intelligence test score of prenatal exposure to ionizing radiation in Hiroshima and Nagasake: a comparison of the T65 and DS86 dosimetry systems. Hiroshima: Radiation Effects Research Foundation. TR 3–88.

[165] Otake M, Schull W, Fujikoshi Y, et al. Effect on school performance of prenatal exposure to ionizing radiation in Hiroshima: a comparison of the T65DR and DS86 dosimetry systems. Hiroshima: Radiation Effects Research Foundation. TR 2–88.

[166] Miller R. Severe mental retardation and cancer among atomic bomb survivors exposed in utero [discussion]. Teratology 1999;59:234–5.

[167] Dunn K, Yoshimaru H, Otake M, et al. Prenatal exposure to ionizing radiation and subsequent development of seizures. Am J Epidemiol 1990;131(1):114–23.

[168] United Nations Scientific Committee on the Effects of Atomic Radiation. 1993 Annex H. New York: United Nations; 1993. p. 805–67.

[169] Yokota S, Tagawa D, Otsuru S, et al. Dissection examination of an individual with Down's syndrome exposed in utero to the atomic bombing. Med J Osaka Univ 1963;38:92–5.

[170] Neriishi S, Matsumura H. Morphological observations of the central nervous system in an in-utero exposed autopsied case. J Radiat Res (Tokyo) 1983;24:18.

[171] Schull W. Radiation-induced mental retardation: an update. REFR Update 1991;3(4):3–4.

[172] Donoso J, Norton S. The pyramidal neuron in cerebral cortex following prenatal X irradiation. Neurotoxicology 1982;3:72–84.

[173] Tsutsui Y, Nagahama M, Mizutani A. Neuronal migration disorders in cerebral palsy. Neuropathology 1999;19:14–27.

[174] Crino P, Miyata H, Vinters H. Neurodevelopmental disorders as a cause of seizures: neuropathologic, genetic, and mechanistic considerations. Brain Pathol 2002;12:212–33.

[175] Little M. A comparison of the risks of leukaemia in the offspring of the Japanese bomb survivors and those of the Sellafield workforce with those in the offspring of the Ontario and Scottish workforces. J Radiol Prot 1993;13:161–75.

[176] Schultheiss T, Kun L, Ang K, et al. Radiation response of the central nervous system. Int J Radiat Oncol Biol Phys 1995;31(5):1093–112.

[177] Ang K. Clinical application of laboratory data on neurotoxicity. In: Weigel T, Hinkelbein W, Brock M, et al, editors. Controversies in neuro-oncology. Basel: Karger; 1999. p. 253–64.

[178] Jones A. Transient radiation myelopathy (with reference to Lhermitte's sign of electrical paresthesia). Br J Radiol 1964;37:727–44.

[179] Smith P. Late effects of x-ray treatment of ankylosing spondylitis. In: Boice JD Jr, Fraumeni JF Jr, editors. Radiation carcinogenesis: epidemiology and biological significance. New York: Raven Press; 1984. p. 107–18.

[180] Georgiou A, Grigsby P, Perez C. Radiation-induced lumbosacral plexopathy in gynecologic tumors: clinical findings and dosimetric analysis. Int J Radiat Oncol Biol Phys 1993;26(3):479–82.

[181] Mendes D, Nawalkar R, Eldar S. Post-irradiation femoral neuropathy: a case report. J Bone Joint Surg Am 1991;73(1):137–40.

[182] Olsen N, Pfeiffer P, Johannsen L, et al. Radiation-induced brachial plexopathy: neurological follow-up in 161 recurrence-free breast cancer patients. Int J Radiat Oncol Biol Phys 1993;26(1):43–9.

[183] Stryker J, Sommerville K, Perez R, et al. Sacral plexus injury after radiotherapy for carcinoma of cervix. Cancer 1990;66(7):1488–92.

[184] Powell S, Cooke J, Parsons C. Radiation-induced brachial plexus injury: follow-up of two different fractionation schedules. Radiother Oncol 1990;18(3):213–20.

NEUROLOGIC
CLINICS

Neurol Clin 23 (2005) 599–621

Neurobiological Weapons

Peter J. Osterbauer, MD[a], Michael R. Dobbs, MD[b,c],*

[a]Department of Neurology, Wilford Hall Medical Center, Lackland Air Force Base, TX, USA
[b]Uniformed Services University of the Health Sciences, Bethesda, MD, USA
[c]Wilford Hall Medical Center, Lackland Air Force Base, TX, USA

Biological warfare has been present since ancient times [1–5], and continues to be a threat today. They can be highly potent, be relatively simple to acquire or produce, remain stable under extreme conditions, and be challenging to detect before exacting a significant toll [6–8]. Technologic advances enabling the addition of virulence factors and treatment resistance mechanisms by means of genetic manipulation pose an additional focus of concern [9,10]. Much has been written on the various aspects of biological warfare and its implications for public health and safety. The purpose of this review is to provide the reader with a comprehensive summary of the most significant biological agents from a neurologic perspective.

Recognition of a biological attack is crucial for beginning effective treatment of exposed victims and to prevent further affliction. This can be difficult, however, because the signs and symptoms caused by such agents often are nonspecific and can be confused easily with those of many common illnesses [1,11]. The fundamental concept in differentiating a naturally occurring epidemic from the intentional release of a biological agent lies in recognition of epidemiologic patterns [12,13]. Clues suggesting a biological attack include peculiar clustering of illness [14]; unusual age distribution of seemingly common illnesses, such as a chickenpox-like outbreak in adults [14]; a rapid, rather than gradual, rise in incidence of a suspicious illness [11]; or an increased incidence in illness and death in pets or other animals [15]. Maintaining a high level of suspicion is, of course, mandatory [16].

The opinions expressed herein are those solely of the authors and not necessarily those of the Department of Defense nor the United States Air Force.

* Corresponding author. Wilford Hall Medical Center, 2200 Bergquist Drive, Suite 1/MMCN, Lackland Air Force Base, TX 78236.

E-mail address: michael.dobbs@lackland.af.mil (M.R. Dobbs).

Various methods exist for the deployment of such agents (Fig. 1 and Table 1). The most likely approach is a release of microscopic infectious particles in aerosol form (Fig. 2) [7]. This can be accomplished using simple, inexpensive technology, such as standard spraying devices [7,11]. Depending on weather conditions, the infective particles may remain suspended in the air for several hours, thereby increasing their infective capability [11].

Contamination of food and water supplies is believed by some to be the easiest manner of biological attack [17]. Others argue that, in most cases, the amount of agent necessary to effect a significant impact usually renders this form of deployment impractical [7,18].

Dissemination using bombs or missiles also is possible; however, the effectiveness of this method is limited for several reasons. With such methods, much of the agent is driven into the ground on impact, and much is destroyed by the ensuing explosion. Of the portion that is deployed, particle size can vary widely, and disbursement often is limited and unpredictable [7,19].

Treatment of infirmity resulting from a biological attack involves stabilization and supportive care, although more specific treatments are available in some instances. Prevention of illness sometimes can be achieved by active immunization; vaccines are available for prophylaxis against some of the more likely agents [20–22]. This, however, is not always possible or practical.

Passive immunization of exposed individuals is another viable treatment option, offering the advantages of low toxicity and high specificity [23]. Antibiotics and antiviral agents also are effective in some cases. A variety of

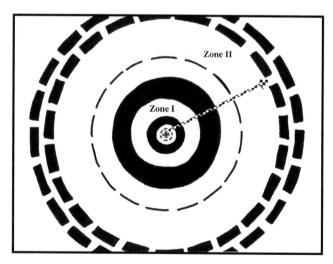

Fig. 1. Characteristics of a biological or toxic agent cloud released from a single point source (*X*). The cloud is seen in black. The arrow emphasizes movement outward over time from point of release. Direction of movement and time to dispersal depend on wind conditions. In Zone I, for the first few hours, the cloud remains intact. The cloud grows in width and length over time, until it begins to break up in Zone II. (Courtesy of Raquel Osterbauer.)

Table 1
Potential routes of infection

Biological agent	Inhalation	Ingestion	Direct contact	Person to person	Other
Botulism	+	+	+	−	
VEEV	+	+	+	−	+[a]
Anthrax	+	+	+	+	
Smallpox	+	−	+	+	
Anatoxin-a	−	+	+	−	
Mycotoxin	+	+	+	+[b]	
Ricin	+	+	−	−	+[c]
Tetrodotoxin	−	+	+	−	
Saxitoxin	−	+	+	−	
Q fever	+	−	−	−	
Tularemia	+	+	+	−	+[d]

A negative indicator does not suggest that the agent cannot be transmitted in the manner indicated, only that it is less likely.

[a] Can be transmitted by mosquito vector.

[b] By direct contact.

[c] Transmissible by injection.

[d] Can be transmitted by bite of infected animal or insect.

other novel treatment options currently are under investigation, such as high-affinity toxin antagonists [24] and topical application of organism-specific lytic enzymes to contaminated mucous membranes [25].

Botulinum toxin

General characteristics

Produced by the anaerobic, gram-positive bacillus, *Clostridium botulinum*, botulinum toxin is one of the deadliest substances known, with estimated lethal doses of the toxin for a 70-kg person only 70 μg if ingested or 0.7 to 0.9 μg if inhaled [25]. Although technically difficult to accomplish, theoretically it is possible for a single gram of toxin to kill more than one million people [26,27]. It is 15,000 times more lethal than the highly potent chemical agent VX and 100,000 times more lethal than sarin [11].

The use of this toxin as a weapon dates back to World War II, when the Japanese biological warfare unit (unit 731) fed *C botulinum* cultures to prisoners of war in Manchuria, with lethal effects. The United States also was researching botulinum toxin as a weapon during World War II. More than one million doses of botulinum toxoid vaccine were prepared for allied troops in preparation for the D-day invasion, out of concern that Nazi Germany had weaponized botulinum toxin.

After the 1972 Biological and Toxin Weapons Convention, the United States halted work on botulinum toxin and other biological weapons, but other countries did not [26]. The former Soviet Union tested weaponized botulinum toxin at Aralsk-7 on the Aral Sea. Iraq had weaponized massive

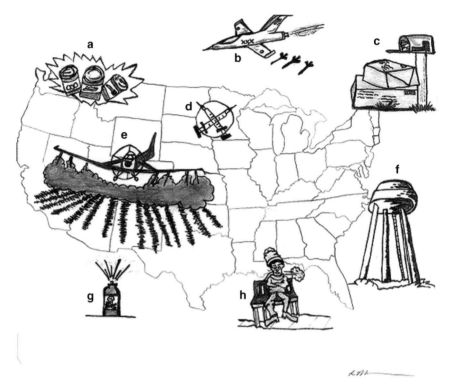

Fig. 2. There are many ways to deploy biological and toxic weapons, several of which might be easy for terrorists to accomplish: (*a*) contamination of food supplies; (*b*) bombs or missiles; (*c*) contamination of mail items; (*d*) direct injection; (*e*) spraying of aerosolized toxin; (*f*) contamination of water supplies; (*g*) setting off small canisters of aerosolized toxin; and (*h*) infiltration of contagious persons. (Courtesy of Raquel Osterbauer.)

amounts of botulinum toxin before the Gulf War [26]. The Aum Shinrikyo cult released botulinum toxin by aerosol at least three times in Japan between 1990 and 1995. These attacks failed, apparently because of poor microbiologic technique [26].

There are seven types of botulinum toxin, A through G, each defined by its absence of cross-neutralization with the others [11,26]. They employ similar mechanisms of action, with essentially the same clinical effects [11]. The toxins are proteins contained within spores produced by the *C botulinum* organism [11,28].

Naturally acquired botulism is contracted by ingesting food that has been contaminated with the spores; however, the spores can be aerosolized for use as a potential weapon [28]. The toxin is absorbed readily by gastrointestinal or respiratory epithelium [29]. It does not penetrate intact skin [25].

In spite of its deadly nature, botulinum toxin is destroyed easily by heat. A temperature of 80°C for 30 minutes, or 85°C for 5 minutes, effectively denatures the protein, inactivating the toxin [18,26]. Direct sunlight can deactivate toxin within 1 to 3 hours [18]. Simple exposure to the open air can deactivate toxin within 12 hours [18]. Decontamination of exposed objects can be accomplished by washing them in a 0.5% sodium hypochlorite solution [6]. These time estimates presume optimal conditions. The actual degradation rate depends on the size of particles released and the ambient atmospheric conditions of the area. The estimated rate of decay of aerosolized toxin is less than 1% to 4% per minute [26]. It could, therefore, take up to 2 days for significant inactivation to occur [26]. Botulism is not known to be contagious, making standard precautions sufficient when caring for exposed individuals [6].

Regarding the mechanism of botulinum toxin, it is necessary to briefly review the physiology of the neuromuscular junction. As a nerve impulse reaches the presynaptic terminal of the neuromuscular junction, vesicles containing the neurotransmitter acetylcholine fuse with the presynaptic membrane, triggering exocytosis of the neurotransmitter molecules into the synaptic cleft, where they then bind with muscle cell receptors, resulting in muscle contraction. Within the presynaptic membranes are complexes of soluble N-ethylmaleimide-sensitive factor attachment protein receptor (SNARE), which act to facilitate fusion of the acetylcholine-containing vesicles with the presynaptic membrane [30]. It is these SNARE proteins that are targeted, and cleaved, by botulinum toxin. Cleavage of these proteins prevents the vesicles from fusing with the membrane, thereby preventing acetylcholine from being released into the synaptic cleft, ultimately inhibiting muscle contraction [11,25,30].

Potential methods of deployment

Aerolization of preformed botulinum toxin is believed the most likely means of deployment of botulinum toxin in a warfare scenario [29]. The toxin is colorless, odorless, and most likely tasteless, making contamination of food supplies possible [26]. Because of its susceptibility to deactivation by heat, it only is of concern in foods that are not heated thoroughly. It also is more commonly expected in foods that have a lower acid content, such as vegetables [26].

Contamination of water supplies, although possible, is more difficult to accomplish. This is because the toxins are inactivated readily by most standard water treatments, such as chlorination, aeration, and even filtration with charcoal, to some extent [18,26]. A large amount of toxin, therefore, is required for any significant amount of contamination to occur, rendering this form of deployment impractical. There are no documented instances of water-borne botulism [26]. The toxin could remain stable for several days, however, in beverages or untreated water supplies [26].

Clinical preparations of botulinum toxin type A are not likely to be used in an attack. A standard vial contains only 0.3% of the estimated lethal inhalational dose and 0.005% of the estimated lethal oral dose, making use of this form expensive and impractical [26].

Clinical aspects

The clinical features of botulism are similar, regardless of the manner in which it is contracted, although onset of symptoms may vary with the route of absorption [11,25,28]. Incubation time is approximately 12 to 36 hours for food-borne botulism, and approximately 24 to 72 hours for the inhaled form [28]. Clinical onset is dose dependent and can begin anywhere from 2 hours to 8 days after exposure [11,25].

Cranial nerves are affected preferentially, making bulbar symptoms, such as ptosis, blurred vision, diplopia, dysarthria, dysphonia, and dysphagia, some of the earliest and most prominent indications of contamination [11,25]. This is followed by a symmetric, descending paralysis of skeletal muscles, which can quickly lead to respiratory failure. The paralysis seen with botulism is a descending paralysis; ascending weakness has not been reported [28].

The neurologic symptoms sometimes can be preceded by gastrointestinal symptoms if the toxin is ingested; however, this is believed caused by other bacterial metabolites in the food and may not manifest if purified toxin is used [26]. Dermatologic abnormalities have not been described in association with botulism [31].

Physical examination may reveal mydriasis, dry mucous membranes, depressed or absent gag reflex, cranial nerve palsies, and even orthostatic hypotension [11,25,26]. Because the toxin does not penetrate the blood-brain barrier, mental status generally is unaffected. Patients can, however, appear lethargic because of diffuse muscle weakness and have difficulty communicating because of bulbar weakness [6,26]. Deep tendon reflexes are intact in the beginning but diminish gradually over a period of days [11,26]. Sensory changes usually are not seen [26]. Electrophysiologic studies, if obtained, are expected to show normal nerve conduction velocities, normal sensory nerve conduction, small motor unit potentials, and an incremental response to repetitive stimulation at 50 Hz [26]. Cerebrospinal fluid and brain imaging studies are normal [25].

Initial diagnosis of botulism is by clinical recognition. A symmetric, descending, flaccid paralysis with significant bulbar palsies in an afebrile patient who has an intact mental status is the characteristic clinical picture [11,26]. Laboratory findings generally are nonspecific and of limited value in the acute setting [6,11]. Antibodies do not develop because the amount of toxin required to initiate a clinical response is not large enough to generate an immunologic response [6,11]. A mouse bioassay is available to detect botulinum toxin in serum, stool, gastric aspirate, or food [6,11,26,32,33,34]. It has been suggested, however, that aerosolized toxin may not be detectable in serum or stool [11].

The differential diagnosis of botulism includes myasthenia gravis, tick paralysis, pontine infarction, diphtheria, and Guillain-Barré syndrome [11,25]. The edrophonium (Tensilon) test may be transiently positive in botulism, limiting its usefulness in differentiating botulism from myasthenia gravis [11]. It has been suggested that, in the United States, botulism is more likely to cause a cluster of acute cases of flaccid paralysis than Guillain-Barré syndrome or poliomyelitis [26].

Initial treatment of botulism should, as in all cases of urgent treatment, focus on the basics of maintaining airway, breathing, and circulation. Mechanical ventilation should be initiated if vital capacity falls below 15 mL/kg or negative inspiratory force below 20 cm H_2O [25]. Placement of a nasogastric tube also should be considered to help prevent aspiration.

The only specific treatment available at this time is a trivalent equine antitoxin, available from the Centers for Disease Control [11,25,26,28]. This antitoxin is active against types A, B, and E, the three most common forms of food-borne toxin [11,25]. Although unable to reverse existing symptoms, the antitoxin may be able to stabilize the deficits and stop progression [25]. Animal studies suggest that, if administered before clinical effects appear, antitoxin might prevent symptoms from occurring [11]. Because the antitoxin is derived from horse serum, skin testing for serum sensitivity is necessary before it is administered. Diphenhydramine and epinephrine should be available during administration of the antitoxin to manage possible hypersensitivity reactions or anaphylaxis [29].

A heptavalent antitoxin has been developed but is not available at this time to the general public [11,25,28]. A pentavalent toxoid (types A through E) is available through the Centers for Disease Control for active immunization but in limited supply [6,11]. It is used to vaccinate high-risk laboratory workers and members of the military [36]. The toxoid is administered subcutaneously at 0, 2, and 12 weeks. This administration schedule produces antibody in 83% of individuals; if an additional fourth dose is given, antibody production rises to 100%. Annual booster doses are recommended. The pentavalent toxoid provides no protection against toxin types F and G. Therefore, if toxin strains F and G are used in an attack, the vaccine would prove useless. Fortunately, however, strains of C botulinum that produce toxins type F and G are difficult to grow in large quantities and, therefore, are unlikely to be used as weapons [35].

Guanidine hydrochloride formerly was given to botulism patients as adjunctive therapy and believed to be of some benefit in recovery [37,38]. Puggiari and Cherington report benefit in 39 of 52 treated cases [37]. A double-blind crossover study of 14 patients who had botulinum toxin type A intoxication, however, showed no benefit [38]. Faich et al, in 1971, reported the lack of beneficial effects from guanidine hydrochloride in their series of four patients who had type A botulinum toxin intoxication [39]. Roblot et al [40] suggest that guanidine is most beneficial in patients who have type B botulism intoxication, particularly when symptoms are mild. They report, in their series, 29 patients treated with guanidine alone and 35 patients treated with guanidine and antitoxin. Two of their patients showed mild signs of intolerance to guanidine [38]. Guanidine hydrochloride is not considered standard of care for botulism.

Antibiotics are of no use because illness is produced by preformed toxin, not by the bacterium itself [6]. Recovery from botulism occurs only by the sprouting of new axons and may require up to a year or longer [25,30].

Venezuelan equine encephalitis virus

General characteristics

Although there are no reported uses of viruses as modern biological weapons, there is potential for the use of viral pathogens as agents of bioterrorism, as suggested by the history of biological warfare. As late as the late 1980s, the Soviet Union had been developing viral pathogens as biological weapons. One pathogen in which they had particular interest was Venezuelan equine encephalitis virus (VEEV), one of many RNA-containing viruses that cause a wide variety of mosquito-transmitted diseases.

Although several arboviral encephalitic agents might be exploited as weapons, there are several factors that make VEEV a likely choice as a bioterrorism agent. First, VEEV, which is an alphavirus that causes an epidemic zoonosis normally limited to the tropical and subtropical Americas, has high infectivity coupled with a low infectious dose. Second, there is no specific treatment for the disease caused by VEEV infection. Finally, few people are vaccinated against infection by the virus.

Immediate recognition of the involvement of VEEV in a bioterrorism attack may be difficult. In nature, Venezuelan equine encephalitis (VEE) epidemics are easily recognizable by the large numbers of equines succumbing to the disease. Because a deliberate aerosol release would likely occur indoors or in areas remote from livestock, however, dead equines may not be a useful barometer for recognition of an attack with VEEV. The most telling indicator of a deliberate VEEV release is a human case occurring anywhere outside of the tropical or subtropical Western hemisphere. Such a sentinel event would require an immediate and detailed investigation.

The time course of VEEV-associated disease also may have an impact on identification of VEEV as a bioterrorism agent and appropriate responses to such an attack. Covert release of VEEV will not have an immediate effect on public health because of the incubation period of 1 to 6 days.

Clinical aspects

VEEV normally causes a bimodal illness in humans (Fig. 3), with an initial severe flu-like illness in nearly everyone exposed, followed several days later by potentially deadly encephalitis in a few patients [40]. The overall human mortality rate in a natural epidemic is less than 1% [41]. Attacks involving

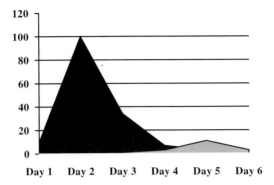

Fig. 3. A typical epidemic curve for a point-source outbreak, as is usual for VEE. The flu-like cases (*black*) are followed days later by a few cases of fulminant encephalitis.

VEEV likely will be performed using aerosolized viral particles, however, because the use of infected vectors may be highly unpredictable and logistically more difficult to accomplish. Studies of VEEV infection using animal models suggest that aerosolized VEEV is highly neurotropic and accesses the central nervous system through the olfactory epithelium [42]. In attacks involving aerosolized viral particles, it is reasonable to expect increased numbers of encephalitis cases after the initial exposure (Fig. 4).

Preventative and postexposure options are limited. Vaccines, which have been shown in limited studies to have protective efficacy [43], are available for laboratory personnel at high risk of exposure. Treatment of the disease subsequent to infection is limited to supportive care. In severe cases, prophylactic, anticonvulsant drugs should be considered. Pegylated interferon-α results in improved survival in mice [44], but implications of these results for humans are unclear. More research is needed to find effective therapies for this and other viral encephalitides, especially in light of the

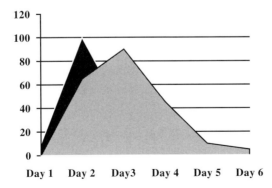

Fig. 4. A possible point-source outbreak curve for a deliberate aerosolized release of VEEV. Because it is believed that the virus is more neurotropic when aerosolized, more cases of encephalitis (*gray*) are seen, and encephalitis cases present earlier than in a natural epidemic.

potential for the use of VEEV and other viral pathogens as agents of bioterrorism.

Anthrax

General characteristics

Anthrax is considered by many an ideal biological weapon; it is a well-known disease of herbivorous animals, dating back to the time of the Biblical plagues of ancient Egypt [45–48]. Anthrax holds a distinguished position in medical history as the prototype disease for Koch's postulate and the target of the first vaccine developed by Pasteur that contained attenuated live organisms [49]. The largest documented outbreak of human infection occurred in 1979 near a Soviet military microbiology facility in Sverdlovsk [46,49]. Deliberate release of anthrax spores in October and November of 2002 led to 18 confirmed, and 4 suspected, cases of disease in the United States [46,48–50].

Clinical anthrax is acquired by infection with spores of the gram-positive organism, *Bacillus anthracis*. The anthrax spores are hearty and can survive in severe environmental conditions for years or even decades [8,18,25,47,48]. The spores are simple and inexpensive to produce, can be stored almost indefinitely, are highly infective, and carry a morbidity rate of 65% to 80% if treatment is not initiated promptly [8]. Although heat resistant, the spores can be inactivated in water if maintained at a temperature of 95°C for 25 minutes. They can be removed by various methods of filtration, provided the filtration pores are smaller than 1 μm. Formaldehyde or 5% to 10% chlorine bleach destroys the spores on contaminated surfaces [18].

Potential methods of deployment

Weaponized anthrax can be produced as insoluble, liquid slurry or as a dry powder [8]. The former is easier to manufacture; however, it is not as stable as the dry form and is more difficult to disburse effectively [8]. The most likely method of deployment is via aerosolization of dry spores [8,32,45,51]. This form of deployment carries an additional risk of secondary aerosolization if the infected area is not decontaminated properly, creating a risk of further exposure [25,51]. Ingestion of spore-contaminated water is known to cause infection in animals; a similar susceptibility in humans can be inferred, and it is known that human ingestion of spore-contaminated foods results in illness [18,52]. Contamination of food and water supplies, therefore, is within the realm of possibility [18,52].

Clinical aspects

Infection is acquired by ingestion, inhalation, or absorption of the spores through breaks in the skin and mucous membranes. Three main forms of illness, therefore, are emphasized: pulmonary, cutaneous, and gastrointestinal [25,45,46,48]. Inhaled spores are transported to pulmonary lymph nodes by alveolar macrophages. Subsequent germination within the lymph nodes leads to a massive release of bacteria and toxins into the blood stream [47].

Serious neurologic manifestations, such as headaches, mental status changes, impaired visual acuity, and visual field defects can occur, regardless of the manner in which the disease is acquired [25]. The most important neurologic manifestation is a hemorrhagic meningitis, which has been associated with the pulmonary form of the disease in up to 50% of cases. Cerebrospinal fluid in such cases shows an elevated leukocyte count, which can be greater than 500/ml; elevated protein, which can be greater than 0.4 g/dL; and an elevated erythrocyte count [25].

Mortality rates of up to 20% for the cutaneous form, 60% to 80% for the gastrointestinal form, and 90% to 99% for the pulmonary form make prompt treatment essential [46,47]. The recommended antibiotic regimen for pulmonary anthrax is ciprofloxacin or doxycycline, plus clindamycin and rifampin [53]. Doxycycline and clindamycin exhibit poor cerebrospinal fluid penetration. The addition of rifampin, therefore, is crucial for the prevention or treatment of neurologic manifestations [25,53]. Regarding a biological attack, resistance to penicillins and tetracyclines should be assumed until proved otherwise by susceptibility testing [51].

A pre-exposure vaccine, consisting of an initial series of six doses, followed by yearly boosters, is available and seems to be effective against pulmonary and cutaneous infection [25]. Vaccination currently is not recommended for the general public [48]. As discussed previously, thorough decontamination of all exposed areas is critical for the prevention of secondary aerosolization and further spread of disease.

Smallpox

General characteristics

Smallpox is a potentially devastating disease caused by variola, a DNA virus of the orthopoxvirus family [54]. It has been used as an agent of biological warfare since the French and Indian wars in the mid-1700s, when Native Americans were given contaminated blankets by British soldiers [54]. It is well known that the disease was declared eradicated in 1980 by the World Health Organization, the last known case having occurred in 1977 [11,54–56]. It also is well known that remnants of this virus have been retained for research purposes at two World Health Organization laboratories: one in the United States and one in the former Soviet Union [11,54,57].

The orthopoxvirus family constitutes one of the largest and most complex of all viruses [54]. Other members of this family include cowpox, monkeypox, camelpox, and vaccinia [54,58]. Although each of these has the capacity to be transmitted between individuals, only smallpox is believed to do so readily [54].

Variola virus first invades mucosal cells of the respiratory system. It then migrates to regional lymph nodes, where it begins to multiply. After 3 to 4 days, an asymptomatic viremia develops, carrying the virus to the bone marrow, spleen, and other lymph nodes, where further replication takes place. After another 3 to 4 days, infected leukocytes transport the virus to the dermis and oropharyngeal mucosa, where neighboring cells are invaded, producing the characteristic skin lesions [54]. From there, the virus particles are released into the environment, enabling them to infect others by droplet exposure or by direct contact with infected persons or contaminated fomites [11,54]. There is thus far no known animal vector, humans being the only recognized reservoir [11,59].

The extent of the threat posed by an outbreak of smallpox is debated. Although recent studies suggest that smallpox transmission may not be as rapid and far-reaching as once believed [56,60], it has been categorized as a Class A bioterrorism threat by the Centers for Disease Control and Prevention [61]. Prudence favors erring on the side of caution.

Potential methods of deployment

Given its capacity for infectivity in droplet form, aerosol release is most likely in an attack situation. Another conceivable scenario is infiltrating crowded areas with infected individuals. Strategic placement of contaminated fomites is a possible approach, although this method is less likely because of its lower propensity for transmission.

Clinical aspects

The course of illness that follows variola infection is well described and fairly predictable. The typical sequence begins with an asymptomatic period of 7 to 17 days (characteristically 12 to 14 days) after the initial exposure [54]. The patient then experiences an abrupt onset of fever, rigors, headache, backache, and malaise [11,54]. Delirium manifests during this phase in approximately 15% of patients [11].

Within 2 to 3 more days, a maculopapular rash begins to develop in a centrifugal fashion, affecting the oropharyngeal mucosa, face, and upper extremities before spreading to the trunk [11,54]. This lesional pattern is a characteristic that helps distinguish variola from varicella. In the latter condition, lesions are more profuse on the trunk than on the extremities [11,54]. The lesions produced by variola tend to present in approximately the same stage of development. In contrast, varicella lesions typically form in waves, a new group appearing every few days, resulting in lesions in various stages of development. A few days after the lesions appear, they begin to crust over, forming scabs. As the scabs fall off, deep, pitting scars form in their place. This residual scarring is another characteristic unique to variola [54].

The greatest period of infectivity occurs during the first week in which the patient becomes symptomatic [54]. From that point on, the smallpox victim is considered contagious until all the scabs have separated [11]. A caveat, however, is that some people can be asymptomatic carriers, shedding infectious virions without ever manifesting the disease themselves [11]. For this reason, during a known smallpox outbreak, prompt identification and isolation of exposed individuals is crucial, whether or not they are symptomatic [11].

One of the most important aspects of management is prevention of further disease spread. All current and potential exposure victims should be isolated immediately, including the initial exposure victim and all persons in his or her household. Everyone with whom he or she had face-to-face contact since the time of exposure should also be quarantined [54]. Vaccination within 4 days of exposure is shown to prevent, or at least attenuate, symptomatic illness [54]. Treatment otherwise is supportive.

One aspect that bears mentioning from a neurologic standpoint is a complication from the vaccine itself. An estimated 1 in 300,000 primary vaccines acquires postvaccinal encephalitis, with a mortality rate of 25% [54]. A constellation of headache, meningismus, fever, drowsiness, and vomiting presents 8 to 15 days after vaccination. A spastic paralysis accompanies some cases. There is no specific treatment other than supportive care, and the reaction can end in seizure, coma, or death [54].

Anatoxin-a

General characteristics

Anatoxin-a, also known as "very fast death factor," is a bicyclic amine produced by *Anabaena flos-aquae*, a filamentous, freshwater bacterium found in pond scum worldwide [18,62,63]. Two mechanisms of action are used by this toxin. First, it acts as an acetylcholine agonist, stimulating muscle contraction by binding to postsynaptic acetylcholine receptors. Unlike acetylcholine, however, anatoxin-a is not released from the receptor. This results in continuous contraction of the affected muscle [63]. Secondly, it inhibits acetylcholinesterase, which leads to an increase of acetylcholine within the synaptic cleft. The combined effect causes a flaccid paralysis, resulting in death if respiratory muscles are affected [63].

Potential methods of deployment

Specific information regarding the use of this toxin as an agent of biological warfare currently is limited. One possible route of deployment is through contamination of water supplies, because many standard methods of water decontamination, including chlorination and carbon filtration, are poorly effective at best [18]. That said, the toxin is converted to a nontoxic form in water within several days [18].

Clinical aspects

When ingested by animals, anatoxin-a is known to produce staggering, gasping, and convulsions, followed by death resulting from respiratory arrest within minutes to hours [18]. Similar symptoms are expected in humans. Symptoms mimicking organophosphate poisoning, such as miosis, excess oral and lacrimal secretions, and muscle fasciculations, are anticipated [63]. Onset of symptoms is approximately 5 minutes or fewer [63]. Currently, there is no known antidote for treatment of antitoxin-a exposure. Animal models suggest that pretreatment with 2-PAM and physostigmine may be effective [63]. Supportive care, including mechanical ventilation if necessary, is the primary focus of treatment.

Trichothecene mycotoxins

General information

Trichothecene mycotoxins, the best known of which is T-2 toxin, are produced by the *Alternaria, Fusarium, Aspergillus, Claviceps, Penicillium,* and *Stachybotrys* species of fungi [18,64,65]. These toxins have tremendous potential for weaponization. They are resistant to autoclaving and ultraviolet light, are fairly simple to obtain, and can be lethal within minutes at proper doses [18,65]. They are believed as potent as the mustard gases but much more readily absorbed through the skin [18].

The tricothecenes are lipophilic and, therefore, quickly absorbed by cell membranes, leading to a fast onset of symptoms [65]. They are highly soluble in organic solvents [65]. They inhibit protein synthesis by interfering with ribosomal peptidyl transferase, with subsequent failure of protein translation [18,65]. They can secondarily affect DNA [65]. The toxins are implicated in disrupting electron transport within mitochondria and in enhancing lipid peroxidation of cell membranes [18].

Potential methods of deployment

Infection is by ingestion, inhalation, or absorption through skin or mucous membranes [18,65]. The toxins, therefore, can be deployed by several methods. They are believed responsible for the "yellow rain" poisonings in Southeast Asia and Afghanistan in the 1970s and 1980s [64,65].

Clinical aspects

Although the principal symptoms of T-2 toxicity are cutaneous (blistering and necrosis) and respiratory (epistaxis, cough, and dyspnea), the toxin can affect the central nervous system, with generalized symptoms of lethargy and incoordination [6,18]. Diagnosis is difficult but should be considered if clinical signs and symptoms consistent with tricothecene toxicity occur in the setting of exposure to a yellowish colored mist or smoke. A rapid diagnostic test currently is not available; however, antigens to toxin metabolites can be detected in blood and urine for up to 1 month after exposure [65].

Treatment of T-2 toxicity is by decontamination and supportive care. Decontamination of skin is accomplished by washing thoroughly with soap and water, and decontamination of exposed surfaces can be achieved with a 1% sodium hypochlorite solution with sodium hydroxide [6,65]. Although no human studies have been performed, treatment with corticosteroids has shown promise in animal models, as has gastric infusion with activated charcoal [6].

Ricin

General characteristics

Ricin is a toxin obtained from the bean of the castor plant and has been known for centuries [18,65]. It consists of an A-chain and a B-chain linked by a disulfide bond [30,65]. Both chains are necessary for cytotoxicity to occur. The B-chain binds to cell surface receptors, triggering internalization of the ricin molecule by the cell membrane [30,65]. Once inside the cell, the A-chain enzymatically inactivates ribosomes. This inhibits DNA replication and protein synthesis, in turn causing cellular necrosis [30,65]. Ricin is inactivated by heat. A temperature of 80°C for 10 minutes or 50°C for approximately 1 hour is sufficient for neutralization the toxin [18].

Potential methods of deployment

Historically, ricin has been used to assassinate individuals rather than as a weapon of mass destruction [1,18,65]. Dispersion of the toxin most likely will occur by means of aerosol or droplet, although it can be injected [65]. Theoretically, it can be used to contaminate food or water supplies; however, the large quantity required to produce a substantial effect makes this method of deployment impractical [30]. Because a considerable amount of aerosolized toxin is required to exact a significant toll on a large population, its use in this manner is believed limited [18].

Clinical aspects

Clinical manifestations depend on the route of exposure but generally are secondary to necrosis of the affected tissue. Ingestion of the toxin results in necrosis of gastrointestinal epithelium and local hemorrhage, with subsequent hepatic, splenic, and renal necrosis [18,30]. Necrosis of upper and lower respiratory epithelium, leading to tracheitis, bronchitis, bronchiolitis, and interstitial pneumonia, occurs if the toxin is inhaled [30,65].

Tissue damage begins within 8 to 12 hours; however, symptoms may not appear for 12 to 24 hours [18]. Death from ricin toxin is dose-dependent, occurring 36 to 72 hours after inhalation [30]. Injection of the toxin produces the most severe symptoms, with the central nervous system affected soon after injection, leading to convulsions and decreased heart function [18].

Diagnosis is by clinical suspicion, although testing for specific antigens and immunohistochemical properties of exposed tissues can be accomplished [30,65]. There currently is no specific treatment for ricin toxicity except for general supportive care [30,65]. Vaccine development is, however, underway [30].

Tetrodotoxin

General characteristics

Widely recognized as the deadly substance produced by fugu, or puffer fish, tetrodotoxin works at the level of the cell membrane. The toxin binds tightly to voltage-gated sodium channels, blocking the influx of sodium necessary for conduction of the action potentials [66]. It affects peripheral nerves, motor and sensory, and causes depression of medullary respiratory and vasomotor centers [67]. The lethal human dose is believed 1 to 2 mg by ingestion [18].

Potential methods of deployment

Tetrodotoxin most likely will be used to contaminate food or water supplies. It is soluble in water that is slightly acidic and is not affected significantly by extremes of temperature [18]. Chlorine readily inactivates the toxin under acidic (pH < 3) and alkalinic (pH > 9) conditions [18].

Clinical aspects

Initial symptoms of oral numbness, gastrointestinal distress, anxiety, headache, and mild peripheral weakness begin to appear within 10 minutes to 4 hours of ingestion. This is followed by an ascending generalized paralysis, hypotension, convulsions, and cardiac arrhythmias, with death occurring in 4 to 6 hours secondary to respiratory failure [18,67]. Distressingly, the victim may remain conscious, although paralyzed, until just before death.

There is no known specific treatment for tetrodotoxin poisoning; treatment is supportive. Empiric gastric lavage with activated charcoal and administration of anticholinergic agents may be beneficial; however, insufficient data are available to assess adequately the efficacy of these options [67].

Saxitoxin

General characteristics

Saxitoxin is produced by the dinoflagellates *Gonyaulax, Alexandrium, Gymnodinium,* and *Pyridodinium* [18,68,69]. Similar to tetrodotoxin, saxitoxin binds to voltage-gated sodium channels within cell membranes, inhibiting membrane depolarization and blocking proliferation of action potentials [70,71]. Because this toxin molecule is not a protein, it is more stable in extremes of temperature and pH [18,72]. It has a lethal human dose of approximately 0.2 mg for the average adult and is approximately one thousand times more toxic than the chemical warfare agent sarin [68].

Clinical aspects

Clinical manifestations of oral numbness, gastrointestinal distress, vertigo, tachycardia, and headache occur within approximately 30 minutes of ingestion [18]. Symptoms may include incoordination, dysarthria, and respiratory distress [68,73]. Death secondary to respiratory failure can occur within 1 to 24 hours [18]. Data regarding routes of exposure are limited; however, inhalation is believed to produce the most severe effects [18]. There currently is no antidote for saxitoxin toxicity, making supportive care the only available treatment.

Q fever

General characteristics

Q fever is a febrile zoonosis associated with exposure to infected sheep, cattle, goats, or other livestock [11]. It is caused by the obligate intracellular coccobacillus, *Coxiella burnetii* [11,74]. Its usefulness as a biological warfare agent comes from its spore-like form, which is resistant to heat and desiccation, allowing it to persist in an area for weeks or even months [11]. This form can be distributed for miles by wind [11] and is highly infective, with as few as one organism necessary to produce disease (range 1–100) [74]. Decontamination of exposed surfaces is by saturation with 5% hydrogen peroxide or 70% ethyl alcohol for 30 minutes [74].

Clinical aspects

The actual illness caused by *C burnetii* is mild compared with that caused by many of the agents discussed previously. Even without treatment, mortality and chronic morbidity are low [11]. Flu-like symptoms with or without cough are normal [11]. Neurologic symptoms of severe retrobulbar headache, meningitis, and encephalitis are reported in up to one fourth of patients who have Q fever [75].

Standard treatment of Q fever is a course of tetracycline or doxycycline, although macrolide antibiotics can be used [11]. Use of a fluoroquinolone should be considered in cases of Q fever meningitis [76]. Treatment is continued until the patient has been afebrile for 1 week [74]. Postexposure prophylaxis with a 5-day course of tetracycline or doxycycline can be efficacious if initiated within 8 to 12 days of exposure [74]. Effective vaccines have been developed but are under investigation in the United States [11,74].

Tularemia

General characteristics

Francisella tularensis is a nonmotile, aerobic, facultative intracellular, gram-negative coccobacillus most commonly associated with zoonoses in rural areas [11,77]. Introduction of only 10 to 50 organisms is sufficient to cause illness in humans, making *F tularensis* one of the most infectious bacteria known [11,77]. It was first studied as a potential biological warfare agent in the 1930s and is considered a prime candidate for such because of its high rate of infectivity and its significant capability to cause disease [77]. The most likely method of deployment is via aerosol, although contamination of food and water sources also is possible [11,77]. Human-to-human transmission has not been documented. The organism is destroyed by heat (55°C for 10 minutes) or standard disinfectant solutions, such as 10% bleach [11,74].

Clinical aspects

The expected presentation of inhaled, or typhoidal, tularemia is similar to that of an atypical pneumonia, with abrupt onset of constitutional symptoms and a nonproductive cough [77]. A local, suppurative skin lesion with subsequent spread to regional lymph nodes characterizes the ulceroglandular form of the disease, which would be anticipated from direct inoculation of the organism to exposed skin or mucous membranes [11,77]. Neurologic manifestations of meningitis or encephalopathy are rare and expected to occur only with widespread dissemination of the organism sufficient to cause sepsis [77].

Initial diagnosis of deliberate infection is difficult because of the nonspecific symptoms. A rapid test involving fluorescent-labeled antibodies to the organism is available if the diagnosis is suspected [77]. Definitive diagnosis is by culture of oropharyngeal specimens or fasting gastric fluid; rarely is it isolated from blood [77]. A variety of other methods, such as enzyme-linked immunoassay, polymerase chain reaction, antigen detection assays, and others can be used [77]; however, these are likely to be employed in a retrospective fashion.

Recommended treatment is a 10-day course of streptomycin or gentomycin [11,53,77]. Alternatives are doxycycline, chloramphenicol, or

Table 2
Neurologic symptoms and signs

Biological agent	Headache or meningitis	Vision change	Incoordination	Paralysis	Encephalopathy	Sensory symptoms	Seizure	Miscellaneous
Botulism	–	+[a,b]	+	+[c]	–	–	–	Normal CSF
VEEV	+	+/–	–	–	+	–	+/–	
Anthrax	+	+[d,f]	–	–	+/–	–	+/–	Possible hemorrhagic meningitis
Smallpox	+	–	+	+/–[e]	+/–	–	+/–	
Anatoxin-a	–	–	+	+[f]	+	–	+/–	Possible hypercholinergic symptoms
Mycotoxin	–	–	–	–	+	–	–	
Ricin	–	–	–	–	–	–	+[g]	
Tetrodotoxin	+	–	+	+[h]	+	+[i]	+	Can affect central nervous system respiratory centers
Saxitoxin	+	–	+	+	–	+[i]	+	
Q fever	+	–	–	–	+	–	–	
Tularemia	+/–	–	–	–	+/–	–	–	

Abbreviations: +, sign/symptom is known to be associated with respective agent; –, sign/symptom typically is not seen with infection by respective agent, or a definite association has not yet been documented.

  [a] Blurring.
  [b] Diplopia.
  [c] Bulbar/descending.
  [d] Visual field defect.
  [e] Spastic.
  [f] Flaccid.
  [g] More likely if injected.
  [h] Ascending.
  [i] Perioral paresthesias.

Table 3
Non neurological symptoms and signs

Biological agent	Fever	Flu-like symptoms	Gastrointestinal	Pulmonary	Cardiac	Cutaneous
Botulism	−	−	+	+[a]	−	−
VEEV	+	+	+	+	−	−
Anthrax	+	+	+	+	−	+[b]
Smallpox	+	+	+	+	−	+[c]
Anatoxin-a	−	−	−	+[a]	−	−
Mycotoxin	−	−	+	+	−	+[d]
Ricin	+	+	+[e]	+	+[f]	−
Tetrodotoxin	−	−	+	+[g]	+	−
Saxitoxin	−	−	+	+	+	−
Q fever	+	+	+[h]	+	+[i]	−
Tularemia	+	+	−	+	−	+

Abbreviations: +, sign/symptom is known to be associated with respective agent; −, sign/symptom typically is not seen with infection by respective agent, or a definite association has not yet been documented.

[a] If respiratory muscles are affected.

[b] Nontender, pruritic papules.

[c] Centrifugal pattern, affecting face and extremities more than trunk. Also with late scarring.

[d] Severe blistering and necrosis.

[e] Hemorrhagic.

[f] More likely if injected.

[g] Works centrally by affecting central nervous system respiratory centers.

[h] Possible mild hepatitis.

[i] Can produce chronic endocarditis.

ciprofloxacin [11,53,77]. Use of alternative medications is associated with considerable potential for relapse, however; thus, an extended course of treatment, 14 to 21 days, is required [11,53]. Postexposure prophylaxis with a 14-day course of doxycycline or ciprofloxacin is shown effective if initiated within 24 hours of exposure [11,53]. A live, attenuated vaccine also exists [11,77].

Summary

Biological warfare is a potential threat on the battlefield and in daily life. It is vital for neurologists and other health care practitioners to be familiar with biological and toxic agents that target the nervous system. Most illnesses caused by biological warfare agents are not commonly considered neurologic diseases, however. Many of these agents (such as anthrax) may present with headache, meningitis, or mental status changes in addition to fever and other symptoms and signs (Tables 2 and 3). Thus, a neurologist may be consulted acutely to aid in diagnosis. Because of the incubation time of many biological agents and their protean manifestations, it is likely that health care workers will be on the front lines in the event of a bioterrorist attack. We must be prepared.

References

[1] Christopher GW, Cieslak TJ, Pavlin JA, et al. Biological warfare: a historical perspective. JAMA 1997;278:412–7.

[2] Jacobs MK. The history of biological warfare and terrorism. Dermatol Clin 2004;22:231–46.

[3] Lesho ME, Dorsey MD, Bunner D. Feces, dead horses, and fleas: evolution of the hostile use of biological agents. West J Med 1998;168:512–6.

[4] Ongradi J. Microbial warfare and bioterrorism. Orv Hetil 2002;143:1935–9.

[5] Wheelis M. Biological warfare at the 1346 siege of Caffa. Emerg Infect Dis 2002;8:971–5.

[6] Blazes DL, Lawler JV, Lazarus AA. When biotoxins are tools of terror: early recognition of intentional poisoning can attenuate effects. Postgrad Med 2002;112:89–92,95–6,98.

[7] Simon JD. Biological terrorism: preparing to meet the threat. JAMA 1997;278:428–30.

[8] Ziliniskas RA. Iraq's biological weapons: the past as future? JAMA 1997;278:418–25.

[9] Daly MJ. The emerging impact of genomics on the development of biological weapons: threats and benefits posed by engineered extremophiles. Clin Lab Med 2001;21:619–29.

[10] Whitby S, Millett P, Dando M. The potential for abuse of genetics in militarily significant biological weapons. Med Confl Surviv 2002;18:157–60.

[11] Franz DR, Jahrling PB, Friedlander AM, et al. Clinical recognition and management of patients exposed to biological warfare agents. JAMA 1997;278:399–411.

[12] Atlas RM. The medical threat of biological weapons. Crit Rev Microbiol 1998;24:157–68.

[13] Berns KI, Atlas RM, Cassell G, et al. Preventing the misuse of microorganisms: the role of the American Society of Microbiology in protecting against biological weapons. Crit Rev Microbiol 1998;24:273–80.

[14] Recognition of illness associated with the intentional release of a biologic agent. MMWR 2001;50:893–7.

[15] Tjaden JA, Lazarus AA, Martin GJ. Bacteria as agents of biowarfare: how to proceed when the worst is expected. Postgrad Med 2002;112:57–60.

[16] Horn JK. Bacterial agents used for bioterrorism. Surg Infect 2003;4:281–7.

[17] Khan AS, Swerdlow DL, Juranek DD. Precautions against biological and chemical terrorism directed at food and water supplies. Public Health Rep 2001;116:3–14.

[18] Burrows WD, Renner SE. Biological warfare agents as threats to potable water. Environ Health Perspect 1999;107:975–84.

[19] Cieslak TJ, Christopher GW, Kortepeter MG, et al. Immunization against potential biological warfare agents. Clin Infect Dis 2000;30:843–50.

[20] Greenfield RA, Bronze MS. Current therapy and the development of therapeutic options for the treatment of diseases due to bacterial agents of potential biowarfare and bioterrorism. Curr Opin Investig Drugs 2004;5:135–40.

[21] Hassani M, Patel MC, Pirofski LA. Vaccines for the prevention of diseases caused by potential bioweapons. Clin Immunol 2004;111:1–15.

[22] Casadevall A. Passive antibody administration (immediate immunity) as a specific defense against biological weapons. Emerg Infect Dis 2002;8:833–41.

[23] Paddle BM. Therapy and prophylaxis of inhaled biotoxins. J Appl Toxicol 2003;23:139–70.

[24] Fischetti VA. Novel method to control pathogenic bacteria on human mucous membranes. Ann N Y Acad Sci 2003;987:207–14.

[25] Martin CO, Adams HP. Neurological aspects of biological and chemical terrorism: a review for neurologists. Arch Neurol 2003;60:21–5.

[26] Arnon SS, Schechter R, Inglesby TV, et al. Botulinum toxin as a biological weapon: medical and public health management. JAMA 2001;285:1059–71.

[27] Gill MD. Bacterial toxins: a table of lethal amounts. Microbiol Rev 1982;46:86–94.

[28] Learning about bioterrorism and chemical warfare: medical students explore key threats. West J Med 2002;176:58–60.

[29] Robinson RF, Nahata MC. Management of botulism. Ann Pharmacother 2003;37:127–31.

[30] Greenfield RA, Brown BR, Hutchins JB, et al. Microbiological, biological, and chemical weapons of warfare and terrorism. Am J Med Sci 2002;323:326–40.

[31] Cieslak TJ, Talbot TB, Harstein BH. Biological warfare and the skin I: bacteria and toxins. Clin Dermatol 2002;5:138–41.

[32] Leggiadro RJ. The threat of biological terrorism: a public health and infection control reality. Infect Control Hosp Epidemiol 2000;21:53–7.

[33] Robinson-Dunn B. The microbiology laboratory's role in response to bioterrorism. Arch Pathol Lab Med 2002;126:291–4.

[34] Burda AM, Sigg T. Pharmacy preparedness for incidents involving weapons of mass destruction. Am J Health Syst Pharm 2001;43:87–9.

[35] Ellison DH. Handbook of chemical and biological warfare agents. Boca Raton (FL): CRC Press; 2000.

[36] Drugs and vaccines for biological weapons. Med Lett Drugs Ther 2001;46:25–34.

[37] Puggiari M, Cherington M. Botulism and guanidine: ten years later. JAMA 1978;240: 2276–7.

[38] Kaplan JE, Davis LE, Narayan V, et al. Botulism type A and treatment with guanidine. Ann Neurol 1979;6:69–71.

[39] Faich GA, Graebner RW, Sato S. Failure of guanidine therapy in botulism A. N Engl J Med 1971;285:773–6.

[40] Roblot P, Roblot F, Fauchere JL, et al. Retrospective study of botulism in Poitiers, France. J Med Microbiol 1994;40(6):379–84.

[41] Paredes A, Alwell-Warda K, Weaver SC, et al. Structure of isolated nucelocapsids from Venezuelan equine encephalitis virus and implications for assembly and disassembly of enveloped virus. J Virol 2003;77:659–64.

[42] Steele KE, Davis KJ, Stephan K, et al. Comparative neurovirulence and tissue tropism of wild-type and attenuated strains of Venezuelan equine encephalitis virus administered by aerosol in C3H/HeN and BALB/c mice. Vet Pathol 1998;35:386–97.

[43] Bronze MS, Huycke MM, Machado LJ, et al. Viral agents as biological weapons and agents of bioterrorism. Am J Med Sci 2002;323:316–25.

[44] Lukaszewski RA, Brooks TJ. Pegylated alpha interferon is an effective treatment for virulent Venezuelan equine encephalitis virus and has profound effects on the host immune response to infection. J Virol 2000;74:5006–15.

[45] Wenner KA, Kenner JR. Anthrax. Dermatol Clin 2004;22:247–56.

[46] Zajkowska J, Hermanowska-Szpakowicz T. Anthrax as a biological warfare weapon. Med Pr 2002;53:167–72.

[47] Schuch R, Nelson D, Fischetti VA. A bacteriologic agent that detects and kills Bacillus anthracis. Nature 2002;418:884–9.

[48] Atlas RM. Responding to the threat of bioterrorism: a microbial ecology perspective—the case of anthrax. Int Microbiol 2002;5:161–7.

[49] Sternbach G. The history of anthrax. J Emerg Med 2003;24:463–7.

[50] Bartlett JG, Inglesby TV Jr, Borio L. Management of anthrax. Clin Infect Dis 2002;35: 851–8.

[51] Whitby M, Ruff TA, Street AC, et al. Biological agents as weapons 2: anthrax and plague. Med J Aust 2002;176:605–8.

[52] Erickson MC, Kornacki JL. Bacillus anthracis: current knowledge in relation to contamination of food. J Food Prot 2003;66:691–9.

[53] Gilbert DN, Moellering RC Jr, Sande MA. In: The Sanford guide to antimicrobial therapy. 33rd edition. Hyde Park (NY): Antimicrobial Therapy, Inc; 2003. p. 46.

[54] Henderson DA, Inglesby TV, Bartlett JG, et al. Smallpox as a biological weapon: clinical and public health management. JAMA 1999;281:2127–37.

[55] Beeching NJ, Dance DA, Miller AR, et al. Biological warfare and bioterrorism. BMJ 2002; 324:336–9.

[56] Pennington H. Smallpox and bioterrorism. Bull World Health Organ 2003;81:762–7.

[57] Breman JG, Henderson DA. Poxvirus dilemmas—monkeypox, smallpox, and biologic terrorism. N Engl J Med 1998;339:556–9.

[58] Georges AJ. Biohazards due to orthopoxvirus: should we re-vaccinate against smallpox? Med Trop 1999;59(4 Pt 2):483–7.

[59] Slifka MK, Hanifin JM. Smallpox: the basics. Dermatol Clin 2004;22:263–74.

[60] Eichner M, Dietz K. Transmission potential of smallpox: estimates based on detailed data from an outbreak. Am J Epidemiol 2003;158:110–7.

[61] Whitley RJ. Smallpox: a potential agent of bioterrorism. Antiviral Res 2003;57:7–12.

[62] Aronstam RB, Witkop B. Anatoxin-a interactions with cholinergic synaptic molecules. Proc Natl Acad Sci USA 1981;78:4639–43.

[63] Fact Sheets on Chemical and Biological Warfare Agents. CBWInfo.com, Ver 2.1. September 2002. Available at: http://www.cbwinfo.com/Biological/Toxins/AnatoxinA.html. Accessed September 4, 2004.

[64] Etzel RA. Mycotoxins. JAMA 2002;287:425–7.

[65] Henghold WB. Other biologic toxin bioweapons: ricin, staphylococcal enterotoxin B, and tricothecene mycotoxins. Dermatol Clin 2004;22:257–62.

[66] Oda K, Araki K, Totoki T, Shibasaki H. Nerve conduction study of human tetrodotoxication. Neurology 1989;39:743–5.

[67] Benzor T. Toxicity, tetrodotoxin; August 5, 2004. Available at:http://www.emedicine.com/emerg/topic576.htm#section-bibliography. Accessed September 25, 2004.

[68] Edwards N. Saxitoxin: from food poisoning to chemical warfare. Availableat The Chemical Laboratories; School of Chemistry, Physics, and Environmental Science; University of Sussex at Brighton Website; 1998: http://www.bris.ac.uk/Depts/Chemistry/MOTM/stx/saxi.htm. Accessed September 4, 2004.

[69] Gallacher S, Flynn KJ, Franco JM, et al. Evidence for production of paralytic shellfish toxins by bacteria associated with *Alexandrium* spp. (Dinophyta) in culture. Appl Environ Microbiol 1997;63:239–45.

[70] Narahashi T. Chemicals as tools in the study of excitable membranes. Physiol Rev 1974;54: 813–89.

[71] Strichartz G. Structural determinants of the affinity of saxitoxin for neuronal sodium channels. J Gen Phys 1984;84:281–305.

[72] Cheng HS, Chua SO, Hung JS, et al. Creatine kinase MB elevation in paralytic shellfish poisoning. Chest 1991;99:1032–3.

[73] Hunter B. Paralytic shellfish poisoning: a growing problem. Consumer's Research Magazine 1992;75:8–9.

[74] Rosenbloom M, Leikin JB, Vogel SN, et al. Biological and chemical agents: a brief synopsis. Am J Ther 2002;9:5–14.

[75] Dupuis G, Petite J, Olivier P, et al. An important outbreak of human Q fever in a Swiss alpine valley. Int J Epidemiol 1987;16:282–7.

[76] Gilbert DN, Moellering RC Jr, Sande MA. In: The Sanford guide to antimicrobial therapy. 33rd edition. Hyde Park (NY): Antimicrobial Therapy; 2003. p. 48.

[77] Dennis DT, Inglesby TV, Henderson DA, et al. Tularemia as a biological weapon: medical and public health management. JAMA 2001;285:2763–73.

ELSEVIER
SAUNDERS

NEUROLOGIC
CLINICS

Neurol Clin 23 (2005) 623–641

Nerve Agents

Jonathan Newmark, MD, COL, MC, USAR[a,b,c,*]

[a]United States Army Medical Research Institute of Chemical Defense,
Aberdeen Proving Ground, MD, USA
[b]Office of the Assistant Secretary for Public Health Emergency Preparedness,
United States Department of Health and Human Services, Washington, DC, USA
[c]F. Edward Hebert School of Medicine,
Uniformed Services University of the Health Sciences, Bethesda, MD, USA

The organophosphonate nerve agents are the deadliest of the classical chemical warfare agents. Because terrorist organizations have a proven interest in these agents, it behooves neurologists to know something about them and about the acute treatment of exposed patients.

Since the review by Gunderson et al [1], nerve agents have been used in two terrorist attacks in Japan [2]. New data recently has become available on the battlefield use of these agents by Iraq from 1984 to 1987 [3].

History

The nerve agents are particularly toxic relatives of organophosphate insecticides, which have been used in agriculture since the early twentieth century. In 1938, Gerhard Schrader, a chemist working at IG Farben Industrie in Cologne, Germany, was given the assignment to produce a more toxic insecticide compound than the organophosphates then in use. He synthesized tabun in that year and then sarin in 1940. Under the law in Nazi Germany, all toxins that had potential military use had to be submitted to the government for screening. Although not a Nazi Party member, Schrader obeyed the law, and the military authorities recognized the potential these

The opinions expressed herein are those solely of the author and not necessarily those of the Department of Defense, the Department of the Army, or of the Army Medical Research and Materiel Command.

This article is an update of previously published material, [Newmark J. Nerve agents: pathophysiology and therapy of poisoning. Semin Neurol 2004;24:185–96]; which appears here courtesy of the permission of the editor, Robert Pascuzzi, MD.

* CDR, United States Army Medical Research Institute of Chemical Defense, Attn: MCMR-UV-ZM, 3100 Ricketts Point Road, Aberdeen Proving Ground, MD 21010-5400.
E-mail address: jonathan.newmark@amedd.army.mil

0733-8619/05/$ - see front matter. Published by Elsevier Inc.
doi:10.1016/j.ncl.2004.12.013

compounds had as chemical weapons. Nazi Germany built a large factory in Dyhernfurth, Silesia, now part of Poland, where tabun and sarin were weaponized and stockpiled in large quantities. Later, German-developed compounds, soman and cyclosarin among them, came along too late in World War II for weaponization [4].

Germany never used the tabun and sarin weapons in World War II, for reasons still debated. By the time the weapons were ready in quantity, Germany had lost air superiority and may not have been able to deliver them effectively. Adolf Hitler had been exposed to the unrelated chemical weapon, sulfur mustard, in World War I and did not like chemical weapons. It also is likely that Germany believed, wrongly, that the Allies also had nerve agents. Had the Germans used these weapons, the Allies would have had no antidotal defense.

At the end of World War II, the Soviet Army captured Dyhernfurth, discovered the factory and weapons stocks, dismantled the factory, and moved it and its workers back to Russia, where the Soviet Union began production of nerve agents. British forces captured small stocks of nerve agents near Hannover, Germany, brought them to England, and rapidly recognized that these agents were unlike any fielded previously. During the Cold War, the United States and the Soviet Union maintained large stockpiles of nerve agents, but refrained from their use.

Nerve agents never were used on the battlefield until 1984, when Iraq turned to its chemical arm to achieve victory against Iran. Iraq had invaded Iran in 1981 but the invasion bogged down against the numerically superior Iranian defenders. From 1984 to 1987, Iraq used sulfur mustard and the nerve agents, sarin and tabun, against Iranian soldiers and then later against Iranian cities [5–7]. Infamously, in 1988 Iraq used chemical weapons, probably nerve agents, against Iraqi Kurdish civilians in the Anfal campaign, most notably at Halabja [8]. There were anywhere from 45,000 to 100,000 Iranian chemical casualties in the war, of whom the majority seem to have been caused by nerve agents. Only recently have data from these patients begun to appear in the open literature [3].

The United States has fought two wars with Iraq, in 1991 and 2003. Chemical weapons were used in neither war, but Iraq's record of their use played a role in the justification for these wars. In 1995, Iraq admitted to the United Nations possession of nerve agents and other chemical and biological weapons. A full accounting of the quantities has not been made by Iraq. A few old Iraqi nerve-agent munitions were discovered by United States forces in Iraq in 2004.

The Japanese religious cult Aum Shinrikyo (Divine Truth) used the nerve agent sarin twice in terrorist attacks. In 1994, the cult rigged up a spray tank on a vehicle which circled an apartment house in the city of Matsumoto, Japan, where a judge about to render an adverse judgment against the cult in Land Court was staying. The judge survived this attack, but seven people died and there were close to 300 casualties. This attack was not well publicized outside Japan. Six months later, in March 1995, the cult released a 30% pure preparation of liquid sarin in three subway trains converging on the Kasumigaseki station, below several government ministries in central Tokyo. In this attack, 12 people died and 5500 people sought medical attention, of whom only approximately 1000 were symptomatic. Several of the physicians who cared for these patients have published their experiences [9]. The accounts by patients as retold to the novelist Haruki Murakami is highly recommended for its insight into how people going about their daily business experience chemical terrorism [10].

The Chemical Weapons Convention came into force in 1997. The United States signed this treaty in 1995. Under its terms, all nations possessing certain chemical weapons, including the nerve agents, agreed to divest themselves of these stocks. Nerve agents, unlike, for example, biological agents, such as anthrax, cannot simply be burned in the open but must be destroyed chemically in specially designed facilities. The United States has completed the destruction of its former overseas stockpile, which was originally housed in Okinawa, Japan, and Germany. The destruction was completed at a specially built plant on Johnston Atoll in the Pacific Ocean. The so-called "continental stockpile" of chemical warfare agents, maintained at eight sites in the United States, is being destroyed gradually at on-site plants. Rarely, cases of nerve-agent poisoning occur among workers at the six sites housing old nerve-agent munitions. These sites are located at Tooele, Utah; Umatilla, Oregon; Anniston, Alabama; Newport, Indiana; Pine Bluff, Arkansas; and Richmond, Kentucky. The Convention gives the United States 10 years to destroy all of its chemical munitions. Although the United States may not meet this deadline, the destruction process has accelerated since September 11, 2001.

Iraq is the only country to have used nerve agents in warfare and the United States, the former Soviet Union, and the United Kingdom have declared their stocks. It is not known how many other countries have clandestine programs involving these agents. Al Qaeda and other terrorist groups have expressed varying degrees of interest in these agents. United States armed forces found literature on these agents in captured Al Qaeda facilities in Afghanistan in 2002.

Physical characteristics

Chemical weapons have common chemical names and North Atlantic Treaty Organisation [NATO] codes, internationally accepted one- or two-letter abbreviations. The classical military nerve agents include tabun (GA), sarin (GB), soman (GD), cyclosarin (GF), and VX (no common name). Their structures are illustrated in Fig. 1. The NATO codes beginning with the letter G are named for Germany. VX was developed in Britain after World War II. A similar compound, developed in the former Soviet Union, goes by the name VR or Russian VX. GC was omitted from the numbering

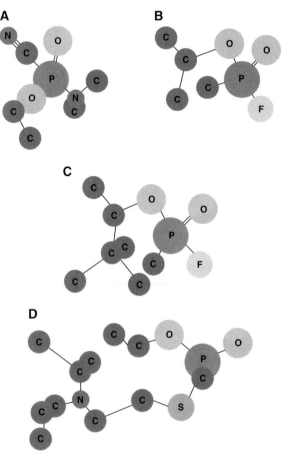

Fig. 1. Molecular models of (*A*) tabun (GA), (*B*) sarin (GB), (*C*) soman (GD), and (*D*) VX. (Courtesy of Offie E. Clark, US Army Medical Research Institute of Chemical Defense, Aberdeen Proving Ground, MD.)

system because it might be confused with gonococcus, which already had an honored place in military medicine, and to avoid confusion with the unrelated compound, phosgene (NATO code CG).

All the classical nerve agents are liquids at standard temperature and pressure. The incorrect term, "nerve gas," arises from a historic misunderstanding. The first chemical warfare agents, World War I agents, such as chlorine and phosgene, were true gases at standard temperature and pressure, and popular accounts tended to call all subsequently developed chemical weapons "poison gas." Clinicians must remember that nerve agents are liquids; failure to recognize this may lead to inadequate treatment (described later).

The nerve agents are claimed to be tasteless and odorless, but data are, not surprisingly, scant.

The liquid nerve agents all are spontaneously volatile; that is, they evaporate spontaneously at room temperature. It is easiest to remember this by recalling that in the Tokyo subway attack, liquid sarin deliberately was spilled out on the floor of subway cars. None of the affected patients actually came into physical contact with the liquid. They all were affected by evaporating nerve agent in the vapor phase.

The G agents have the density of water and evaporate at approximately the same rate as does water, with freezing points at approximately 0°C and boiling points at approximately 150°C. A puddle of G agent outdoors in a temperate climate probably evaporates in 24 hours, making these agents, in the military tactical sense, nonpersistent. VX, by contrast, is oily, with a consistency similar to that of motor oil, and evaporates slowly. Thus, although it poses less vapor hazard than the G agents, it is militarily persistent and contaminates an area far longer.

With the exception of certain polypeptide biologic toxins, most notably botulinum, the nerve agents as a group are the most toxic substances known in biology. Because no one would ever synthesize botulinum from scratch, the nerve agents are the most toxic substances that can be synthesized easily. Toxicity data for poisons in the liquid or solid state are given in units of LD_{50}, the amount of the poison that kills 50% of an exposed population. Toxicity data for vapors or aerosols are given in units of LCt_{50}, the amount of the poison, measured as a product of concentration × time, that kills 50% of an exposed population. These data are given for the five classical nerve agents listed in Table 1.

Clinicians are not used to seeing data expressed in mg × min/m³ units. It may be more graphic to point out that an LD_{50} of liquid VX forms a droplet just large enough to cover two columns on the image of the Lincoln Memorial on the back of a United States penny. After placing a droplet of VX this large on the unbroken skin of a group of people, approximately half of them are expected to be dead in approximately 30 minutes or less if not treated. Chemical munitions developed in past decades were capable of delivering approximately 20,000 LD_{50}s per round.

Pathophysiology

Nerve agents act primarily, as do the organophosphate insecticides, as cholinesterase inhibitors. Antidotal blockade of cholinesterase inhibition by nerve agents can save exposed animals or patients, proving that this is the major pathophysiology of these agents, although they may have additional effects on the nervous system. In summary, nerve agents, then, cause a life-threatening cholinergic crisis.

It sometimes comes as a surprise to civilian physicians that all service members in NATO, most having no medical training, nevertheless are trained to recognize and treat acute cholinergic crisis in themselves or in buddies. This is because the cholinergic crisis caused by nerve agents must

Table 1
Chemical, physical, environmental, and biologic properties of nerve agents

Properties	Tabun (GA)	Sarin (GB)	Soman (GD)	VX
Chemical and physical				
Boiling point	230°C	158°C	198°C	298°C
Vapor pressure	0.037 mm Hg at 20°C	2.1 mm Hg at 20°C	0.40 mm Hg at 25°C	0.0007 mm Hg at 20°C
Density				
Vapor (compared to air)	5.6	4.86	6.3	9.2
Liquid	1.08 g/mL at 25°C	1.10 g/mL at 20°C	1.02 g/mL at 25°C	1.008 g/mL at 20°C
Volatility	610 mg/m^3 at 25°C	22,000 mg/m^3 at 25°C	3900 mg/m^3 at 25°C	10.5 mg/m^3 at 25°C
Appearance	Colorless to brown liquid	Colorless liquid	Colorless liquid	Colorless to straw-colored liquid
Odor	Fairly fruity	No Odor	Fruity; oil of camphor	Odorless
Solubility				
In water	9.8 g/100 g at 25°C	Miscible	2.1 g/100 g at 20°C	Miscible < 9.4°C
In other solvents	Soluble in most organic solvents	Soluble in all solvents	Soluble in some solvents	Soluble in all solvents
Environmental and biologic detectability				
Vapor	M8A1, M256A1, CAM, ICAD	M8A1, M256A1, CAM, ICAD	M8A1, M256A1, CAM, ICAD	M8A1, M256A1, CAM ICAD
Liquid	M8, M9 Paper	M8, M9 Paper	M8, M9 Paper	M8, M9 Paper
Persistency				
In soil	Half-life 1–1.5 d	2–24 h at 5°C–25°C	Relatively persistent	2–6 d
On material	Unknown	Unknown	Unknown	Persistent
Decontamination of skin	M258A1, diluted hypochlorite, soap and water, M291 kit	M258A1, diluted hypochlorite, soap and water, M291 kit	M258A1, diluted hypochlorite, soap and water, M291 kit	M258A1, diluted hypochlorite, soap and water, M291 kit
Biologically effective amount				
Vapor	LCt_{50}: 400 mg × min/m^3	LCt_{50}: 100 mg × min/m^3	LCt_{50}: 50 mg × min/m^3	LCt_{50}: 10 mg × min/m^3
Liquid	LD_{50} (skin): 1.0 g/70-kg man	LD_{50} (skin): 1.7 g/70-kg man	LD_{50} (skin): 350 mg/70-kg man	LD_{50} (skin): 10 mg/70-kg man

Abbreviations: CAM, chemical agent monitor; ICAD, individual chemical agent detector; LCt_{50}, vapor or aerosol exposure necessary to cause death in 50% of the population exposed; LD_{50}, dose necessary to cause death in 50% of the population with skin exposure; M8A1, chemical alarm system; M256A1, detection card; M258A1, self-decontamination kit; M291, decontamination kit; M8 and M9, chemical detection papers.

be treated quickly and cannot wait until patients reach the care of a physician [11,12].

To understand the pathophysiology of nerve-agent poisoning, recall that the cholinergic synapses, those using acetylcholine (ACh) as their neurotransmitter, carry acetylcholinesterase (AChE) on their postsynaptic membrane. AChE functions at cholinergic synapses as the turn-off switch for cholinergic transmission and can be understood as the governor that prevents cholinergic transmission from getting out of control. AChE blockade produces precisely this effect of uncontrolled cholinergic transmission.

AChE is an enzyme with only one active site. Blockade of AChE by any of the organophosphates or nerve agents essentially is irreversible, unless an oxime, a specific reactivator, is administered. AChE molecules inhibited by a nerve agent must be replaced by normal cell synthesis of AChE, which can take several months.

The cholinergic system divides classically into muscarinic and nicotinic cholinergic synapses, named for the false neurotransmitters that were originally found to trigger them. Nerve-agent poisoning turns all of these on, of course, because AChE is invariant between the two major classes of synapses, but, because antidotes work differentially, it is helpful to remember that certain cholinergic synapses, notably those in bronchial smooth muscle, exocrine neuroglandular synapses, and the vagus nerve, are muscarinic, whereas others, particularly sympathetic cholinergic synapses and skeletal neuromuscular junctions, are nicotinic. The brain is an approximately 9:1 mixture of cholinergic muscarinic and nicotinic synapses. The cholinergic system is the most widely distributed in the human brain.

It is helpful to work through the pathophysiology of nerve-agent poisoning by considering two routes of exposure: exposure to vapor and exposure to liquid on the skin. The clinical syndromes differ in speed and order of symptoms and, consequently, the treatment of the syndromes is somewhat different.

Exposure to nerve agent vapor is overwhelmingly more likely in terrorist and battlefield scenarios. In this situation, the most vulnerable cholinergic synapses on the outside of patients' bodies are those in the pupillary muscles, part of the parasympathetic nervous system. Small vapor molecules of nerve agent pass unaltered through the cornea and interact directly with the pupillary muscle, causing miosis. Military medics commonly assume that miosis is the sine qua non of nerve-agent poisoning; this probably is true for the vapor route. Patients complain of dim or blurred vision; approximately 10% of them may have nausea. In the Japanese subway attack, patients described looking at a cloudless sky and wondering why everything seemed dark [10].

The next most accessible cholinergic synapses are those exocrine glands in the nose and mouth. Activating these causes rhinorrhoea and salivation, usually the next symptoms noticed.

Once patients inhale nerve-agent vapor, exocrine glands in the respiratory passages pour excess secretions into those passages, for which the technical term is bronchorrhea. Simultaneously, cholinergically innervated smooth muscle in respiratory passages constrict (bronchoconstriction). The result is respiratory distress strongly resembling that caused by an acute asthmatic attack.

Unhappily for the patients, however, nerve agent easily crosses the alveolar-capillary barrier and enters the circulating blood from the lung. Blood passively carries the nerve agent everywhere in the body. For unclear reasons, the first symptoms of systemic or blood-borne nerve-agent poisoning tend to be gastrointestinal. Cholinesterase inhibition there causes parasympathetic hyperstimulation, leading to abdominal cramping, abdominal pain, nausea, vomiting, diarrhea, and increased bowel movements.

A blood-borne nerve agent more or less simultaneously causes cholinergic overstimulation in the heart and brain. In the heart, the effects are unpredictable, because each individual possesses a specific balance of vagal and sympathetic inputs to the heart, and muscarinic vagal inputs may cancel out nicotinic sympathetic inputs. In many patients, there is an initial tachycardia, but this may not occur; in fact, either tachycardia or bradycardia and either hypotension or hypertension may occur.

In peripheral muscles, nerve-agent poisoning causes cholinergic overload at neuromuscular junctions, which clinically manifests first as fasciculations, then as frank twitching, which moves joints. Untrained, and sometimes trained, observers may mistake this clinical sign for grand mal seizures, and only an electroencephalogram distinguishes them definitively. Eventually, if twitching persists, ATP is depleted and patients may develop flaccid paralysis. Crucially, in contrast to the situation with botulinum toxin, which causes flaccid paralysis early because of the failure of the presynaptic neuron to secrete ACh, flaccid paralysis in nerve-agent poisoning never is the first sign observed but develops only after a period of hyperstimulation. The peripheral neuromuscular effect of nerve agents also can worsen respiratory distress as the diaphragm becomes involved.

Nerve-agent poisoning in the brain essentially simultaneously activates all cholinergic synapses. Because the cholinergic system is widespread within the human brain, a large nerve-agent challenge causes almost immediate loss of consciousness, effectively multicentric seizure activity, and then central apnea.

Death from nerve-agent poisoning almost always is respiratory, resulting from a combination of bronchorrhea and bronchospasm from direct muscarinic effects, central apnea from mixed muscarinic and nicotinic effects in the brain, and paralysis of the muscles of respiration, notably the diaphragm, from direct nicotinic effects on neuromuscular junction.

In a vapor challenge of sufficient magnitude, probably 0.5 LCt_{50} or greater, the sequence of symptoms just described can be so fast as to seem clinically almost simultaneous.

Casualties of nerve agent vapor, if removed from the source of contamination, or masked, and treated aggressively, either die or improve. Humans metabolize circulating nerve agent quickly if it does not kill them. No depot effect is observed with vapor casualties.

The situation is quite different in patients who get a drop of liquid nerve agent on the skin. Nerve agent is not irritating to skin, an important point, in that patients do not, unless they suspect its presence, necessarily perform the most important decontaminating action, which is physical removal. That proportion that does not evaporate, and which varies according to temperature, humidity, and degree of skin moisture, retains its chemical integrity and begins its passage through the skin. First it encounters sweat glands in the skin, causing localized sweating, which may escape patients' notice. Then, it travels through a subcutaneous layer whose depth, and thus transit time, varies greatly from location to location in the body; for example, it take less time from directly behind the ear than it does from the soles of the feet. In women, the layer is thicker; hence, it requires a longer time; in small children, the stratum corneum is thinner and transit time is expected to be much shorter [13]. Beneath the skin, it encounters neuromuscular junctions in the underlying muscles, producing localized fasciculations, which, again, may escape notice. Because muscle is well vascularized, nerve agent enters the bloodstream readily. Systemic involvement first causes gastrointestinal, then brain, smooth and skeletal muscle, heart, and respiratory symptoms. Only at the end of the sequence does the nerve agent diffuse through the aqueous humors of the eye and involve the pupillary muscle, causing miosis to appear last.

The development of the full-blown cholinergic crisis after liquid-on-skin nerve-agent challenge takes much longer than with the vapor challenge. Even a lethal drop may require 30 minutes, rather than seconds, to manifest clinically, and a small, nonlethal drop may develop symptoms over 18 hours. As a result, if this route of exposure is suspected, the physician must treat for a longer time and more aggressively than with uncomplicated vapor exposure, because the subcutaneous tissue forms a "depot" from which the agent is absorbed into the bloodstream, causing symptoms for hours after exposure. Decontamination of the skin, if delayed more than a few minutes, does not catch all of the agent, and clinical symptoms then must be anticipated for hours after exposure.

Special mention must be made of a delayed neurobehavioral syndrome that has been seen in a small proportion of nerve-agent survivors. The development of this syndrome is not correlated with dose. Some patients who have otherwise recovered clinically report new headache syndromes, difficulty sleeping, difficulty concentrating, mood disorders, and even changed personalities lasting 3 to 6 weeks in most industrial cases but for several months in a few of the Tokyo survivors. This neurobehavioral syndrome overlaps with posttraumatic stress disorder and in some patients may in fact be posttraumatic stress disorder [14]. The pathophysiology is not understood and may involve hypoxia or direct neurotoxicity [15,16]. Individual case reports emphasize the treatment of symptoms with the expectation of full recovery [17].

Before the Tokyo subway attack, it was assumed that few patients who had not been pretreated with a cholinesterase inhibitor, such as pyridostigmine bromide, would go into status epilepticus after nerve-agent poisoning. Pyridostigmine bromide was given to troops in the 1991 Gulf War. This assumption proved false in Tokyo, where a small number of patients who had no previous history of epilepsy went into prolonged seizures upon nerve-agent vapor challenge.

Differential diagnosis

Only two potential classes of chemical warfare or terrorist agents have the potential to cause a person not injured directly by the weapon to fall suddenly, lose consciousness, and seize. These are the nerve agents and cyanides. In cyanide poisoning, miosis typically is not seen. Although both can cause seizures, cyanide classically does not cause the huge increase in secretions seen in nerve-agent poisoning. In ingestion or in liquid exposure on skin, the cholinergic crisis seen in nerve-agent poisoning is nearly identical to that caused by insecticides or any other cholinesterase inhibitor. Luckily, the treatment is identical, at least initially.

Therapy

The basic principles of the treatment of nerve-agent casualties were worked out by British researchers at Porton Down, England, during one weekend in 1945, after the initial discovery of German nerve-agent munitions. The major principles are decontamination, supportive care (particularly respiratory), two antidotal strategies (anticholinergic and oxime therapy), and anticonvulsant therapy [12].

Decontamination

An important principle to emerge from animal studies [18] is that physical removal trumps all known decontamination solutions. In the civilian context, copious amounts of water, ideally used with soap and applied as quickly as possible, is the preferred decontamination method, as long as it is accompanied by physical scrubbing.

In the Tokyo subway attack, where all affected patients were exposed to vapor only, patients were not disrobed before entering the hospital, and 10% of the emergency room staffs in some hospitals became miotic [19]. This almost certainly was not because of actual liquid contamination, rather because of vapor that had become trapped in the patients' clothing, because the patients were not, in fact, exposed to liquid sarin at all.

Supportive care

Nerve-agent casualties are most likely to die of respiratory distress. Intubation and oxygen may be required. The period of support is likely to be longer for liquid casualties than for vapor casualties. Respiratory support can prevent hypoxic encephalopathy from complicating the picture [17].

Even in a liquid casualty, for which support is required longer than for vapor casualties, the period of support is far shorter than for the far less toxic organophosphate insecticides. This may seem counterintuitive, because these poisons are less toxic, but the explanation lies in the greater lipid solubility of insecticides, such as malathion and parathion. In patients poisoned with these agents off-gas insecticide for days and often require days in the ICU with respiratory support. Because the military nerve agents generally are water soluble rather than lipid soluble, the period of support required usually is hours rather than days.

Antidotal therapy

The two antidotal strategies used in nerve-agent casualty care are synergistic and are used simultaneously.

Atropine

Atropine competes with ACh for the postsynaptic muscarinic receptor. A high enough dose of atropine, even in the face of the huge excess of ACh produced by cholinergic crisis, prevents the excess ACh from having deleterious effects by binding to the postsynaptic muscarinic receptor; even though there is too much ACh around, it does not have its life-threatening effects. Atropine does not work at nicotinic sites, but can be life saving because the life-threatening effects, particularly respiratory, are mediated mostly by muscarinic synapses. Of all the anticholinergics in medicine, atropine has been adopted universally for this purpose because of its extremely good uptake via the intramuscular (IM) route and its effectiveness over a wide temperature range. Field treatment is given via an IM auto-injector. In the United States, the IM autoinjector in the commonly fielded MARK I kit (Meridian Medical Technologies, Columbia, Maryland; used by military and by civilian agencies and approved by the Food and Drug Administration [FDA]) (Fig. 2) gives a dose of 2 mg atropine. In 2003, the FDA also approved pediatric doses of 0.5 mg and 1 mg.

The field doctrine in a severely nerve-agent–poisoned adult is to use three autoinjectors or 6 mg of atropine to start, then to retreat every 5 to 10 minutes. Retreatment may be given either IM or intravenously (IV). There is no upper limit to atropine use. Endpoint for atropine administration should be that patients are able to breathe comfortably on their own, without the complication of increased secretions.

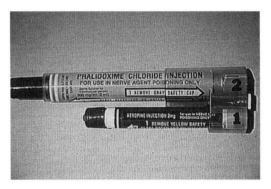

Fig. 2. MARK I set as presently fielded, containing two autoinjectors. Autoinjector 1 contains 2 mg of atropine sulfate. Autoinjector 2 contains 600 mg of 2-PAM Cl.

Patients have been saved with the use of atropine alone. In the Iran-Iraq War, the Iranians had only limited amounts of oximes available at aid stations and no far-forward oxime therapy. They reported using much higher doses of atropine, sometimes as much as 50 to 100 mg at once in a severe casualty [20]. With good availability of oximes, United States doctrine states that probably only 15 to 20 mg of atropine is necessary for a severe casualty, either IM or IV.

In patients severely poisoned with a nerve agent who still have a beating heart, giving an IM atropine autoinjector before taking the time to intubate probably is the best advice. Ventilation of patients who have severe nerve-agent poisoning probably is ineffective because of bronchospasm and bronchorrhoea. Atropine, by contrast, works quickly IM, within 1 minute in nonhuman primates.

Dosage recommendations for children are not universally accepted. One set of recommendations is available [13]. In children who weigh less than 20 kg, autoinjectors may not be practical and IV access must be achieved to treat patients.

Oximes

Oximes are a class of drugs that react with the AChE nerve agent. The result of this reaction is to cleave the nerve agent into two harmless and rapidly metabolized fragments and restore normal, catalytic AChE. Because oximes, unlike atropine, react directly with AChE and not with the postsynaptic receptor, they work equally well, in theory, at nicotinic and muscarinic sites.

In the United States, the licensed oxime is pralidoxime chloride (2-PAM Cl). 2-PAM Cl usually is found only at poison control centers. The 2-PAM Cl injector in the MARK I kit contains 600 mg of 2-PAM Cl. No pediatric injector has been fielded. The loading dose can be up to three MARK I kits or 1800 mg of 2-PAM Cl. At doses of 2000 mg or greater (IM or IV), there is a substantial chance of triggering dangerous hypertension, so the general rule in United States doctrine is to give no more than 1800 mg via autoinjector or 2000 mg IV per hour [21]. If treatment must be continued during that time, atropine alone is used. Pediatric use of 2-PAM Cl is entirely IV in children too small to be treated with the autoinjector [13].

All oximes have the same limitation, a side-reaction misleadingly entitled, "aging," which constrains their use greatly. After a nerve agent has bound to AChE, unless it is reactivated by oxime, and after a characteristic period of time has elapsed, this side-reaction occurs, during which the nerve agent moiety loses a side chain. The result is to charge the remaining complex negatively. Oximes cannot reactivate negatively charged nerve-agent–AChE complexes. The effect of the aging side-reaction is to render AChE essentially impossible for oxime to reactivate. Clinically, aging is most relevant for nerve agents, such as soman, which age rapidly ($t\frac{1}{2}$ = 2 min).

In 2003, the FDA approved a multichambered autoinjector combining 2 mg atropine and 600 mg 2-PAM Cl. Once this product is available generally, it will reduce the time required to treat a nerve agent casualty acutely by about 50%.

Anticonvulsant therapy

Nerve-agent–induced status epilepticus does not resemble other form of status epilepticus in its response to anticonvulsant medications. Animal experiments clearly show [22] that these seizures do not stop without industrial-strength doses of phenytoin, phenobarbital, lamotrigine, carbamazepine, or valproic acid. The reason for this may reside in the wide anatomic distribution of the cholinergic system within the human brain. Status in nerve-agent poisoning may be considered multicentric; thus, drugs that work, at least in part, by dampening the spread of seizure discharges are not effective. Although anticholinergic medications actually are anticonvulsant in animal models of nerve-agent–induced seizures, they retain this activity only temporarily, for approximately 20 minutes in guinea pigs, presumably because other neurotransmitter systems are recruited [23,24].

The only class of anticonvulsant drugs effective in nerve-agent–induced seizures is the benzodiazepines. Because the United States military must use only FDA-approved drugs on-label (for the approved indications), it can use only a benzodiazepine for nerve-agent–induced seizures that carries the indication for seizures, and the only benzodiazepine so labeled is diazepam. For this reason, the United States military fields 10-mg autoinjectors of diazepam (labeled as Convulsive Antidote for Nerve Agent) to all its service members. Animal studies show that for full-blown nerve-agent status epilepticus, 10 mg probably does not suffice. Extrapolation to humans leads to the expectation that the actual anticonvulsant dose of diazepam is 30 to 40 mg.

Licensed physicians are not constrained to use the benzodiazepines only for their on-label indication. A study of the entire benzodiazepine class shows that the member of this class that stops the seizures fastest and at the lowest blood level administered IM, against all of the nerve agents, is midazolam [24]. For a civilian physician, it is best to remember that all the benzodiazepines are effective and that midazolam probably is the best, based on animal data. It has not yet been approved specifically for this specific indication.

It has been shown in animal models that stopping seizures in nerve-agent poisoning is crucial for preventing neuronal loss, which can proceed through either apoptotic or frankly necrotic pathways [25]. It may be necessary to check the electroencephalogram of patients emergently to make sure that seizures are not continuing, masked by flaccid paralysis. Once patients are in the hospital and proper respiratory control is established, it probably is safer to overmedicate with an anticonvulsant than to undermedicate, although clinical experience with this condition is fragmentary.

Chronic neurologic sequelae

Attention has focused classically on the acute treatment of nerve-agent poisoning, for the good reason that immediate treatment is the only thing that saves patients from death. The United Nations team that was invited to Iran to document chemical weapons use by Iraq probably underestimated the impact of the nerve agents precisely because, by the time the team arrived, the nerve-agent casualties largely were either dead or well [3].

There is no indication that survivors of nerve-agent poisoning who have seized are at any greater risk for epilepsy than the general population, although data are fragmentary [26].

There is, likewise, no indication that survivors of nerve-agent poisoning are at increased risk for neuromuscular problems. One patient who survived the Tokyo attack has had documented neuropathy [27], but causality is not proved.

As discussed previously, a proportion of nerve-agent survivors complain of nonspecific neurobehavioral changes, in some cases allegedly lasting for months. In some studies, this affected a majority of patients. Most of the data is from the 1950s, when offensive munitions still were being tested. In one series of accidental exposures [28], 51% of patients accidentally exposed to small doses of sarin or tabun (49 patients, 53 exposures) reported central nervous system effects ranging from sleep disturbances to mood changes and easy fatigueability. In another series of 72 workers exposed accidentally to sarin, 16 reported difficulty in concentration, mental confusion, giddiness, or insomnia [29]. This seems to be idiosyncratic, not dose related, and may overlap with posttraumatic stress disorder.

The most significant long-term neurologic effect of nerve-agent exposure is hypoxic encephalopathy, which can complicate nerve-agent exposure because of the respiratory depression seen in nerve-agent poisoning. Dissecting how much of the neuropathologic picture seen in nerve-agent exposure is the result of hypoxic encephalopathy is difficult.

It was believed previously that nerve-agent intoxication in humans produced only short-lived convulsions [30,31]. In the Tokyo subway attack, however, a few patients were found to seize clinically for prolonged periods after exposure [32]. The possibility of lasting status epilepticus added to hypoxic encephalopathy makes it even more difficult to distinguish between nerve-agent direct toxicity to the brain, hypoxic encephalopathy, and status epilepticus as causative in neurologic dysfunction.

Patients who survive nerve-agent attack presumably are at greater risk for severe problems in a subsequent exposure to a cholinesterase inhibitor, because of the time that it takes for synapses to replace AChE. In one Tokyo survivor, the circulating red blood cell AChE level did not return to normal for 6 months [17].

Pyridostigmine bromide

Because neurologists are the physicians most familiar with pyridostigmine bromide from its use in myasthenia gravis, they are likely to receive inquiries regarding the use of this medication as a pretreatment for nerve-agent poisoning.

During the late 1980s, the United States military became concerned about rapidly aging nerve agents, such as soman. It was known that Iraq was interested in obtaining the starting materials for the synthesis of soman. Iraq, however, did not use soman during the 1984–1987 war with Iran. Animal studies were performed showing that the MARK I autoinjector kit containing atropine and 2-PAM Cl did not confer sufficient protection to soldiers exposed to soman, because of the rapid aging of this toxin. Within 10 minutes after exposure, or five half-lives, one of the two legs of this standard treatment, the oxime, was rendered useless by aging.

To solve this problem, the military turned to the carbamate, pyridostigmine, a reversible cholinesterase inhibitor. Pyridostigmine had a long safety record, having been approved by the FDA for myasthenia gravis in 1951. Because humans have a large excess of AChE, the reasoning went, if there were a strong likelihood of exposure to a rapidly aging nerve agent, pretreatment with enough pyridostigmine to inhibit a fraction of the AChE reversibly would allow a soldier to survive what would have been a lethal challenge of agent, because that fraction would be unavailable for the agent to inhibit permanently and would become available if patients were supported through the clinical crisis by the standard antidotes. Animal data was submitted to the FDA in 1991 showing that the protective ratio against soman was increased from 1.6 to 40 using pyridostigmine pretreatment, and on the basis of this data the FDA waived informed consent. The result of this was the issuance of pyridostigmine tablets to 100,000 coalition forces in the 1991 Gulf War. The data underlying this choice and the resultant side-effect profile reported by unit physician assistants are summarized [33]. The waiver was withdrawn in 1992, but in 2003, with a new war with

Iraq looming, the FDA finally approved pyridostigmine for the specific purpose of pretreatment against soman. In the 2003 war with Iraq, however, pyridostigmine was not used. In the event of a future war with an adversary equipped with a rapidly aging nerve agent, it is United States and NATO doctrine to issue pyridostigmine.

The dose of pyridostigmine usually taken for myasthenia is 60 mg every 8 hours and may go much higher. The nerve-agent pretreatment dose is 30 mg every 8 hours. Military doctrine allows commanders to decide to use this drug; the decision is not a medical one, as it is technically not a medication but a defensive weapons system. Once patients are exposed to nerve agent, of course, pyridostigmine is contraindicated. Pyridostigmine does not obviate standard antidotes; it merely converts what would have been dead patients into living but very sick patients.

Neuroprotection

The microscopic damage caused to brain tissue by nerve agents resembles ischemic penumbra. Necrotic and apoptotic neurons are observed. This apparent similarity has stimulated interest in adapting neuroprotectants for patients who survive nerve-agent exposure, to optimize the eventual neurologic recovery. None of the neuroprotectants investigated so far is yet established for this indication. Preliminary work shows proof of concept using the experimental drug HU-211, or dexanabinol, a nonpsychotropic analog of tetrahydrocannabinol [34]. In a rat model, dexanabinol reduced the size of the lesion produced in highly cholinergic cortex by 90% after exposure to a high dose of soman and subsequent status epilepticus. Dexanabinol, however, could not exert this effect in the thalamus. Dantrolene, a ryanodine agonist commonly used against malignant hyperthermia, synergized with diazepam in the same rat model [35]. It also showed protection in the thalamus, which dexanabinol did not. Ongoing work aims to delineate the parameters of protection with dantrolene, which may turn out to be a useful postexposure neuroprotectant in survivors of nerve-agent poisoning.

Bioscavengers

A substantial research effort is under way in the medical chemical defense community to develop a circulating bioscavenger. Such a compound, either a human cholinesterase molecule or an altered human cholinesterase with one or two amino acids substituted so as to alter the active site, detoxifies a nerve agent entering the circulation so that it is unable to reach the tissue AChE and produce clinical symptoms. Several putative bioscavengers are shown to be effective against multiple LD_{50}s of many of the nerve agents in animal models, including rodents and nonhuman primates [36]. Of these, a plasma-derived human butyrylcholinesterase preparation probably is closest to submission to the FDA as an Investigational New Drug.

Summary

Nerve agents cause a rapidly fatal cholinergic crisis, but rapid, appropriate antidotal treatment saves lives. Survivors of nerve-agent poisoning generally are healthy, unlike survivors of some other chemical agent attacks. Neurologists can assist first responders and mass casualty planners materially by serving as resources for information on nerve agents and the syndromes they cause. They also can help their communities by reinforcing that treatment for nerve-agent poisoning is effective.

Appendix: Where to go for information

Most of the standard references, including treatment protocols and a procedure for processing biologic samples for the nation's reference laboratory, are available on the Chemical Casualty Care Division website, http://ccc.apgea.army.mil. Refs. [4,11,12,33] are available in their entirety. Non–United States government clinicians and agencies are welcome to use this website but must register to gain access to the reference materials. If the reader has an urgent need to access this material, the reader is strongly encouraged to register in advance. Clinical advice may be obtained from the US Army Medical Research Institute of Chemical Defense 24 hours a day at Tel. 410-436-3276.

References

[1] Gunderson CH, Lehmann CR, Sidell FR, et al. Nerve agents: a review. Neurology 1992;42: 946–50.
[2] Yokoyama K, Yamada A, Nobuhide M. Clinical profiles of patients with sarin poisoning after the Tokyo subway attack. Am J Med 1996;100:586.
[3] Foroutan SA. Medical notes on chemical warfare, part I–XI. Kowsar Med J; Fall 1996– Spring 1999:1(1)–4(1) [in Farsi].
[4] Sidell FR. Nerve agents. In: Sidell FR, Takafuji ET, Franz DR. Medical aspects of chemical and biological warfare. Washington, DC: Office of the Surgeon General and Department of the Army, and Borden Institute; 1997. p. 129–80.
[5] Pelletiere SC, Johnson DV. Lessons learned: the Iran-Iraq War. Carlisle Barracks (PA): Strategic Studies Institute, US Army War College; 1991.
[6] Cordesman AH, Wagner AP. The lessons of modern war, vol. II: the Iran-Iraq War. Boulder (CO): Westview Press; 1990.
[7] Dingeman A, Jupa R. Chemical warfare in the Iran-Iraq conflict. Strategy and Tactics Magazine 1987;113:51–2.
[8] Barnaby F. Iran-Iraq War: the use of chemical weapons against the Kurds. Ambio 1988;17: 407–8.
[9] Okumura T, Takasu N, Ishimatsu S, et al. Report on 640 victims of the Tokyo subway sarin attack. Ann Emerg Med 1996;28:129–35.

[10] Murakami H. Underground. New York: Vintage Books; 2001. [Gabriel P, Trans.].

[11] Headquarters: Departments of the Army, Navy, and Air Force, and Commandant, Marine Corps. Field manual: treatment of chemical agent casualties and conventional military chemical injuries. Serial numbers: Army FM 8–285; Navy NAVMED P-5041; Air Force AFJMAN 44–149; and Marine Corps FMFM 11–11. Washington, DC; December 1995.

[12] Chemical Casualty Care Division, US Army Medical Research Institute of Chemical Defense. Medical management of chemical casualties handbook. 3rd edition. Aberdeen Proving Ground (MD); July 2000.

[13] Rotenberg JS, Newmark J. Nerve agent attacks on children: diagnosis and management. Pediatrics 2003;112:648–58.

[14] Kawana N, Ishimatsu S, Kanda K. Psycho-physiological effects of the terrorist sarin attack on the Tokyo subway system. Mil Med 2001;166(Suppl 2):23–6.

[15] Murata K, Araki S, Yokoyama K, et al. Asymptomatic sequelae to acute sarin poisoning in the central and autonomic nervous system six months after the Tokyo subway attack. J Neurol 1997;244:601–6.

[16] McDonough JH. Performance effects of nerve agents and their pharmacological counter-measures. Mil Psychol 2002;14:93–119.

[17] Hatta K, Miura Y, Asukai N, et al. Amnesia from sarin poisoning. Lancet 1996;347:1343.

[18] Van Hooidonk C, Ceulen BI, Bock J, et al. Chemical warfare agents and the skin: penetration and decontamination. In: Proceedings of the International Symposium on Protection against Chemical Warfare Agents. Stockholm (Sweden): National Defence; 1983. p. 153–60.

[19] Rodgers JC. Chemical incident planning: a review of the literature. Accid Emerg Nurs 1998; 6:155–9.

[20] Newmark J. The birth of nerve agent warfare: lessons from Syed Abbas Foroutan. Neurology 2004;62:1590–6.

[21] Sidell FR. Clinical considerations in nerve agent intoxication. In: Somani SM, editor. Chemical warfare agents. New York: Academic Press; 1992. p. 181.

[22] Shih T, McDonough JH, Koplovitz I. Anticonvulsants for soman-induced seizure activity. J Biomed Sci 1999;6:86–96.

[23] Shih TM, McDonough JH. Neurochemical mechanisms in soman-induced seizures. J Appl Toxicol 1997;17:255–64.

[24] McDonough J, McMonagle J, Copeland T, et al. Comparative evaluation of benzodiaepines for control of soman-induced seizures. Arch Toxicol 1999;73:473–8.

[25] Shih TM, Duniho SM, McDonough JH. Control of nerve agent-induced seizures is critical for neuroprotection and survival. Toxicol Appl Pharmacol 2003;188:69–80.

[26] Duffy FH, Burchfiel JL, Bartels PH, et al. Long-term effects of an organophosphate upon the human electroenecephalogram. Toxicol Appl Pharmacol 1979;47:161–76.

[27] Himuro K, Murayama S, Nishiyama K, et al. Distal sensory neuropathy after sarin intoxication. Neurology 1995;51:1195–7.

[28] Craig AB, Freeman G. Clinical observations on workers accidentally exposed to "G" agents. Medical laboratory research report 154. Edgewood Arsenal (MD): Medical Research Laboratory; 1953.

[29] Brody BB, Gammill JF. Seventy-five cases of accidental nerve gas poisoning at Dugway. Medical investigational branch special report 5. Dugway Proving Ground (UT): Medical Investigational Branch; 1954.

[30] Sidell FR. Soman and sarin: clinical manifestations and treatment of accidental poisoning by organophosphates. Clin Toxicol 1974;7:1–17.

[31] Grob D. The manifestations and treatment of poisoning due to nerve agents and other organic phosphate anticholinesterase compounds. Arch Intern Med 1956;98:221–39.

[32] Ohbu S, Yamashina A, Takasu N, et al. Sarin poisoning on Tokyo subway. South Med J 1997;90:587–92.

[33] Dunn MA, Hackley BE, Sidell FR. Pretreatment for nerve agent exposure. In: Sidell FR, Takafuji ET, Franz DR. Medical aspects of chemical and biological warfare. Washington, DC: Office of the Surgeon General and Department of the Army, and Borden Institute; 1997. p. 181–96.

[34] Filbert MG, Forster JS, Smith CD, et al. Neuroprotective effects of HU-211 on brain damage resulting from soman-induced seizures. Ann N Y Acad Sci 1999;890:505–14.

[35] Newmark J, Ballough GPH, Filbert MG. Dantrolene plus diazepam: a viable strategy for neuroprotection following soman-induced status epilepticus. Neurology 2003;60(Suppl 1): A385.

[36] Cerasoli DM, Lenz DE. Nerve agent bioscavengers: protection with reduced behavioral effects. Mil Psychol 2002;14:121–43.

ELSEVIER
SAUNDERS

Neurol Clin 23 (2005) 643–654

NEUROLOGIC CLINICS

Index

Note: Page numbers of article titles are in **boldface** type.

Changing Your Address?

Make sure your subscription changes too! When you notify us of your new address, you can help make our job easier by including an exact copy of your Clinics label number with your old address (see illustration below.) This number identifies you to our computer system and will speed the processing of your address change. Please be sure this label number accompanies your old address and your corrected address—you can send an old Clinics label with your number on it or just copy it exactly and send it to the address listed below.

We appreciate your help in our attempt to give you continuous coverage. Thank you.

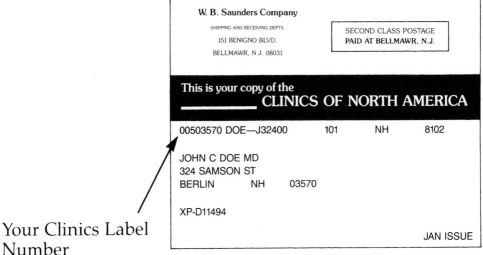

W. B. Saunders Company

SHIPPING AND RECEIVING DEPTS.

151 BENIGNO BLVD.

BELLMAWR, N.J. 08031

SECOND CLASS POSTAGE
PAID AT BELLMAWR, N.J.

This is your copy of the
_____ **CLINICS OF NORTH AMERICA**

00503570 DOE—J32400   101   NH   8102

JOHN C DOE MD
324 SAMSON ST
BERLIN   NH   03570

XP-D11494

JAN ISSUE

Your Clinics Label Number

Copy it exactly or send your label
along with your address to:
W.B. Saunders Company, Customer Service
Orlando, FL 32887-4800
Call Toll Free 1-800-654-2452

Please allow four to six weeks for delivery of new subscriptions and for processing address changes.